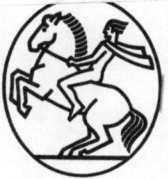

# Muscle Transplantation

Edited by G. Freilinger, J. Holle,
and B. M. Carlson

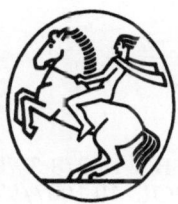

Springer-Verlag Wien NewYork

Prof. Dr. Gerhard Freilinger
Doz. Dr. Jürgen Holle
Department of Plastic and Reconstructive Surgery,
Second Surgical University Clinic of Vienna, Austria

Prof. Dr. Bruce Martin Carlson
Department of Anatomy, University of Michigan,
Ann Arbor, Michigan, U.S.A.

With 161 partly colored figures

ISBN-13:978-3-7091-8620-6    e-ISBN-13:978-3-7091-8618-3
DOI: 10.1007/978-3-7091-8618-3

# Preface

It was a long and troublesome history but an inspiring and exciting one too—from the time of Zielonko, a Russian pathologist who in 1874 first transplanted muscles, to the present day microneurovascular muscle graft.

Today we know that for functional recovery of muscle tissue vascularisation and neurotisation are of equal importance. With the establishment of microsurgery of small vessels and nerves, its application for myoplastic operations has gained increasing interest.

It was my intention to bring together leading authorities from all over the world in the field of muscle transplantation. Open questions and unsolved problems had to be discussed between research workers in the basic medical sciences and our clinical colleagues; in this way progress can best be accomplished.

This publication is the result of the "Vienna Muscle Symposium" (June 13–14, 1980). It gives an up-to-date viewpoint and should act as a stimulus to all who are interested in this particular field. I wish to express my sincere thanks to those who have contributed to this publication, to the two co-editors J. Holle and B. M. Carlson for their effective cooperation, and to Springer-Verlag Wien for their prompt and most efficient work.

Vienna, June 1981                                                G. Freilinger

# Preface

It was ... and ...
...

# Contents

## Muscle Transplantation and Regeneration

## Muscle Transplantation in Experimental Surgery

## Myoplastic Operations in Facial Palsy

## Myoplastic Operations for Sphincter Reconstruction, Upper Extremity and Other Regions

# Muscle Transplantation and Regeneration

# The Biology of Muscle Transplantation

## B. M. Carlson

Departments of Anatomy and Biological Sciences,
University of Michigan,
Ann Arbor, Michigan, U.S.A.

With 6 Figures

## Introduction

After a long history of unsuccessful attempts, the free grafting of entire mammalian muscles has been accomplished in both the research laboratory (Bosova, 1962; Studitsky, 1963, 1977; Carlson, 1978) and in clinical practice (Thompson, 1971). Although working completely independently of one another, Thompson and Studitsky devised similar grafting techniques. After considerable experience with various regeneration models, Studitsky (1963) elaborated the concept of the "plastic state", a condition to which mammalian muscle must be reduced in order for massive amounts of regeneration to occur. Treatments leading to the plastic state are denervation or slicing trauma prior to whole muscle grafting, or mincing a fresh muscle into small (one mm³) fragments. According to Studitsky, the plastic state facilitates regeneration, which he considered to be the basis for the success of muscle grafts.

The Thompson (1971) procedure also relied upon preliminary denervation as the basis for successful muscle grafting, but the theoretical basis behind his procedure was quite different. Thompson believed that predenervation reduces the metabolism of a muscle to a lower level and shifts it toward anerobiasis, allowing the muscle fibers within a free graft to survive intact during the initial avascular period. The possibility of muscle fiber regeneration in free grafts has not been considered in Thompson's reports.

The clinical application of free muscle grafting has been beset by a number of real or apparent contradictions in working hypotheses. Since a number of aspects of muscle transplantation surgery depend upon an exact knowledge of the biology of transplanted muscle, a number of important theoretical considerations and the experimental evidence behind them will be examined here. The intent of this article is to clarify what we now know and what we still need to know in order to establish a firm scientific basis for muscle transplantation.

## The Basis for Grafting Success–Muscle Fiber Survival or Regeneration?

As was outlined in the introduction, the first successful models of muscle grafting were based upon radically different proposed mechanisms–the survival of the muscle fibers within the graft or their breakdown and regeneration. Experiments on laboratory animals have shown that both phenomena occur in free muscle grafts. A typical early muscle graft is characterized by a thin peripheral rim of surviving muscle fibers and a large central core of muscle fibers in a state of ischemic necrosis (Fig. 1). As ingrowing blood vessels penetrate into

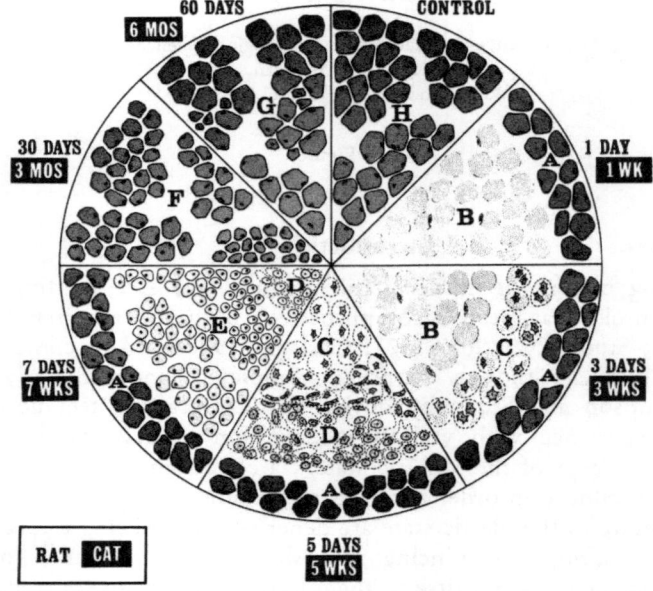

Fig. 1. Diagram illustrating typical cellular reactions at various intervals within a cross-section of a grafted extensor digitorum longus muscle in the rat and cat. As a general rule what takes a day in the rat takes a week in the cat. *A* Surviving muscle fibers. *B* Original muscle fibers in a state of ischemic necrosis. *C* Muscle fibers invaded by macrophages that are phagocytizing the necrotic cytoplasm. *D* Myoblasts and early myotubes within the basal lamina of the original muscle fibers. *E* Early cross-striated muscle fibers. *F* Maturing regenerating muscle fibers. *G* Mature regenerated muscle fibers. *H* Normal control muscle fibers. [From Carlson, B. M., *et al.,* 1979, in: Muscle Regeneration (Mauro, A., ed.). New York: Raven Press]

---

Fig. 2. Summary drawings of major phases in the degeneration and regeneration of a single muscle fiber in the rat. *A* Early ischemic damage. The nucleus is becoming pycnotic with chromatin clumping inside the nuclear membrane. The mitochondria are swollen and the bundles of contractile filaments are breaking apart throughout the muscle fiber. *B* Fragmentation phase. Macrophages *(M)* associated with the ingrowing vasculature enter the degenerating muscle fibers and remove bundles of contractile filaments and other cytoplasmic debris. Beneath the basal lamina (arrows), spindle-shaped myoblasts *(Mb)* line up in preparation for the formation of new muscle fibers. *C* Myotube. Beneath original basal lamina myoblasts have fused to form a multinucleated fiber with bundles of newly forming contractile filaments at the periphery. *D* Muscle fiber. The mature segmented muscle fiber is in most respects indistinguishable from a normal muscle fiber [From Foster, A. H., Carlson, B. M., Anesthesia and Analgesia *59*, 727 (1980)]

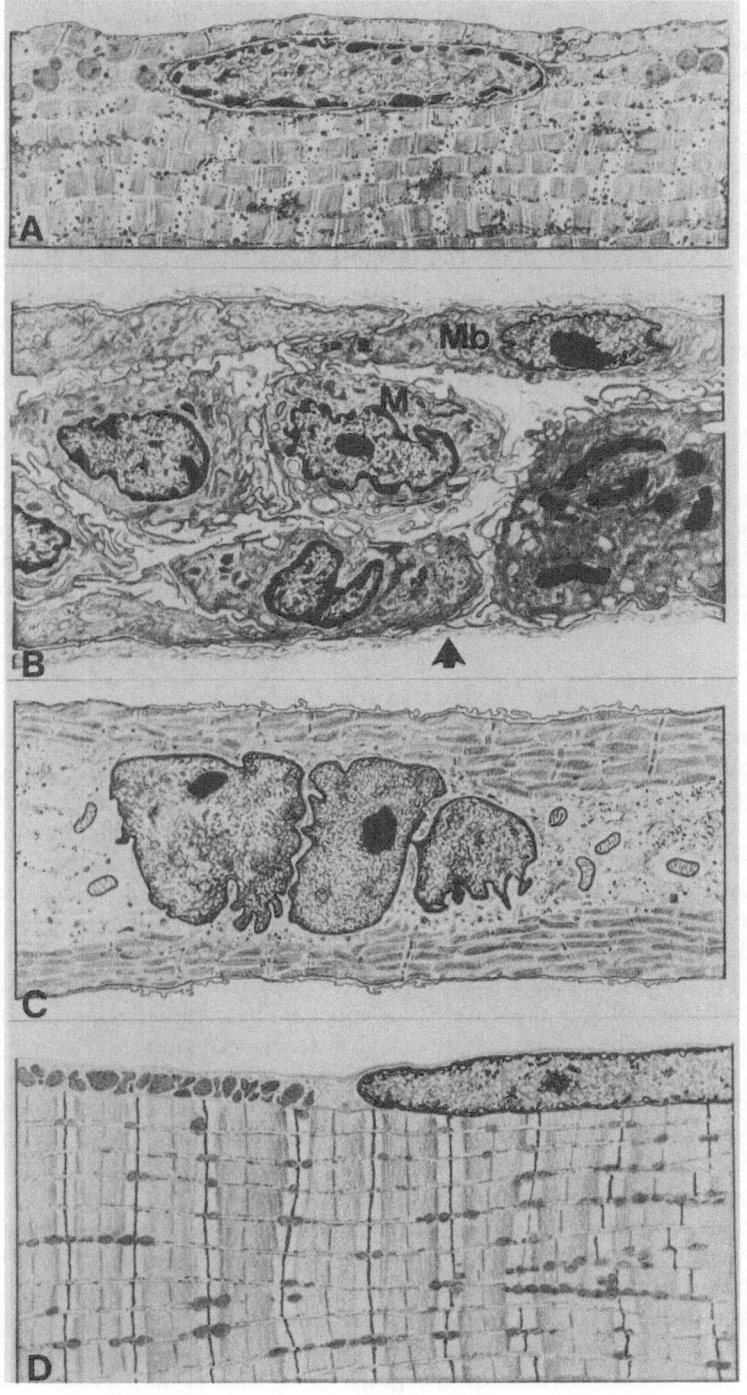

the interior of the graft, the ischemic muscle fibers are broken down by invading macrophages, and within the persisting basal laminae of the original muscle fibers new muscle fibers regenerate (Fig. 2), presumably from satellite cells (Snow, 1977). This pattern of peripheral survival and internal breakdown and regeneration of muscle fibers has been documented in grafts of mouse, hamster, rat and cat muscles. Regeneration has also been seen in grafts of monkey palmaris longus muscles, but not enough grafts have been examined to ascertain the extent of muscle fiber regeneration in relation to survival. There is almost no information on the histology of human muscle grafts.

Within a single type of graft, the proportions of surviving and regenerating muscle fibers differ widely with varying treatments of the muscles. Such experiments can provide considerable insight into the relative importance of survival versus regeneration in accounting for the long-term success of a graft. If the extensor digitorum longus (EDL) muscle of the rat is grafted without any pretreatment, only a small percentage (2–4%) of muscle fibers survive, whereas after predenervation the number of surviving muscle fibers increases to almost 25% (Carlson, 1976). By injecting the muscle with the myotoxic local anesthetic, Marcaine, it is possible to eliminate almost all surviving muscle fibers from the graft. Regardless of the number of surviving muscle fibers, the number of muscle fibers in mature grafts in the rat differs little from the normal number. This means that regeneration of new muscle fibers can compensate for any number of muscle fibers that fail to survive the grafting procedure.

## The Predenervation Question

With increasing experimental evidence demonstrating that predenervation is not critical for the successful free grafting of muscles in many laboratory animals, it is appropriate to examine the known effects of denervation on muscle before (Gutmann, 1962) and after grafting. The histochemical alterations in denervated muscle (Romanul and Hogan, 1965) are well known in the transplantation literature, as is the well-documented increase in the percentage of satellite cells after denervation (Ontell, 1974). A gross change which may be of considerable importance is the reduction in cross-sectional area of a denervated muscle. The suggested increase in vascularity of denervated muscle is probably related more to the atrophy of muscle fibers rather than an absolute increase in the number of muscle fibers in a denervated muscle. After grafting there is a more rapid breakdown of ischemic muscle fibers in muscles that have been predenervated and, in the rat, an acceleration of the early stages of regeneration by about 24 hours. The latter is probably the result of the increase in number of satellite cells, which may reduce the time required to generate a critical population of proliferating myoblastic cells.

In larger laboratory mammals and in humans, the relative merits of predenervation remain unclear. In the case of the cat, Hakelius (1977) finds predenervation necessary in the case of the peroneus longus or tertius muscles grafted over the intercostal muscles, whereas for orthotopically grafted EDL muscles, predenervation results in no long-term advantage, despite some difference in the early course of the grafts (Faulkner et al., 1980; Faulkner,

Markley and White, this volume). Bosova (1976) has reported on the need for predenervation in the free grafting of the gastrocnemius muscle in dogs. In palmaris longus grafts of the monkey, predenervation does not seem to alter long-term results, but further confirmatory work would be useful. At present there is no basis for commenting upon the relative merits of predenervation versus no predenervation in human muscle grafting, but this is an extremely important question.

From the perspective of a laboratory researcher, what are the potential advantages and disadvantages of predenervation in clinical muscle grafting? The most apparent disadvantage is that predenervation involves an extra operation which, if not required, would involve the expenditure of extra time and money by the patient, as well as a small risk of complications. A potential advantage of predenervation is a reduction in the cross-sectional area of the muscle In the relatively large muscles used in human transplantation, this would reduce the distance that ingrowing blood vessels would have to travel to reach the center of the graft and it could lead to the survival and/or regeneration of more cells in the center of the graft than might otherwise be the case. In small muscles, such considerations may not be relevant because blood vessels get to the center of the graft before permanent necrosis sets in, but in grafts of muscles that show a tendency to form a central core of dense connective tissue, a possible beneficial effect of predenervation should be carefully investigated.

In summary, it is now well established that predenervation results in no long-term improvement in the size or functional capacities of grafted muscles weighing less than 6 gm. More experimentation is needed to establish the degree of effectiveness of predenervation in larger muscles.

## The Revascularization of Muscle Grafts

Very little is yet known about the revascularization of free muscle grafts. A recent electron microscopic study (Hansen-Smith et al., 1980) has shown that in rat muscle grafts the capillaries break down within 24 hours. In larger vessels the endothelium disappears and the smooth muscle undergoes at least partially reversible degenerative changes. By two days new blood vessels begin to grow into the grafts at many sites along the periphery (Fig. 3). Most of the ingrowing vessels occupy completely new sites, but some grow into the remains of pre-existing vascular channels, utilizing the persisting basal lamina and possibly some of the smooth muscle elements of the original vessels. Later aspects of vascular reintegration have been studied by White et al. (in press).

Little, if anything, is known about the stimulus leading to the ingrowth of blood vessels into a muscle graft. Little is also known about factors leading to the maturation of vascular pattern and function.

From the clinical standpoint, the most important aspect of revascularization is the rate of ingrowth of blood vessels in relation to the length of time that the central regions of the graft can be repopulated by regenerating muscle fibers. At this time it is not known whether myogenic cells in the center of even a small muscle graft survive or whether they die from ischemia and are later replaced by myogenic cells migrating in from the peripheral region of the graft. The recent studies by Lipton and Schultz (1979) and Jones (1979) on the selective penetration of myoblastic cells into the basal laminae of mature muscle fibers *in vivo* lend some credence to the latter possibility.

From the practical standpoint, if a mature muscle graft contains muscle fibers throughout its cross-section, neither the rate nor the extent of revascularization are likely factors limiting the success of the graft. In contrast, if a mature graft

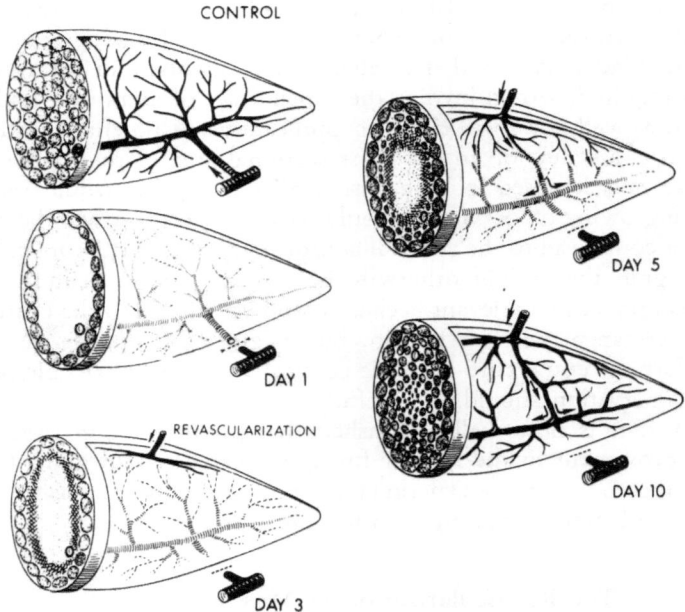

Fig. 3. Diagrams illustrating the revascularization of grafted EDL muscles in the rat. Day 1) The larger vessels in the graft are severely ischemic and most capillaries have degenerated. The cut face of the muscle shows surviving muscle fibers (dark circles) and ischemic muscle fibers (central stippling). Day 3) New blood vessels begin to grow into the graft. Correlated with this, a zone of muscle fiber degeneration and regeneration (cross-hatching in cut surface) is established. Day 5) Ingrowing blood vessels occupy a greater portion of the graft. Some new vessels are growing into the lumens of old, degenerating ones, and some larger original vessels are re-utilized as vascular channels. The flow of blood is indicated by arrows. Day 10) The graft is revascularized throughout, with an amalgamation of old and new blood vessels. Within the peripheral zone of surviving muscle fibers, the central part of the graft is filled with thin regenerating muscle fibers [From Hansen-Smith, F. M., *et al.*, Am. J. Anat. *158*, 65 (1980)]

contains a central core of dense connective tissue, surrounded by a ring of surviving and/or regenerating muscle fibers (Fig. 4), it is likely that blood vessels have not reached the center rapidly enough to prevent the takeover of the part of the graft by fibroblasts and their secretions. The formation of a central core of connective tissue in a given type of graft would be an indication for the use of microvascular anastomoses between graft and host. If a central core of connective tissue does not form, then vascular anastomosis is probably unnecessary.

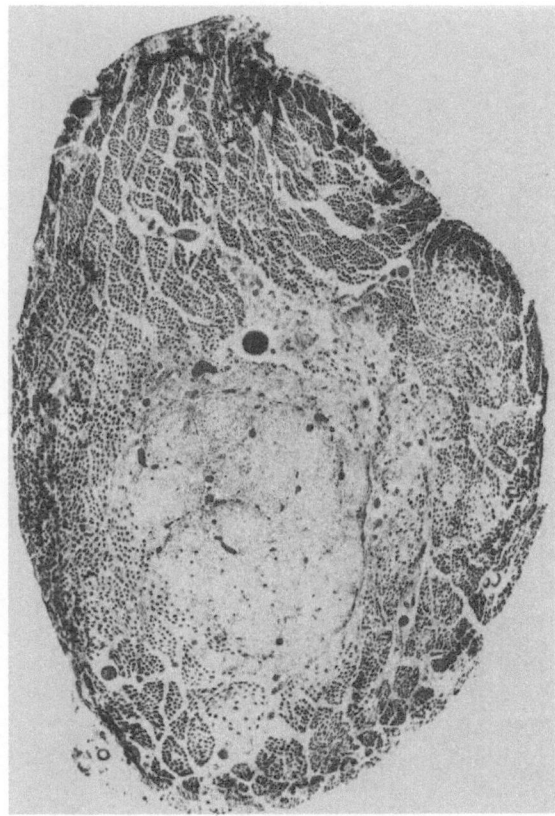

Fig. 4. Cross-section through an 83-day orthotopic palmaris longus muscle transplant in the monkey. Bundles of regenerating muscle fibers surround a central core of dense fibrous connective tissue. Palmgren's silver stain. 20X

## The Reinnervation of Muscle Grafts

Depending upon the experimental or clinical model, a grafted muscle can become innervated either by nerve fibers which grow out from the cut end of a nerve (neural neurotization) or by nerve fibers which sprout from muscles adjacent to the grafted muscle (muscular neurotization). Although many surgical models of muscle grafting involve muscular neurotization (Holle, 1976), little laboratory investigation has yet been performed in this area.

The most extensively studied model of reinnervation has been the orthotopically grafted extensor digitorum longus muscle of the rat. If no attempt is made to reconnect the severed nerve to the graft, the first regenerating nerve fibers enter the graft early in the second week after transplantation (Carlson *et al.*, 1979). At this time the muscle fibers in the graft are already capable of contraction when directly stimulated (Carlson and Gutmann, 1975). Despite their relatively early penetration into the muscle graft, the regenerating nerve

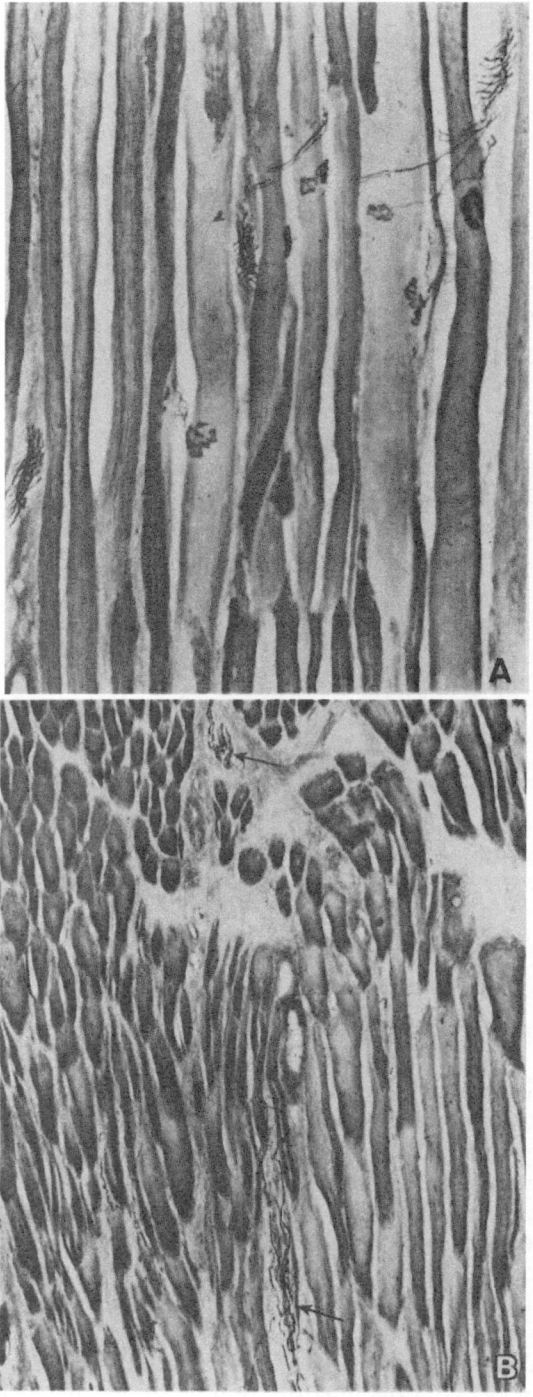

fibers do not form functional neuromuscular synapses until early in the fourth postoperative week (Fig. 5A). After neuromuscular transmission has been established, the regenerating muscle fibers undergo histochemical differentiation into fast and slow types, and the final nerve-dependent maturation of contractile properties takes place (Fig. 6).

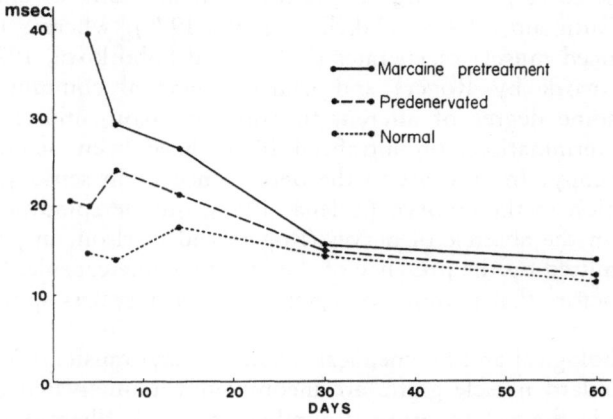

Fig. 6. Comparison of the time-course of development of the full contraction time (time to peak tension) in normal, predenervated and Marcaine-treated rat EDL grafts. In normal grafts the first contractions (4 and 7 days) are due to surviving muscle fibers. The contribution of the more slowly contracting, regenerating muscle fibers is added to this at 14 days. In predenervated grafts the surviving predenervated muscle fibers begin to contract earlier and more slowly than surviving muscle fibers in normal grafts. The slow contractions of regenerating muscle fibers are added on as early as 7 days. Marcaine-treated grafts contain no surviving muscle fibers. The curve of contraction times in these grafts represents a pure population of regenerating muscle fibers. In all kinds of grafts, the time to peak tension returns to essentially control values by 60 days [From Carlson, B. M., et al., 1979, in: Muscle Regeneration (Mauro, A., ed.). New York: Raven Press]

One of the major questions regarding reinnervation of muscle grafts is the mechanism of formation of new synaptic connections between regenerating axons and muscle fibers. The problem is exemplified by the almost two-week delay between the appearance of nerves and the formation of functional neuromuscular connections in grafts of rat muscles. What are the nerve fibers doing during this period? There is evidence from experiments on regenerating muscle in both the frog (Marshall et al., 1977) and the rat (Bader, 1980) that ingrowing axons seek out and settle down preferentially at sites of former neuromuscular junctions. More specifically, characteristics of the persisting original basal lamina that surrounds a regenerating muscle fiber at the neuromuscular junction appear to be critical (Sanes et al., 1978; Sanes and Hall, 1979), since the nerve fibers do not ever make direct contact with the muscle

Fig. 5. A Nerve fibers and motor end plates in a 30-day EDL muscle graft in the rat. Goshgarian combined silver-acetylcholinesterase stain. 145 X. B Innervated muscle spindles (arrows) from the same graft as that in part A. 88 X

fibers. Despite the apparent specificity in the above systems, small numbers (1–3%) of new neuromuscular junctions do form in soleus grafts in the rat. According to some reports (Hakelius and Nyström, 1979), new motor endplates are commonly seen in grafted cat muscles. This indicates the possibility of species differences in the specificity of motor reinnervation in regenerating muscle.

Muscle spindles (Fig. 5B) are commonly seen in grafts of entire muscles (Carlson and Gutmann, 1975a; Hakelius *et al.*, 1975), whereas they do not reappear in minced muscle regenerates (Zelená and Sobotková, 1971; Carlson, 1972). Recent work by Rogers and Quick (personal communication) has demonstrated some degree of afferent function in mature muscle grafts, and sensory nerve terminations on intrafusal fibers have been demonstrated by electron microscopy. In contrast to the dependence upon sensory innervation for their induction in the embryo (Zelená, 1957), muscle spindles in the adult can regenerate in the absence of nerves (Rogers and Carlson, in press). This is apparently permitted by the presence of the intact spindle capsule, but the exact nature of the factors that permit the regeneration of nerveless spindles remains obscure.

Both morphological and biochemical (choline acetyltransferase) studies have shown that standard muscle grafts are incompletely reinnervated despite their having, at least in the rat, the normal number of muscle fibers (Carlson *et al.*, 1979; Bader, 1980). Standard muscle grafts have a considerably smaller mass (35–50% of normal) and a correspondingly weaker contractile strength. In laboratory experiments a dramatic improvement in the functional mass of a muscle graft can be obtained by leaving the motor nerve intact (Carlson *et al.*, 1979) or by anastomosing the nerve stumps of the graft and host bed (Markley and Faulkner, in press). Ongoing experiments suggest that the better the anatomical distribution of regenerating nerve fibers among the muscle fibers of the graft, the better will be the mass and functional capacity of the muscle.

## Concluding Remarks

Free muscle grafting brings up a number of important questions of relevance to both laboratory scientists and clinicians. One of the first questions to arise concerns the problem of reinnervation of existing paralyzed muscles versus grafting. Making this decision requires considerable clinical experience and, ideally, concrete information at the cellular and molecular level on conditions that must be met in order for regenerating nerve fibers to re-establish synaptic connections in long-term denervated muscle. The latter information is not yet at hand.

If a muscle is to be grafted, it is of considerable practical importance to know the cellular basis that accounts for the success of a graft. The relationship of muscle fiber survival to degeneration and regeneration is well defined in several laboratory models. Predenervation of the muscle to be grafted is not necessary in most laboratory models of muscle transplantation. Yet we know little about the cellular reactions in human muscle grafts. To what extent do they follow the rules laid out by those who study muscle transplantation in the laboratory?

In order for any muscle graft to be successful, it must become well integrated with the vascular and nervous systems of the host and also establish origin and insertion points that will permit the effective transmission of mechanical tension. Vascular reintegration is the first critical step, because in the prolonged absence of direct vascularization the deprived portions of the graft will become filled in with dense connective tissue. We do not now know the size beyond which spontaneous revascularization will fail to supply the entire graft effectively before terminal necrosis of the central region sets in. There may be considerable species variations in this regard. Knowledge of this point is important in making a decision concerning whether or not to employ vascular anastomosis.

There are many important questions concerning neural integration. We know little about the relative effectiveness of muscular as opposed to neural neurotization of transplanted muscle. We do not know what causes nerves (or blood vessels) to sprout and enter a graft. More is known about what causes nerves to settle down and establish functional connections, but we still do not know if knowledge gained from studies on rats and amphibians can be applied to human muscle. Almost nothing is known about the return of sensory function in muscle grafts. There is now considerable evidence that the quality of a graft can be improved by guiding regenerating nerve fibers into old nerve channels leading into the muscle.

The object of muscle grafting is, of course, to restore function. Assuming that the conditions of grafting have been the best possible, it is still necessary for the muscle to be efficiently connected to its desired insertion point and that volitional contraction be accomplished as soon as possible. Although there is ample evidence of effective mechanical integration of a grafted muscle with the associated structures of the host bed, there has been little rigorous documentation of this phenomenon. Likewise, there has been little work done on the response of regenerating muscle to training programs or the facilitation of recovery of human muscle grafts by physical therapy or training.

The field of free muscle transplantation is still in its infancy. Much more well controlled work in both the research laboratory and the clinic is necessary before any real appreciation of the potential and limitations of this technique can be realized.

## Acknowledgements

Original research was supported by grants from the Muscular Dystrophy Association and NIH.

## References

Bader, D.: Reinnervation of motor endplate-containing and motor endplate-less muscle grafts. Devel. Biol. 77, 315–327 (1980).

Bosova, N. N.: Free autoplastic transplantation of whole muscles. (Russian.) Byull. Exp. Biol. Med. 53, 88–92 (1962).

Bosova, N. N.: Restorative processes in dog muscles after free auto- and homografting. (Russian.) Byull. Exp. Biol. Med. 82, 1377–1379 (1976).

Carlson, B. M.: The Regeneration of Minced Muscles. Basel: Karger. 1972.

Carlson, B. M.: A quantitative study of muscle fiber survival and regeneration in normal, predenervated, and Marcaine-treated free muscle grafts in the rat. Exp. Neurol. 52, 421–432 (1976).

Carlson, B. M.: A review of muscle transplantation in mammals. Physiol. Bohemoslov. *27*, 387–400 (1978).

Carlson, B. M., Gutmann, E.: Regeneration in free grafts of normal and denervated muscles in the rat: Morphology and histochemistry. Anat. Rec. *183*, 47–62 (1975a).

Carlson, B. M., Gutmann, E.: Regeneration in grafts of normal and denervated rat muscles. Contractile properties. Pflügers Arch. *353*, 215–225 (1975b).

Carlson, B. M., Hník, P., Tuček, S., Vejsada, R., Bader, D.: Comparison between standard free muscle grafts and grafts with intact nerves in the rat EDL muscle. (Abstr.) Anat. Rec. *193*, 498 (1979).

Carlson, B. M., Wagner, K. R., Max, S. R.: Reinnervation of rat extensor digitorum longus muscles after free grafting. Muscle & Nerve *1979*, 304–307.

Faulkner, J. A., Niemeyer, J. H., Maxwell, L. C., White, T. P.: Contractile properties of transplanted extensor digitorum longus muscles of cats. Am. J. Physiol. *238*, C 120–C 126 (1980).

Gutmann, E.: The denervated muscle. Prague: Publishing House of the Czechoslovak Academy of Sciences. 1962.

Hakelius, L.: Free muscle and nerve grafting in the face, in: Reanimation of the Paralyzed Face (Rubin, L., ed.), pp. 279–293. St. Louis: Mosby. 1977.

Hakelius, L., Nyström, B.: Histochemical studies of end-plate formation in free autologous muscle transplants in cats. Scand. J. Plast. Reconstr. Surg. *9*, 9–14 (1975).

Hakelius, L., Nyström, B., Stålberg, E.: Histochemical and electrophysiological studies of autotransplanted cat muscle. Scand. J. Plast. Reconstr. Surg. *9*, 15–24 (1975).

Hansen-Smith, F. M., Carlson, B. M., Irwin, K. L.: Revascularization of the freely grafted extensor digitorum longus muscle in the rat. Am. J. Anat. *158*, 65–82 (1980).

Holle, J.: Die muskuläre Neurotisation in der rekonstruktiven Chirurgie. Wien. klin. Wschr. *88*, Suppl. 48, 1–21 (1976).

Jones, P. H.: Implantation of cultured regenerate muscle cells into adult rat muscle. Exp. Neurol. *66*, 602–610 (1979).

Lipton, B. H., Schultz, E.: Developmental fate of skeletal muscle satellite cells. Science *205*, 1292–1294 (1979).

Markley, J. M., Faulkner, J. A.: Transplanted skeletal muscle regeneration in primates, with clinical correlation. In: Proceedings of the Fourth International Facial Nerve Symposium, Los Angeles, 1980. New York: Raven Press. In press.

Marshall, L. M., Sanes, J. R., McMahan, U. J.: Reinnervation of original synaptic sites on muscle fiber basement membrane after disruption of muscle cells. Proc. Nat. Acad. Sci. USA *74*, 3073–3077 (1977).

Ontell, M.: Effects of denervation on satellite cell population of rat striated muscle. Anat. Rec. *178*, 211–228 (1974).

Rogers, S. L., Carlson, B. M.: A quantitative assessment of muscle spindle formation in reinnervated and non-reinnervated grafts of the rat extensor digitorum longus muscle. Neuroscience (in press).

Romanul, F. C. A., Hogan, E. L.: Enzymatic changes in denervated muscle. I. Histochemical studies. Arch. Neurol. *12*, 263–273 (1965).

Sanes, J. R., Hall, Z. W.: Antibodies that bind specifically to synaptic sites on muscle fiber basal lamina. J. Cell Biol. *83*, 357–370 (1979).

Sanes, J. R., Marshall, L. M., McMahan, U. J.: Reinnervation of muscle fiber basal lamina after removal of myofibers. J. Cell Biol. *78*, 176–198 (1978).

Snow, M. H.: Myogenic cell formation in regenerating rat skeletal muscle injured by mincing. II. An autoradiographic study. Anat. Rec. *188*, 201–218 (1977).

Studitsky, A. N.: Dynamics of the development of myogenic tissue under conditions of explantation and transplantation, in: Cinemicrography in Cell Biology (Rose, G. G., ed.), pp. 171–200. New York: Academic Press. 1963.

Studitsky, A. N.: The Transplantation of Muscles in Animals. (Russian.) Moscow: Izd. Meditsina. 1977.

Thompson, N.: Autogenous free grafts of skeletal muscle. Plast. Reconstr. Surg. *48*, 11–27 (1971).

White, T. P., Sosin, D. M., Maxwell, L. C., Faulkner, J. A.: Blood flow of autotransplanted extensor digitorum longus muscles of cats. Am. J. Physiol.: Heart and Circ. Physiol. (in press).

Zelená, J.: The morphogenetic influence of innervation on the ontogenetic development of muscle spindles. J. Embryol. Exp. Morphol. 5, 283–292 (1957).

Zelená, J., Sobotková, J.: Absence of muscle spindles in regenerated muscles of the rat. Physiol. Bohemoslov. 20, 433–439 (1971).

Author's address: Dr. B. M. Carlson, Department of Anatomy, 4622 Medical Sciences II, University of Michigan, Ann Arbor, MI 48109, U.S.A.

## Discussion

*Freilinger:* I am very grateful that you brought up the question about Studitsky's research. The question, I have to you is: Would you think that Studitsky's minced muscles, as far as functional recovery is concerned, have any relevance in the clinical use?

*Carlson:* I don't think so. Minced muscle regeneration, at least in my hands, is a very good experimental model, and I used it in some early work on morphogenesis of regenerating muscles. But in the main, functional recovery has not been very good because of a large number of adhesions. Therefore it would not be a very good clinical technique. Prof. Maréchal later on this morning may have some different opinions on that, because he has used minced muscle regeneration with better functional success. This technique has been used in muscular dystrophy research–by exchanging minced muscles between dystrophic and normal mice. Here they regenerate very well. I know of only one case, in which minced muscle regeneration have been attempted in humans, and this has not been published. A number of years ago a man had a severe injury to his leg and the tibialis anterior muscle was badly damaged and was essentially minced. The decision was made to mince it up in fine pieces. The patient's leg was then placed in a cast for three weeks. This particular muscle ended up as a sheet of connective tissue with no obvious muscle fibres. So I myself, if I had a damaged muscle, would not want anyone to mince mine.

*Benetar:* You showed in your slide that muscles that have been denervated for 14 days seem to have a higher rate of regeneration in terms of the number of fibres, in comparison with muscles that have not been denervated. Why did you use just 14 days instead of 6 weeks?

*Carlson:* The reason we used 14 days is that this was the time that Studitsky originally used. There is no significant difference between amount of muscle fiber regeneration, in fact there is actually less. Because, if you look at the number of muscle fibers in a mature graft, there is no statistical difference–at least in our hands–in any of these techniques. But yet the pre-denervated muscles start out with a 1000 more surviving fibers than in a standard muscle graft. This means that in a pre-denervated muscle there are approximately 3000 regenerating muscle fibres, whereas in a standard muscle graft there are 4000. Pre-denervation in our hands greatly increases the number of surviving muscle fibres; thus there is a corresponding decrease in the amount of regeneration. The Michigan group does quite a lot of work on larger animals. But counting muscle fibers in grafts of cat muscles is very difficult for topographical reasons. In the rat we can easily dissociate at a certain period of time the surviving from the regenerating muscle fibres. In cases, in which we have attempted to do in the cat, it has not been possible.

*Holle:* I think, the most important questions for us plastic surgeons is: Does the same regeneration as you have showed us in the rat muscle, take part in a big human muscle?

*Carlson:* This is a very important question. In Michigan we have looked at larger muscles in cats and in monkeys. In cat muscle regeneration occurs within the transplant in exactly the same sequence as we find it in the rats, but the time is greatly prolonged. What takes one day in the rat, takes one week in the cat. This is the rule–Dr. Faulkner will be showing this later. In a transplant of the EDL-muscle in a cat, you still see original muscle fibres and ischemic necrosis as late as six weeks after grafting. Ischemic muscle fibres disappear in six days in the rat. Innervation is correspondingly delayed in this model. We have done not enough work on monkeys, to get a good sequence, but I do know that muscles thus break down and regenerate. One of the critical things that must be done is to demonstrate a sequence of degeneration and regeneration under controlled circumstances in a human. To my knowledge this information does not exist, but it would be very important, in terms of understanding how to apply a human muscle graft.

Question: About motor endplates in free grafts. Do they degenerate completely and are replaced by new motor end-plates? This is contradictory to what you have just told us. What do you think about that?

*Carlson:* Yes, I know. I would like to ask Prof. Hakelius. Do you really know that the new end-plates are new motor end-plates and not persisting original ones? We thought that we knew, but it is very difficult by using only cholinesterase to be sure that a motor end-plate is in fact reinnervated. It may also be that there are species differences–We have not carefully studied reinnervation in the cat.

*Hakelius:* Yes, I think, we are quite sure that there are new motor end-plates instead of reinnervated ones, because a lot of them are not in the normal motor end band, but are scattered throughout the muscle. So it is not like before. There is only a small band before grafting.

*Carlson:* Do you have any idea what percentage of the muscle fibres in your grafts are reinnervated?

*Hakelius:* No, we have not counted it.

*Carlson:* There is some new formation of motor end-plates in rat grafts as well, but a very small percentage.

*Hakelius:* Yes, but I think, you have a lot of reinnervation in the muscle-transplant and you get a contraction of the muscles with this new motor end plate, which is quite good.

*Carlson:* Do you know if the contraction comes from the nerves? It could be a muscle to muscle contact. In your model of taking a muscle and putting it into the intercostal space you saw a contraction, with electromyographic evidence of activity corresponding with breathing movements. Is there a possibility that there could be muscle ingrowth from the intercostal muscles into your graft as a secondary connection? We find this very common in our grafts.

*Hakelius:* I don't think so, because there is a quite good fascial plane between the donor muscle and the recipient and the fibres are at right angles against each other when we made the transplantation. So it is quite easy to dissect it.

*Carlson:* Of course it may be that there are species-specific differences.

*Brunelli:* We did experiments in rabbits and rats and we take the experiments in human beings. We were able to demonstrate that if you take of all the tibial nerves and transplant the peroneal nerve into the gastrocnemius, into a zone in the proximal part of the muscle, where there are no existing motor plates, you can see motor end-plates by both the optical and electron microscope. Then we translated this experiment in human beings, for instance, who had lost all proximal parts of the forearm extensor muscle, bone, skin and nerve. We did direct neurotisation of the muscle and had good results also after some years. I will show you some slides in the afternoon.

*Carlson:* This is very interesting and this is why I think that there are pronounced differences right now in some of these experimental models. I will be very curious in the next two or three years to see how recent work on the immunology of the basement membrane is going to relate to our experiments, which we have been conducting on grafted muscles. There are many interesting experiments, not yet published, which indicate that there are antigenic specifities at the site of the former neuromuscular junction. Right now my feeling is that there is a great gap between some of these works and some of the classical works in the neurotisation of muscles. And I doubt that we are going to be able to solve this problem in this meeting.

*Thompson:* On the question of the production of motor end-plates, I think it was the Australian Hoffman working on the Australian opossum, who produced hyperneurotisation in a normal muscle by implanting a motor nerve into it. I worked on dogs transplanting denervated skeletal muscles to the myocardium. The denervated muscle transplant failed to survive in all cases in 30 or 40 animals, unless the phrenic nerve was implanted into it. And once the phrenic nerve was implanted into it, we saw a routine survival. The histologic examination did show a picture of degenerating motor end plates and surviving end plates and the interpretation is that reinnervation of existing motor end plates takes place.

*Carlson:* One of the important aspects of reinnervation is to separate also the stimuli which cause the nerves to sprout from those which cause nerves to settle down. And you have brought up the work of Hoffman. Much of this work was involved with the simulation of nerve-sprouting and it is in many respects a completely different biological problem.

*Hakelius:* How do the motor end-plates look in minced muscles of the rat? Have you studied it?

*Carlson:* I have not spent to much time studying that. Zhenevskaya in Russia has done that extensively, and in one period she talked about hyperneurotisation of minced muscle regenerates. But they were using only morphological techniques and their impression was based upon examination of silver-stained nerves distributed throughout the muscle. I think it would be worthwhile to examine this with some of the newer techniques.

*Mayr:* I feel, in the discussion concerning end-plates also the myomyous junctions that you mentioned might have some importance. We found myomyous junctions in normal muscles with a very complicated muscle architecture, especially in extra-ocular muscles. And there on both sides of the myomyous junction were always motor end-plates or multiple endings. You have mentioned in connection with the myomyous junction, that you found them in quite a high number, associated with electrical coupling. It seems that one of the explanations of the functional myomyous junction could be the coupling of fibres, so that not each part should have its own motor ending. In normal muscles, where myomyous junctions do occur, this is not the case. We were always thinking that those junctions have merely a mechanical function and that they are there in extraocular muscles, because of the need for a very, very fast contraction. This would allow a faster contraction of the whole system than if there were long fibres with single motor end-plates. But still in this connection it would be interesting to know the relation of the number of motor end-plates to the number of muscle fibres.

*Carlson:* This is what we are just doing now and I think it would be at least six months before we have the information.

*Freilinger:* For us clinicians it would be most important to know the question: is muscular neurotisation versus neural neurotisation more effective? I think, in our hands muscular neurotisation brings much more for reinnervation in facial cases if it works. It would be very interesting, if anybody in the auditorium could tell us something more about these two differences.

*Carlson:* This is one of the most important questions of clinical relevance. Especially there are two aspects. How effective is this mode of operation from the clinical sense and what is the mechanism of restoration of function? Is it through motor nerves; is it through muscle contact? How many nerves are required to grow into the graft to make it functional in the clinical sense? I don't know the answer of any of these.

# The Muscle Satellite Cell and Its Role in Muscle Transplantation (A Short Review)*

### R. Mayr

Department of Anatomy 2,
University of Vienna, Austria

With 3 Figures

Successful *free autologous muscle transplantation* is highly dependent on the regenerative capacity of skeletal muscle. Because of transient ischemia, only a thin superficial layer of muscle fibres was found to survive free muscle transplantation, as shown by the Vienna group (Holle *et al.*, 1974; Lischka *et al.*, 1977) and in more detail by Carlson and Gutmann (1975 a, b), Schiaffino *et al.* (1975), and Hansen-Smith and Carlson (1979). Even after prior denervation of the transplanted muscle, as first recommended by Thompson (1971), the number of surviving superficial muscle fibres is only moderately increased (Carlson, 1978). Thus, a process of degeneration and regeneration governs the events resulting in the structural and functional recovery of the transplanted muscle. Of course, modern research in muscle transplantation aims to avoid ischemic necrosis as far as possible by immediate reconstitution of the muscle's vascular supply (Harii *et al.*, 1976), but still under such favorable conditions damage to the transplant will not be avoidable, and a good result will still be dependent on the regenerative capacity of striated muscle.

The *regeneration of muscle* (for review see Carlson, 1973; Mauro, 1978) and thus also the success of free muscle transplantation is fundamentally dependent on the presence and the activation of *myogenic cells.* Such cells are found as mononucleated cells between the degenerating muscle fibre and its basal lamina. They are able to undergo mitosis, to fuse with each other or with preexisting muscle fibres, and to produce myofilaments. If recognizable myofilaments are already present, these cells are called myoblasts; if their organelles resemble those of myoblasts except the presence of myofilaments, the term 'presumptive myoblasts' has been adopted (Carlson, 1973). The *origin of these mononuclear myoblastic cells* has been the subject of much controversy for many decades,

* Supported by the "Fonds zur Förderung der wissenschaftlichen Forschung in Österreich" (Project 2618).

2*

especially however since the early sixties, when Alexander Mauro (1961) described a hitherto unknown cell, the *satellite cell of skeletal muscle fibres* or *myosatellite cell,* as it is now often called, and put forward in his short and concise first communication on that cell the hypothesis of its possible importance for the ability of skeletal muscle to regenerate.

I want to recall the characterization of this cell by Mauro's (1961) description in frog muscle, as it has proved to be generally valid by confirmation in many other species (compare Figs. 1 and 2):

". . ., the striking paucity of cytoplasm relative to its nucleus results in the cell assuming the shape of the nucleus. In fact, it is virtually impossible to discern the cellular nature of this entity in the light microscope, as it appears to be indistinguishable from a peripheral nucleus proper. In electron micrographs the cell is seen 'wedged' between the plasma membrane of the muscle fiber and the basement membrane, which invests the fiber throughout its length in close association with the plasma membrane. The intimacy of this satellite cell with respect to the multinucleate muscle cell is further revealed in the fact that, in general, the surface of the muscle fiber is not distorted outward but instead the satellite cell protrudes inward pushing the myofibrils of the muscle cell aside. On the inner side, the plasma membrane of the satellite cell is in apposition with the plasma membrane of the muscle cell."

Speculating about the origin and the role of these cells, Mauro already suggested in this first publication that his satellite cells "might be pertinent to the vexing problem of skeletal muscle regeneration", and proposed three hypothetical functions, which are nourishing the controversy on the origin and function of this myosatellite cell up to today:

1. ". . ., that in the resting state some (of these) cells are being produced at a slow rate by the above mechanism" (i.e. by splitting from multinucleate muscle cells) "and reside just outside the plasma membrane of the muscle cell, and that upon being stimulated by trauma, e.g. ischemia, mechanical compression, toxic agents etc., the rate of production of such cells is increased."–2. ". . . that the satellite cells are remnants from the embryonic development of the multinucleate cell which results from the process of fusion of individual myoblasts. Thus the satellite cells are merely dormant myoblasts that failed to fuse with the other myoblasts and are ready to recapitulate the embryonic development of skeletal muscle fiber when the main multinucleate muscle fiber is damaged."–3. ". . . satellite cells (might be) 'wandering' cells that have penetrated the basement membrane and are lying underneath it ready to be mobilized into activity under the proper conditions."–And in a footnote Mauro gives another hint to the eventual importance of satellite cells for skeletal muscle regeneration, speculating "whether the apparent inability of cardiac muscle cells to regenerate is related to the absence of satellite cells".

Twelve years after the discovery of the myosatellite cell Carlson (1973), in his review on the regeneration of skeletal muscle, included a critical survey of the literature on that cell in the decade after its first description. Controversial data and interpretations had been published by different authors adhering either to the first or to the second of Mauro's hypothetical suggestions (cf. also Mauro *et al.,* 1970). One group (Reznik, 1969, 1970; Elyakova, 1972; Walker, 1972;

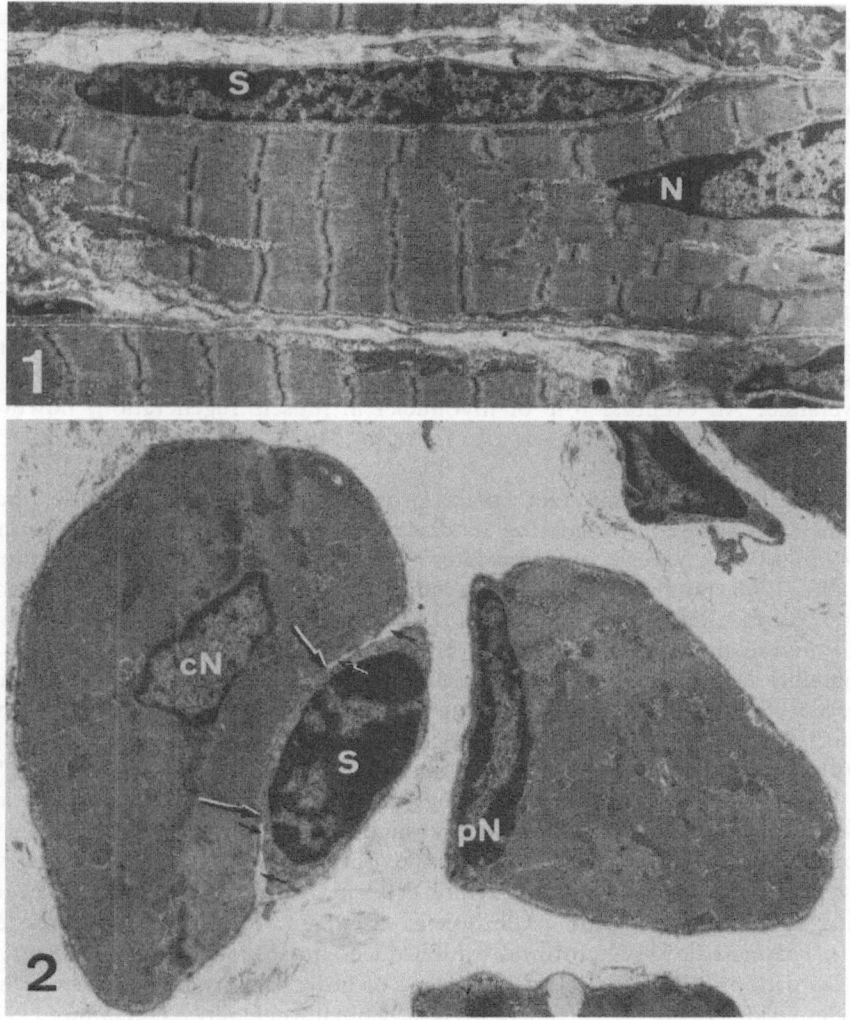

Fig. 1. Longitudinally sectioned myosatellite cell *(S)* of a guinea pig stapedius muscle fibre of typically small diameter with a centrally located myonucleus *(N)*. × 4500. Length of satellite cell nucleus about 17 μm (From Burgener and Mayr 1980, by kind permission of the Springer-Verlag)

Fig. 2. Cross-sectioned myosatellite cell (S) of a guinea pig stapedius muscle fibre. × 9000. Small diameters of satellite cell nucleus about 3 and 1.5 μm. Compare satellite cell nucleus *(S)* with its more condensed chromatin with a centrally located myonucleus *(cN)* of the same muscle fibre and a peripheral myonucleus *(pN)* of an adjacent muscle fibre. All muscle fibres are extremely thin in guinea pig stapedius muscle. As in other muscles, the myosatellite cell typically protrudes into a depression of the muscle cell proper without distorting the contour of the muscle fibre. In this case, as often found in others, the basal lamina invests a part of the adjacent plasmalemmas of both the muscle cell and satellite cell (small arrows) which are more distant from each other in these areas than in the zone of the usual 200 Å space without intervening basal lamina (between large arrows).

(Figs. 2–3 are unpublished material from joint work of the author with J. Burgener)

Aloisi *et al.*, 1973) assumed that myosatellite cells originate by separation of myonuclei from degenerating or injured muscle fibres. According to Reznik (1969), satellite cells are not even present in normal adult muscle. Other studies presented evidence that myogenic cells of regenerating muscle are direct descendants of satellite cells which are, according to these authors, remnants from embryonic development and represent dormant myoblasts permanently present in skeletal muscle fibres constituting a small percentage of the "muscle nuclei" (Church *et al.*, 1966; Shafiq *et al.*, 1967; Reger and Craig, 1968; Church, 1969, 1970b; Shafig, 1970; Moss and Leblond, 1971).

In the last 7 years evidence has been accumulating more and more in favour of the hypothesis that satellite cells, as dormant myoblasts, are the source of myogenic cells for regenerative processes in the adult stage, and against a possible involvement of myonuclei whose postmitotic state is widely held to be irreversible. An eventual role of myonuclei in muscle regeneration, however, cannot be completely ruled out (Aloisi *et al.*, 1973; Aloisi and Mussini, this symposium).

In the following some data on the properties of myosatellite cells, whose presence has been confirmed after its discovery in frog skeletal muscle (Mauro, 1961) in a wide variety of vertebrates (Muir *et al.*, 1965: fruit bat, mouse; Venable, 1966: rat Shafiq *et al.*, 1967: man; Reger and Craig, 1968: man; Flood, 1971: axolotl; Kahn and Simpson, 1974: lizard; Kryvi, 1975: shark; Trupin, 1976: anuran muscle, etc.), shall be briefly summarized:

Satellite cells of normal adult muscle have been reported to be mitotically quiescent (Schultz *et al.*, 1978), making up about 1–5% of all intrasarcolemmal nuclei (Ontell, 1974; Schultz, 1974; Schultz *et al.*, 1978; cf. also Table 4 in: Castillo de Maruenda and Franzini-Armstrong, 1978); a value of 4% (± 2%) has been found in normal human skeletal muscle (Schmalbruch and Hellhammer, 1976). An exceptionally high amount of 12–20% has been reported for adult fruit bat web muscle (Church, 1970a). A characteristic decrease of the proportion of satellite cells in relation to myonuclei occurs during the postnatal period (Allbrook *et al.*, 1971; Hellmuth and Allbrook, 1973). Fast and slow twitch fibres exhibit different proportions and amounts of satellite cells and myonuclei, the incidence of both being higher in slow twitch muscles (Aloisi *et al.*, 1973; Kelly, 1978a). Schmalbruch and Hellhammer (1977) reported the presence of 900 myosatellite cells per mm³ of muscle tissue in rat tibialis anterior muscle as compared to about 5000 in soleus and diaphragm muscles. The distribution of satellite cells along a muscle fibre is not equal; their higher perisynaptic incidence has been mentioned by Kelly (1978b) and can be confirmed by our own observations in rat extraocular and guinea pig stapedius muscles (Fig. 3a, unpublished observations).

Concerning the structure of myosatellite cells, the presumably metabolically inactive cells exhibiting a high nucleo-cytoplasmic ratio and a reduced complement of organelles (Schultz *et al.*, 1978) have been shown, in a freeze-fracture study of rat skeletal muscle (Schmalbruch, 1978), to be not simply fusiform in shape, but to possess long and thin cytoplasmic processes which are also often seen in EM sections. In the stage of muscle development, satellite cells can be only distinguished from others after the formation of the

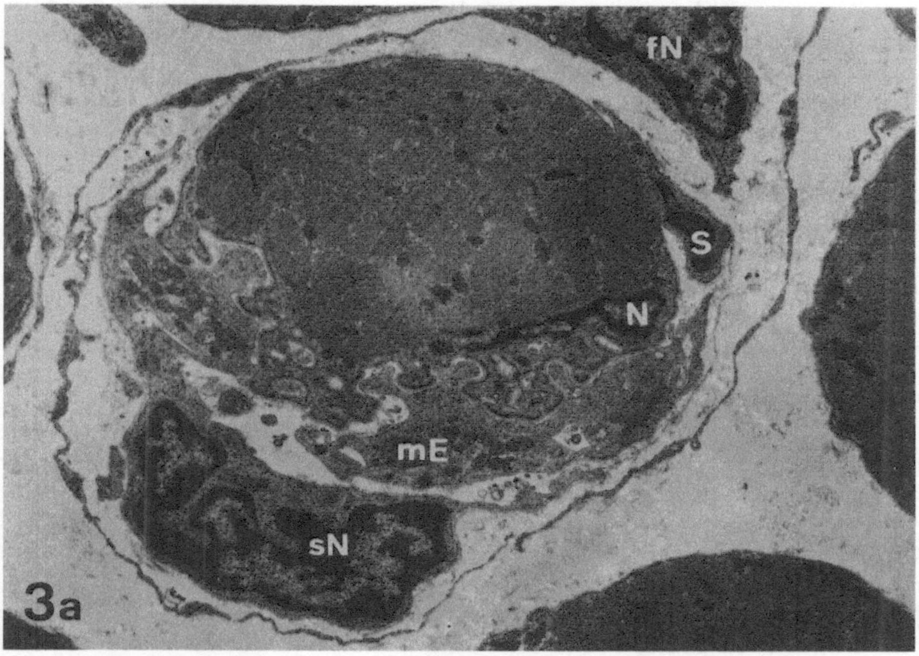

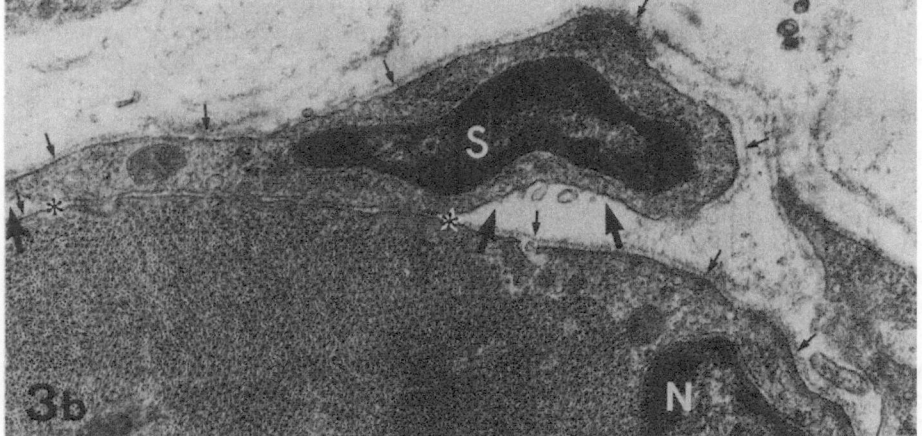

Fig. 3. *a* Myosatellite cell *(S)* in the vicinity of a motor endplate *(mE)* in a guinea pig stapedius muscle fibre. × 9000. Myonucleus of the sole plate *(N)*, fibrocyte nucleus *(fN)*, and Schwann cell nucleus *(sN)*. *b* Detail of Fig. 3 a. × 27.000. Cross sectioned myosatellite cell *(S)*, lying typically beneath the basal lamina of the muscle fibre (small arrows), however in this case partially lifted from the muscle fibre (large arrows) with basal lamina between the plasmalemmas of muscle and satellite cells. Normal relations with 200 Å extracellular space between asterisks

basal lamina; they are present in high numbers and exhibit a cytology indicating high mitotic and metabolic activity (Ishikawa, 1966; Conen and Bell, 1970; Schultz, 1976). A return to this "active state" with a higher incidence of mitotic figures, more cytoplasm, ribosomes, and other cytoplasmic organelles, as well as more prominent cytoplasmic processes, was reported after different kinds of trauma and activating conditions of muscle, such as mechanical compression (Teräväinen, 1970), denervation (Hess and Rosner, 1970; Ontell, 1974, 1975; Schultz, 1978; Verma, 1978), and compensatory hypertrophy (Schiaffino et al., 1972, 1976; Hanzlíková et al., 1975). In such cases the "budding off" of satellite cells from the multinucleate muscle fibre (Hess and Rosner, 1970) and an eventual migration (Kelly and O'Donoghue, 1974) has been suggested. Partial lifting of satellite cells from the surface of the muscle cell can, however, also be observed in uninjured muscle (Fig. 3b, own observations).

The presence of myosatellite cells and their similar behaviour in muscle spindles in the case of denervation as compared to those of extrafusal muscle fibres is well documented (Katz, 1961; Karlsson et al., 1966; Rumpelt and Schmalbruch, 1969; Maynard and Cooper, 1973; Milburn, 1976).

The role of satellite cells in the growth of normal muscle and for the increase of the number of myonuclei is well established, most convincingly by .autoradiographic evidence after H³-thymidine incorporation (Shafiq et al., 1968; Venable and Lorenz, 1970; Moss and Leblond, 1970, 1971; Cardasis and Cooper, 1975): Satellite cells divide mitotically and fuse with the adjacent multinucleated muscle fibre. According to Moss and Leblond (1971), H³-thymidine injection in growing rats resulted in exclusive labelling of satellite cells within 1–10 hours, but in increasing numbers of labelled myonuclei and decreasing label in satellite cells 24–72 hours after injection.

Concerning the role of satellite cells during the regeneration of mammalian skeletal muscle, a contribution of satellite cells to muscle fibre regeneration has been well documented by in vivo and in vitro experiments (Bischoff, 1974, 1975; Konigsberg et al., 1975; Snow, 1977b, c). Pronase and/or trypsin treatment leading to destruction of the basal lamina results in the liberation of cells which are capable of in vitro myogenesis (Bischoff, 1974); these cells are held to be satellite cells. In vivo studies of Snow (1978) in young rats gave evidence, after the transplantation of muscles containing 31% labelled satellite cells but no labelled myonuclei, that satellite cells can differentiate into multinucleated myotubes after the trauma of transplantation. However an exclusion of a participation of myonuclei in muscle regeneration (Aloisi and Mussini, this symposium) is extremely difficult, although recent studies strongly suggest this exclusion. Using labelled myonuclei according to a proposition by Carlson in his 1973 review, Pullman and Yeoh (1978) could demonstrate in their tissue culture experiments that myonuclei remain postmitotic; when muscle is disrupted, such nuclei cannot reenter the mitotic cycle to contribute to the formation of myotubes. Also in in vivo experiments new evidence in favour of the view has been presented that myonuclei are not involved in the formation of new myotubes; Lipton and Schultz (1979) showed by implantation of pellets of pure labelled satellite cells into the living animal that satellite cells are able to migrate rather far in the host muscle, to invade the muscle fibres (i.e. to penetrate the basal lamina), and to contribute by fusion to the myonuclei of preexisting fibres, to create satellite fibres, or to create new myotubes in the interstitium. Former authors maintaining in contrast to the above that myogenic cells in muscle grafts are formed by a process of nuclear sequestration within degenerating muscle fibres, and that satellite cells are more or less inactive (Mastaglia *et al.*, 1975), seem nowadays to be less supported.

In conclusion it may be stated that there is more and better evidence now than 5–10 years ago that myosatellite cells are responsible for the capacity of skeletal muscle to regenerate and thus also to survive free muscle transplantation, without, however, having completely excluded a possible role of myonuclei.

## References

Allbrook, D. B., Han, M. F., Hellmuth, A. E.: Population of muscle satellite cells in relation to age and mitotic activity. Pathology *3*, 233–243 (1971).

Aloisi, M., Mussini, I., Schiaffino, S.: Activation of muscle nuclei in denervation and hypertrophy. In: Basic Research in Myology (Kakulas, B. A., ed.). Amsterdam: Excerpta Medica I.C.S. No. 294. 1973.

Bischoff, R.: Enzymatic liberation of myogenic cells from adult rat muscle. Anat. Rec. *180*, 645–662 (1974).

Bischoff, R.: Regeneration of single muscle fibers in vitro. Anat. Rec. *182*, 215–236 (1975).

Burgener, J., Mayr, R.: Guinea pig stapedius muscle. A histochemical, light and electron microscopic study. Anat. Embryol. *161*, 65–81 (1980).

Cardasis, C. A., Cooper, G. W.: An analysis of nuclear numbers in individual muscle fibers during differentiation and growth: a satellite cell muscle fiber growth unit. J. exp. Zool. *191*, 347–356 (1975).

Carlson, B. M.: The regeneration of skeletal muscle – A review. Am. J. Anat. *137*, 119–150 (1973).

Carlson, B. M.: A review of muscle transplantation in mammals. Physiol. Bohemoslov. *27*, 387–400 (1978).

Carlson, B. M., Gutmann, E.: Regeneration in free grafts of normal and denervated muscles in the rat. – Morphology and histochemistry. Anat. Rec. *183*, 47–61 (1975 a).

Carlson, B. M., Gutmann, E.: Regeneration in grafts of normal and denervated rat muscles. – Contractile properties. Pflügers Arch. ges. Physiol. *353*, 215–225 (1975 b).

Castillo de Maruenda, E., Franzini-Armstrong, C.: Satellite and invasive cells in frog sartorius muscle. Tissue Cell *10*, 749–772 (1978).

Church, J. C. T.: Satellite cells and myogenesis; a study in the fruit-bat web. J. Anat. *105*, 419–438 (1969).

Church, J. C. T.: Cell quantitation in regenerating bat web muscle. In: Regeneration of Striated Muscle and Myogenesis (Mauro, A., Shafiq, S. A., Milhorat, A. T., eds.), pp. 101–117. Amsterdam: Excerpta Medica. 1970 a.

Church, J. C. T.: A model for myogenesis using the concept of the satellite cell segment. In: Regeneration of Striated Muscle and Myogenesis (Mauro, A., Shafiq, S. A., Milhorat, A. T., eds.), pp. 118–121. Amsterdam: Excerpta Medica. 1970 b.

Church, J. C. T., Noronha, R. F. X., Allbrook, D. B.: Satellite cells and skeletal muscle regeneration. Brit. J. Surg. *53*, 638–642 (1966).

Conen, P. E., Bell, C. D.: Study of satellite cells in mature and fetal human muscle and rhabdomyosacroma. In: Regeneration of Striated Muscle and Myogenesis (Mauro, A., Shafiq, S. A., Milhorat, A. T., eds.), pp. 194–211. Amsterdam: Excerpta Medica. 1970.

Elyakova, G. V.: Electron microscopic investigation of the formation of myoblasts in regenerating muscular tissue (Russian). Doklady Akad. Nauk SSSR *202*, 1196–1198 (1972).

Flood, L.: The three-dimensional structure and frequency of myosatellite cells in trunk muscle of the Axolotl *(Siredon mexicanus)*. J. Ultrastruct. Res. *36*, 523–524 (1971).

Hansen-Smith, F. M., Carlson, B. M.: Cellular responses to free grafting of the extensor digitorum longus muscle of the rat. J. Neurol. Sci. *41*, 149–173 (1979).

Hanzlíková, V., Macková, E. V., Hník, P.: Satellite cells of the rat soleus muscle in the process of compensatory hypertrophy combined with denervation. Cell Tissue Res. *160*, 411–421 (1975).

Harii, K., Ohmori, K., Torii, S.: Free gracilis muscle transplantation with microneurovascular anastomosis for the treatment of facial paralysis. Plast. Reconstr. Surg. *57*, 133–143 (1976).

Hess, A., Rosner, S.: The satellite cell bud and myoblast in denervated mammalian muscle fibers. Am. J. Anat. *129*, 21–40 (1970).

Holle, J., Freilinger, G., Gruber, H., Lischka, A., Mayr, R.: Tierexperimentelle Untersuchungen zur freien autologen Muskeltransplantation. Langenbecks Arch. Chir., Suppl. Chir. Forum *1974*, 235–239.

Ishikawa, H.: Electron microscopic observations of satellite cells with special reference to the development of mammalian skeletal muscles. Z. Anat. Entw. Gesch. *125*, 43–63 (1966).

Kahn, E. B., Simpson, S. B., Jr.: Satellite cells in mature uninjured skeletal muscles of the lizard tail. Develop. Biol. *37*, 219–233 (1974).

Karlsson, U., Andersson-Cedergren, E., Ottoson, D.: Cellular organization of the frog muscle spindle as revealed by serial sections for electron microscopy. J. Ultrastruct. Res. *14*, 1–35 (1966).

Katz, F. R. S.: The termination of the afferent nerve fibre in the muscle spindle of the frog. Phil. Trans. R. Soc. (London) *B 243*, 221–240 (1961).

Kelly, A. M.: Satellite cells and myofiber growth in the rat soleus and extensor digitorum longus muscles. Develop. Biol. *65*, 1–10 (1978a).

Kelly, A. M.: Perisynaptic satellite cells in the developing and mature rat soleus muscle. Anat. Rec. *190*, 891–904 (1978b).

Kelly, A. M., O'Donoghue, J. L.: "Wandering" satellite cells in skeletal muscle. J. Cell Biol. *63*, 164a (1974).

Konigsberg, U. R., Lipton, B. H., Konigsberg, I. R.: The regenerative response of single mature muscle fibers isolated in vitro. Develop. Biol. *45*, 260–275 (1975).

Kryvi, H.: The structure of the myosatellite cells in axial muscles of the shark *Galeus melastomus*. Anat. Embryol. *143*, 35–44 (1975).

Lipton, B. H., Schultz, E.: Developmental fate of skeletal muscle satellite cells. Science *205*, 1292–1294 (1979).

Lischka, A., Holle, J., Freilinger, G.: Lichtmikroskopische Untersuchungen der morphologischen Veränderungen bei autologer Muskeltransplantation. Acta anat. (Basel) *97*, 450–458 (1977).

Mastaglia, F. L., Dawkins, R. L., Papadimitriou, J. M.: Morphological changes in skeletal muscle after transplantation. A light- and electron-microscopic study of the initial phases of degeneration and regeneration. J. neurol. Sci. *25*, 227–247 (1975).

Mauro, A.: Satellite cell of skeletal muscle fibers. J. biochem. biophys. Cytol. *9*, 493–495 (1961).

Mauro, A. (ed.): Muscle Regeneration. New York: Raven Press. 1979.

Mauro, A., Shafiq, S. A., Milhorat, A. T. (eds.): Regeneration of Striated Muscle and Myogenesis. Amsterdam: Excerpta Medica. 1970.

Maynard, J. A., Cooper, R. R.: Two unusual satellite cell-intrafusal muscle fiber relationships. Z. Anat. Entw. Gesch. *140*, 1–9 (1973).

Milburn, A.: The effect of the local anaesthetic bupivacaine on the muscle spindle of rat. J. Neurocytol. *5*, 425–446 (1976).

Moss, F. P., Leblond, C. P.: Nature of dividing nuclei in skeletal muscle of growing rats. J. Cell. Biol. *44*, 459–462 (1970).

Moss, F. P., Leblond, C. P.: Satellite cells as the source of nuclei in muscles of growing rats. Anat. Rec. *170*, 421–436 (1971).

Muir, A. R., Kanji, A. H. M., Allbrook, D.: The structure of the satellite cells in skeletal muscle. J. Anat. (London) *99*, 435–444 (1965).

Ontell, M.: Muscle satellite cells: a validated technique for light microscopic identification and a quantitative study of changes in their population following denervation. Anat. Rec. *178*, 211–228 (1974).

Ontell, M.: Evidence for myoblastic potential of satellite cells in denervated muscle. Cell Tiss. Res. *160*, 345–353 (1975).

Pullman, W. E., Yeoh, G. C. T.: The role of myonuclei in muscle regeneration: An in vitro study. J. Cell Physiol. *96*, 245–252 (1978).

Reger, J. F., Craig, A. S.: Studies on the fine structure of muscle fibers and associated satellite cells in hypertrophic human deltoid muscles. Anat. Rec. *162*, 483–500 (1968).

Reznik, M.: Origin of myoblasts during skeletal muscle regeneration. Lab. Invest. *20*, 353–363 (1969).

Reznik, M.: Satellite cells, myoblasts and skeletal muscle regeneration. In: Regeneration of Striated Muscle and Myogenesis (Mauro, A., Shafiq, S. A., Milhorat, A. T., eds.), pp. 133–156. Amsterdam: Excerpta Medica. 1970.

Rumpelt, H.-J., Schmalbruch, H.: Zur Morphologie der Bauelemente von Muskelspindeln bei Mensch und Ratte. Z. Zellforsch. *102*, 601–630 (1969).

Schiaffino, S., Bormioli, S. P., Aloisi, M.: Cell proliferation in rat skeletal muscle during early stages of compensatory hypertrophy. Virchows Arch. B. Cell Path. *11*, 268–273 (1972).

Schiaffino, S., Bormioli, S. P., Aloisi, M.: The fate of newly formed satellite cells during compensatory hypertrophy. Virchows Arch. B. Cell Path. *21*, 113–118 (1976).

Schiaffino, S., Sjöström, M., Thornell, L. E., Nyström, B., Hakelius, L.: The process of survival of denervated and freely autotransplanted skeletal muscle. Experientia (Basel) *31*, 1328–1330 (1975).

Schmalbruch, H.: Satellite cells of rat muscles as studied by freeze-fracturing. Anat. Rec. *191*, 371–376 (1978).

Schmalbruch, H., Hellhammer, U.: The number of satellite cells in normal human muscle. Anat. Rec. *185*, 279–287 (1976).

Schmalbruch, H., Hellhammer, U.: The number of nuclei in adult rat muscles with special reference to satellite cells. Anat. Rec. *189*, 169–175 (1977).

Schultz, E.: A quantitative study of the satellite cell population in postnatal mouse lumbrical muscle. Anat. Rec. *180*, 589–596 (1974).

Schultz, E.: Fine structure of satellite cells in growing skeletal muscle. Am. J. Anat. *147*, 49–69 (1976).

Schultz, E.: Changes in the satellite cells of growing muscle following denervation. Anat. Rec. *190*, 299–312 (1978).

Schultz, E., Gibson, M. C., Champion, T.: Satellite cells are mitotically quiescent in mature mouse muscle: an EM and radioautographic study. J. exp. Zool. *206*, 451–456 (1978).

Shafiq, S. A.: Satellite cells and fiber nuclei in muscle regeneration. In: Regeneration of Striated Muscle and Myogenesis (Mauro, A., Shafiq, S. A., Milhorat A. T., eds.), pp. 122–132. Amsterdam: Excerpta Medica. 1970.

Shafiq, S. A., Gorycki, M. A., Milhorat, A. T.: An electron microscopic study of regeneration and satellite cells in human muscle. Neurology *17*, 567–575 (1967).

Shafiq, S. A., Gorycki, M. A., Mauro, A.: Mitosis during postnatal growth in skeletal and cardiac muscle of the rat. J. Anat. *103*, 135–141 (1968).

Snow, M. H.: The effects of aging on satellite cells in skeletal muscles of mice and rats. Cell Tiss. Res. *185*, 399–408 (1977a).

Snow, M. H.: Myogenic cell formation in regenerating rat skeletal muscle injured by mincing. I. A fine structural study. Anat. Rec. *188*, 181–199 (1977b).

Snow, M. H.: Myogenic cell formation in regenerating rat skeletal muscle injured by mincing. II. An autoradiographic study. Anat. Rec. *188*, 200–218 (1977c).

Snow, M. H.: An autoradiographic study of satellite cell differentiation into regenerating myotubes following transplantation of muscles in young rats. Cell Tiss. Res. *186*, 535–540 (1978).

Teräväinen, H.: Satellite cells of striated muscle after compression injury so slight as not to cause degeneration of the muscle fibers. Z. Zellforsch. *103*, 320–327 (1970).

Thompson, N.: Autogenous free grafts of skeletal muscle. Plast. Reconstr. Surg. *48*, 11–27 (1971).

Trupin, G. L.: The satellite cells of normal anuran skeletal muscle. Develop. Biol. *50*, 517–524 (1976).

Venable, J. H.: Morphology of the cells of normal, testosterone-deprived and testosterone-stimulated levator ani muscles. J. Anat. *119*, 271–302 (1966).

Venable, J. H., Lorenz, M. D.: Trial analysis of the cytokinetics of a rapidly growing skeletal muscle. In: Regeneration of Striated Muscle and Myogenesis (Mauro, A., Shafiq, S. A., Milhorat, A. T., eds.), pp. 271–278. Amsterdam: Excerpta Medica. 1970.

Verma, V.: Satellite cells in denervated muscles. Experientia (Basel) *35*, 40–42 (1978).

Walker, B. E.: Skeletal muscle regeneration in young rats. Am. J. Anat. *133*, 369–378 (1972).

Author's address: Prof. Dr. R. Mayr, Institut für Anatomie (2), Universität Wien, Währinger Strasse 13, A-1090 Wien, Austria.

# Number of Satellite Cells and Muscle Regeneration[*]

## M. Aloisi and I. Mussini

National Research Council Unit for Muscle Biology and Physiopathology,
Institute of General Pathology,
University of Padova, Italy

With 6 Figures

During the last 30 years the possibilities and mechanisms of muscle regeneration have been thoroughly studied, particularly in mammals, and the occurrence of complete muscle reconstruction from minced muscle fragments has been demonstrated since the experiments made by Studitsky (for the past literature, see Carlson, 1972, 1973).

However, the mechanisms underlying the regeneration of muscle fibres have not yet been completely clarified. After the discovery of satellite cells (Mauro, 1961) and of their capacity for division and myoblastic transformation, the problem of the source of regenerating elements was almost completely solved. Thus, muscle regeneration appeared to be a process evolving *per discontinuum*, through the proliferation of stimulated satellite cells after severe muscle injury, while the possibility of a regeneration *per continuum* from the stumps of disrupted muscle fibres appeared to be a very improbable process, at least in mammals. The physiopathology of muscle fibres shows that even in the absence of any local complication a severed mammalian muscle fibre is not able to survive, and the great majority of its cytoplasm rapidly undergoes hyalinization and necrosis. This is particularly true for the myoplasm, whereas the peripheral sarcoplasm seems to be more resistent to degeneration after mechanical injury.

Since satellite cells are strictly adjacent to the outer surface and lie underneath the basal membrane of the fibre, muscle regeneration has often been described, before the advent of EM analysis, as starting from nucleated peripheral parts of the sarcoplasm and producing several basophilic protoplasmic growths inside the basal membrane of the muscle fibre remnants. These plurinucleated syncytial growths are often seen as crescent-like formations

---

[*] This work was supported by funds from the Consiglio Nazionale delle Ricerche to the Centro di Studio per la Biologia e Fisiopatologia Muscolare and, in part, by a grant from the Muscular Dystrophy Association of America to Prof. M. Aloisi.

facing and embracing the central bulk of the degenerated myoplasm. Their extension under the connective sarcolemma and self-rebuilding basal membrane increases parallel to the reabsorption of the degenerative material.

With the recognition of the presence of such individualized elements as satellite cells and of the possibility given by EM morphology for the study of

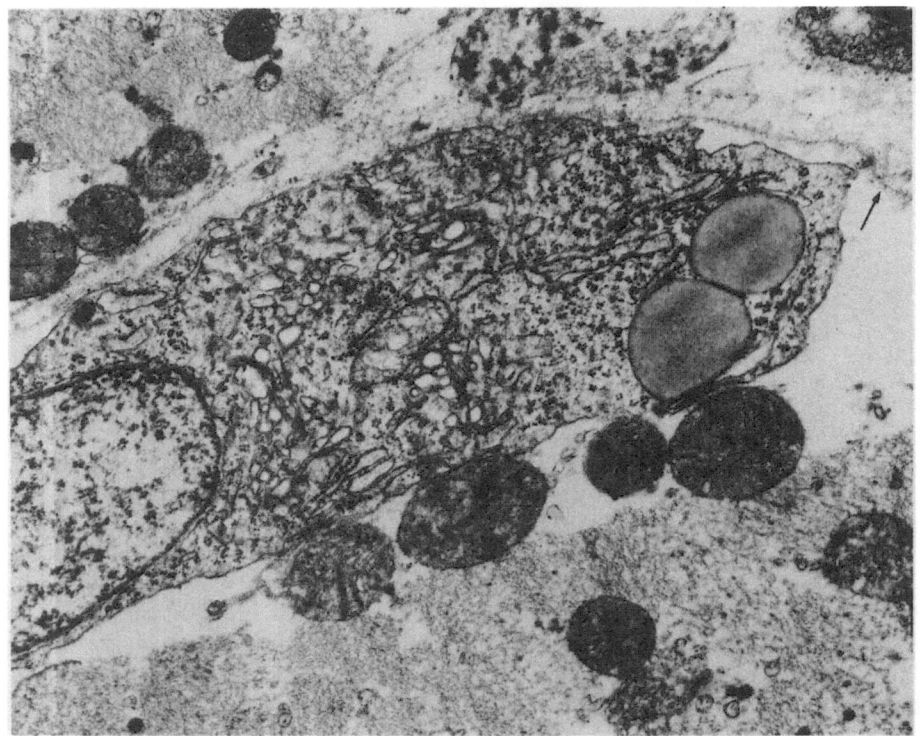

Fig. 1. Two-day culture of minced muscle in a Millipore chamber. It shows the presence of a myoblastic cell adjacent to a remnant of muscle fibre undergoing degeneration. The viable cell, rich in ribosomes and rough endoplasmic reticulum, is clearly located underneath the basement membrane of the fibre (arrow), as is normal for a satellite cell. 18,000 x

their relationship with the adjacent fibres (Fig. 1), it has been almost generally assumed that the true source of regenerating muscle elements is in fact satellite cells and that the first basophilic, not yet myofibrillar (or poorly myofibrillar) symplasts are actually the products of the first fusion of myoblasts derived from activation and transformation of satellite cells (Fig. 2).

In spite of this clarifying achievement, the question of the mechanism of muscle regeneration remains open to discussion, since the very nature, number and reactivity of satellite cells remains still obscure.

The number of satellite cells is greatly variable, not only from birth to adult age (Allbrook et al., 1971), but also as a consequence of a variety of conditions,

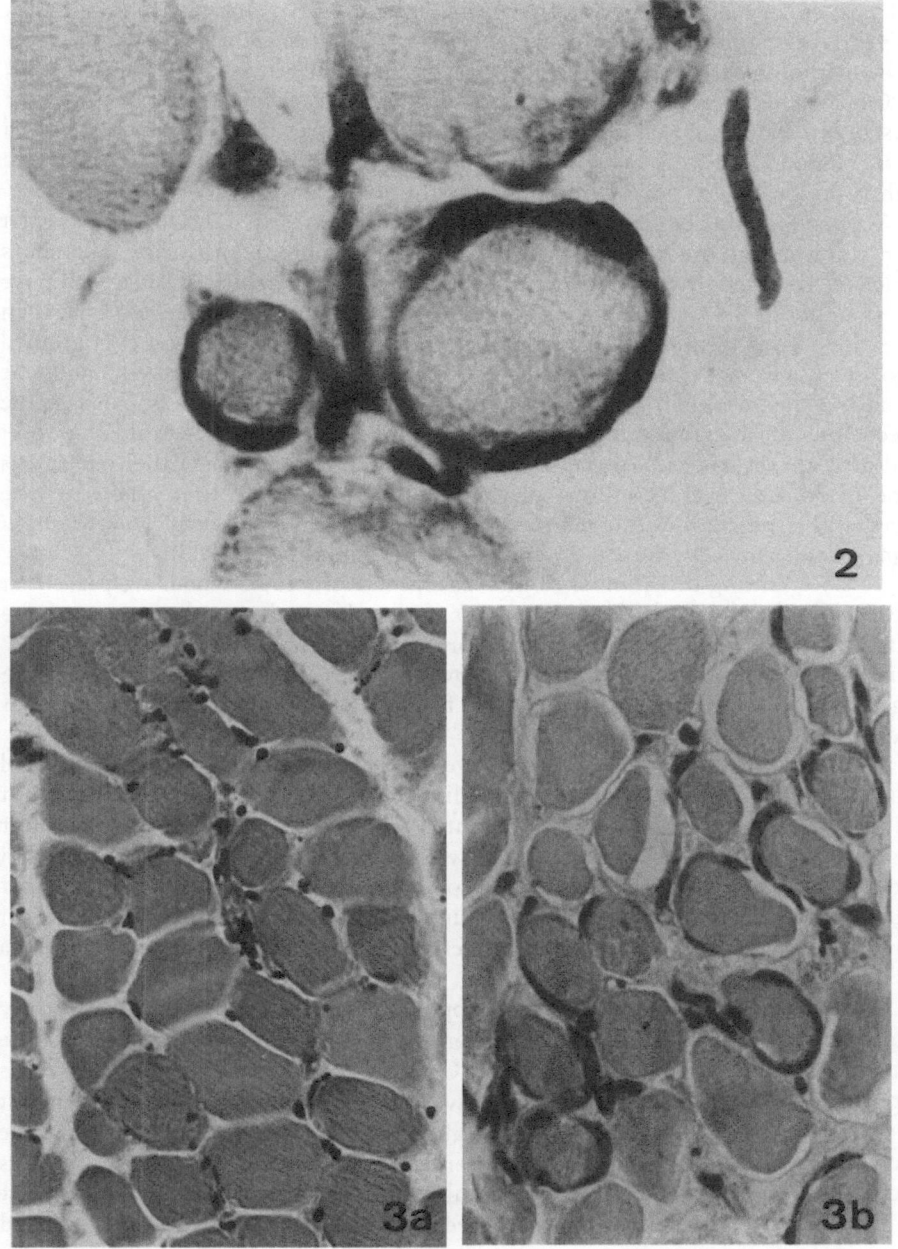

Fig. 2. Light micrograph. Cross-section of two normal muscle fibres after 2 days of culture. The periphery of the fibres is largely occupied by multinucleated symplasts of new viable elements while the parent fibre is completely degenerated. 1,080 x

Fig. 3. Minced fast muscle implanted in Millipore chambers and incubated *in vivo* for 2 days. *a* normal muscle, *b* denervated muscle. The initial process of regeneration is much more advanced in denervated fibres which show several newlyformed crescent-like symplasts. 385 x

and particularly after denervation (Aloisi *et al.*, 1973; Ontell, 1974; Schultz, 1974), hypertrophy (Hanzlìkovà *et al.*, 1975; Schiaffino *et al.*, 1976), or other physiopathological conditions (Hall-Craggs and Lawrence, 1970; Teräväinen, 1970). The number of satellite cells is also variable according to the type of muscle fibre, being much more numerous in slow fibres than in fast ones (Aloisi *et al.*, 1973). This fact may well account for the different initial regenerative ability of the two types of muscle (Mussini *et al.*, 1980).

We have studied many aspects of the initial phases of muscle regeneration from minced rat muscle fragments enclosed in Millipore diffusion chambers which were inserted into the peritoneal cavity of littermates. Using Millipore filters of about 0.45 $\mu$m, we were sure to avoid any entrance of cells others than those belonging to the implanted muscle fragments (which, obviously, contained also mesenchymal cells). Leucocytes from the host are kept outside the chamber; this results in a slowing down of the regenerative process, because the precocious destruction and the lysis of the necrotic material speed up the onset and increase the kinetics of the true regenerating phase. On the other hand, this type of *in vivo* culture allows an easy study of the very first phases of the regenerative process. With this method we have been previously able to show some peculiarities of muscle regeneration (Mussini *et al.*, 1980):

1. By counting the number of new basophilic structures which are present at the periphery of muscle fibre fragments 48 hr after culture, the extent of the initial regenerative ability has been approximately quantified in fast and slow muscles of young adult rats. In slow muscles the lag phase preceding regeneration is much shorter than that found in fast muscles (with a ratio of about 40 to 10).

2. After denervation the regenerative capacity markedly increases, parallel with an increase of the number of satellite cells. This can be an explanation at cellular level of the "plastic state" attributed by Studitsky (1959) to muscles after denervation. In our experiments the activation due to denervation is different in the two types of muscle fibres: much more rapid is the onset in denervated fast muscles (Fig. 3) than in the corresponding slow muscles, while the number of satellite cells increases by a factor greater than 5 in fast muscles and only by a factor of 2 in slow muscles.

Not contrasting with these results appears to be the demonstration (Murray and Robbins, 1979) that after denervation there is a small increase of thymidine incorporation by satellite cell nuclei. On the other hand, Kelly (1978) has reported a marked decline of proliferative activity of satellite cells in both fast and slow muscles of the rat 24 hours after denervation. He suggests that the increased incidence of satellite cells observed 2 or 3 weeks after denervation, as shown by Ontell (1974) and also by Schultz (1974), may be a secondary response to degenerative processes of the fibres. However, while the last quoted experiments on denervation were long-term experiments, where a degenerative process cannot be excluded, in our experiments, in which the denervated state lasted only 3 days, any degenerative process could be ruled out at least at morphological level (conventional and EM observations). Therefore, the variation in satellite cell number should be directly accounted for by the denervation as such.

As we have already mentioned, it appears that not only denervation, but also other different physiopathological alterations of muscle fibre equilibria are able to induce an increase of the satellite cell population in muscle tissue. It is possible that the state of "nucleosis", so common in muscle pathology, is an expression of such a reactivity of satellite cells.

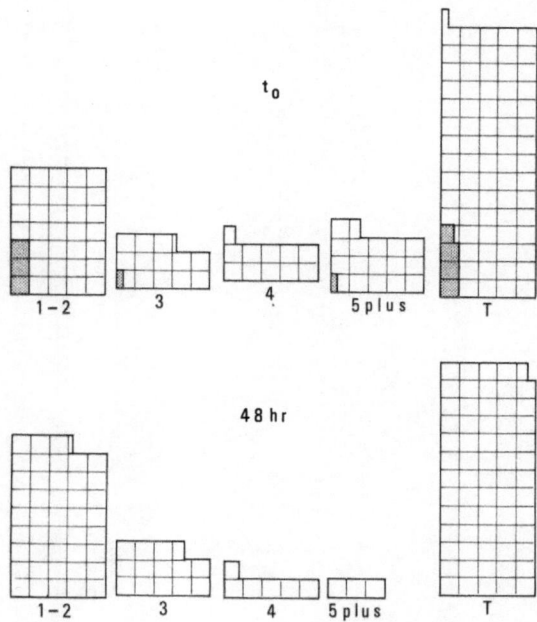

Fig. 4. Distribution of labelling in muscle nuclei before $(t_o)$ and after 48 hr of culture of soleus muscle fragments of a previously labelled rat. $t_o$: the different partial areas represent the number of labelled muscle nuclei as percentage of total labelling. The amount of this labelling in the nuclear population was measured by counting the number of silver grains/nucleus (from 1 to 5 and more). The T area corresponds to the total labelled nuclei. The shaded areas represent the relative proportion of satellite cells before culture. *48 hr:* at this time of culture the number of labelled nuclei of the growing new muscle elements cannot be only accounted for by the proliferation of pre-existing satellite cells (shaded areas in the upper part of the Figure)

By integrating our experience on hypertrophic, atrophic, simply denervated (in a stage preceding atrophy) and regenerating muscle with many of the data already existing in the literature we suggest that the variations in size of the satellite cell population are not always due to a controlled proliferative process. An increase may also be due to segregation (shedding off) of nucleated peripheral portions of sarcoplasm from the rest of the fibre (particularly when it is damaged). On the contrary, satellite cells may decrease as a result of reassimilation by fusion with the parent fibre (hypertrophy): in this way the number of fibre nuclei (true myonuclei) may increase without any apparent mitosis. With this suggestion we extend to physiopathological conditions the process described during post-natal development of growing rats by Moss and Leblond (1971).

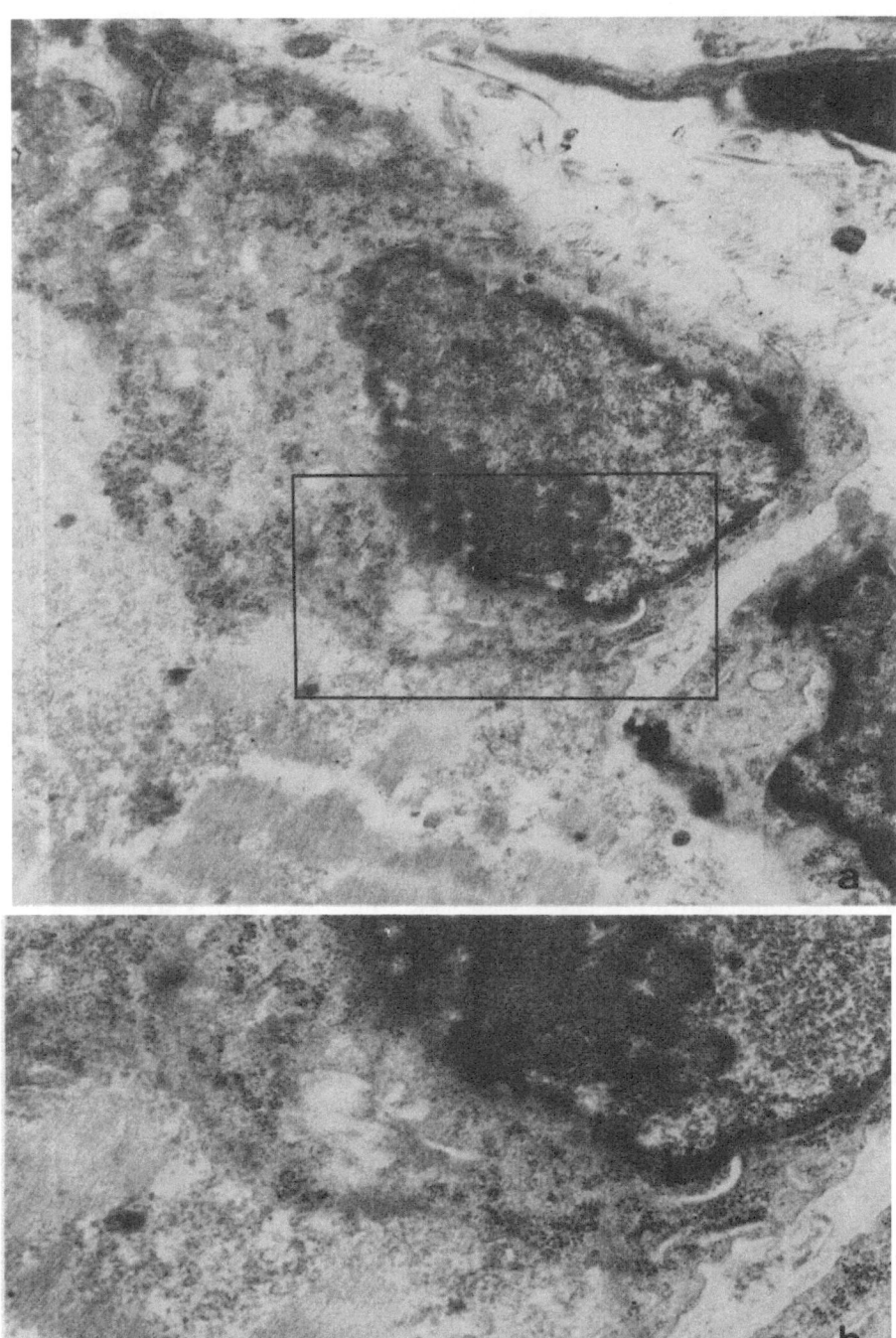

We have morphological evidence of the process of segregation of new satellite cells from the mother fibre (for instance after denervation) although the necessary distinction between two individual membranes at the initial point of shedding is not always easy in the EM analysis, often requiring the use of a goniometer stage.

For this reason we consider particularly interesting the experiments we report here concerning the differentially labeled muscular nuclei and their fate after *in vivo* culture in Millipore chambers inserted in peritoneal cavities of untreated littermates.

Newborn rats were from birth given injections of $^3$H-thymidine (1 $\mu$Ci/g body weight) daily for a week; the animals were then allowed to grow undisturbed for one month. At this time ($t_o$, Fig. 4) we found, as expected, a differential labelling of myonuclei and satellite cell nuclei (as well as of connective tissue nuclei), the latter having greatly diluted their label because of multiplication during post-natal growth (Moss, Leblond 1971). While the percentage of labelled myonuclei was 40.2 % in slow muscles and 46.9 % in fast muscles, the percent of labelled satellite cell nuclei was only 2.2 % and 1.1 % respectively. After 48 hours of culture the majority of the nuclei of new muscle elements (myoblasts and products of their fusion) were labelled (Fig. 4, 48 hr): they represented 34.2 and 23.8 percent in slow and fast muscles respectively, indicating that most of the new elements received their nuclei also from myonuclei and not exclusively from satellite cells. Only a massive proliferation of satellite cells in the short incubation time lapse of our experiments could explain this very large labelling of the new muscle growths.

The data of Bishoff (1970), concerning *in vitro* muscle culture, show that the generation time for embryonic myoblastic cells is about 9.5 hours, followed by a lag phase before fusing of 5–7 hours. On the other hand, during post-natal growth satellite cells are found to undergo two successive divisions in about three days (Moss, Leblond, 1971). However, following a scheme according to which in *in vivo* regeneration experiments a consistent proportion of the daughter cells stop dividing at any cell duplication, the amount of labelled elements found in our growing muscle elements cannot be explained only by the contribution of pre-existing satellite cells.

An accurate electron microscopic investigation of the process of shedding off of some of the nucleated portions of sarcoplasm from muscle fragments gives pictures like those shown in Figs. 5 and 6. A labelled myonucleus is surrounded by a cytoplasmic portion very rich in polysomes. This structure is underneath the basal membrane and actually inside the mother fibre with which still persisting structural cytoplasmic connections can clearly be observed. This very fact excludes the possibility of that cell being a macrophage; in general, in our work we never had difficulties in differentiating at the ultrastructural level macrophages from satellite cells, as claimed by Trupin *et al.* (1979). A later stage

Fig. 5. Electron micrograph of the peripheral part of a minced muscle fibre after 2 days of culture. The bulk of the fibre is clearly degenerated while a nucleated cytoplasmic portion of the fibre is surviving with a viable nucleus and many polysomes. There is no sharp delimitation between this element and the rest of the fibre, as occurs with a satellite cell. For detail see section b). *a* 22,000 x; *b* 36,000 x

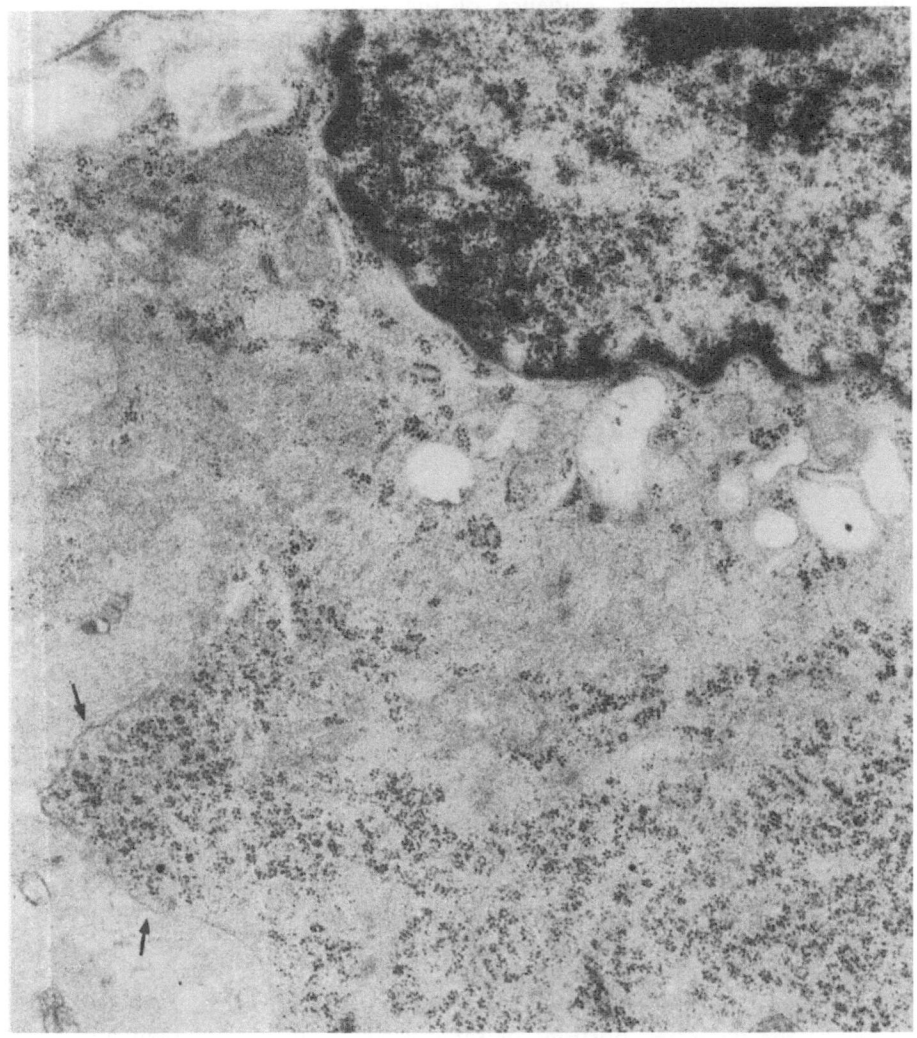

Fig. 6. Micrograph of another EM section of the same material of Fig. 5. It shows in detail the formation of a new cell membrane (arrows) which appears to be still largely discontinuous all around the nucleus. 30,000 x

of shedding off is better shown in Fig. 6, where polysome-rich cytoplasmic material is delimited, although not completely, by a membrane.

### References

Allbrook, D. B., Han, M. F., Hellmuth, A. E.: Population of muscle satellite cells in relation to age and mitotic activity. Pathology 3, 233–243 (1971).

Aloisi, M., Mussini, I., Schiaffino, S.: Activation of muscle nuclei in denervation and hypertrophy. In: Basic Research in Myology, Part I (Kakulas B. A., ed.), ICS 294, pp. 338–342. Amsterdam: Excerpta Medica. 1973.

Bischoff, R.: The myogenic stem cell in development of skeletal muscle. In: Regeneration of Striated Muscle and Myogenesis (Mauro, A., Shafiq, S. A., Milhorat, A. T., eds.), pp. 218–231. Amsterdam: Excerpta Medica. 1970.

Carlson, B. M.: The regeneration of minced muscles. (Monographs in Development Biology, Vol. 4.) Basel: Karger. 1972.

Carlson, B. M.: The regeneration of skeletal muscle. A review. Am. J. Anat. *137*, 119–150 (1973).

Hall-Craggs, E. C. B., Lawrence, C. A.: Longitudinal fibre division in skeletal muscle: A light and electron microscopic study. Z. Zellforsch. *109*, 481–494 (1970).

Hanzlíková, V., Macková, E. V., Hník, P.: Satellite cells of the rat soleus muscle in the process of compensatory hypertrophy combined with denervation. Cell Tiss. Res. *160*, 411–421 (1975).

Kelly, A. M.: Satellite cells and myofiber growth in the rat Soleus and Extensor Digitorum Longus muscles. Develop. Biol. *65*, 1–10 (1978).

Mauro, A.: Satellite cells of skeletal muscle fibers. J. Biophys. Biochem. Cytol. *9*, 493–495 (1971).

Moss, F. P., Leblond, C. P.: Satellite cells as the source of nuclei in muscles of growing rats. Anat. Rec. *170*, 421–436 (1971).

Murray, M. A., Robbins, N.: Cell proliferation in denervated mouse muscle. Soc. Neurosci. Abstr., Vol. 5, p. 769. 1979.

Mussini, I., Aloisi, M., Fidzianska, A.: Increase of satellite cells in fast and slow denervated mammalian muscle fibres and segregation of new cells from parent fibres. J. Submicr. Cytol. (submitted).

Ontell, M.: Satellite cells: A validated technique for light microscopic identification and a quantitative study of changes in their population following denervation. Anat. Rec. *178*, 211–228 (1974).

Schiaffino, S., Pierobon-Bormioli, S., Aloisi, M.: Cell proliferation in rat skeletal muscle during early phases of compensatory hypertrophy. Virchows Arch. B Cell Pathol. *11*, 268–273 (1972).

Schultz, E.: A study of satellite cells in denervated skeletal muscle. Anat. Rec. *180*, 589–597 (1974).

Studitsky, A. N.: Experimental surgery of muscles. (Russian.) Moscow: Izdatel. Akad. Nauk. 1959.

Teräväinen, H.: Satellite cells of striated muscle after compression injury so slight as not to cause degeneration of the muscle fibres. Z. Zellforsch. *103*, 320–327 (1970).

Trupin, G. L., Hsu, L., Hsieh, Y.-H.: Satellite cell mimics in regenerating skeletal muscle. In: Muscle Regeneration (Mauro, A., ed.), pp. 101–114. New York: Raven Press. 1979.

Authors' address: Prof. Dr. M. Aloisi, Istituto di Patologia Generale, Università di Padova, Via Loredan, 16, I-35100 Padova, Italy.

## Discussion

*Carlson:* This would be the right moment to discuss the origin of cells in regenerating muscles.

*Nikolai:* Some authors have mentioned double nuclei after or even before denervation, and one of these nuclei is often a satellite cell lying next to a myonucleus. Did you see these double cells?

*Mussini:* We call this situation coupled nuclei and this is quite frequent—mainly during postnatal development. I think it is the expression of multiplication of satellite cells inside the basal membrane and one of these satellite cells has fused with the myofibre, but one can remain outside and gives the impression of being paired.

*Mayr:* There are reports of double nuclei, but Carlson has interpreted that picture as possibly being identical nuclei, which gave the impression of a double satellite cell nuclei. Double satellite cell nuclei have not yet been found in one cell.

Question: Are there some stains to demonstrate the protein synthesis in satellite cells?

*Mussini:* If myo-fibrillar protein can be demonstrated in the satellite cells, it is then a satellite myofibre. Myofilaments in satellite myofibres can only be seen at electromicroscopic magnification, not by any other light microscopical stainings.

*Brunelli:* What is your definition of satellite myofibre and where do they come from?

*Mussini:* Satellite myofibre means that two satellite cells are coupled and are lying under the same basal lamina. And this is a quite normal situation during postnatal development. Only later on the basal lamina is there more and more detaching of the two fibres, until each fibre has its own basal lamina. This is quite similar to embryologic development.

# The Functional Recovery of Minced Muscles

C. Bertrand, L. Plaghki, and G. Maréchal

Laboratoire de Physiologie Générale,
Université Catholique de Louvain,
Brussels, Belgium

With 5 Figures

## Introduction

The regeneration of muscles minced and grafted orthotopically has been well described by Carlson (1972). Such muscles show a remarkable degree of recovery: they contract; they are supplied with vascularization and innervation within a few weeks after the surgery. They show noticeable morphological, biochemical and mechanical differences in comparison to normal muscles (Carlson and Gutmann, 1972; Galucci et al., 1966; Plaghki and Maréchal, 1976; Plaghki et al., 1980a, b; Rifenberick et al., 1974; Salafsky, 1971; Snow, 1973). Their functional value may be questioned, as there is no available information concerning their use by the animals. This work describes some clinical aspects of the recovery of minced triceps surae of the rat, and establish a correlation with the mechanical recovery of the regenerating muscles.

## Methods

The experiments were performed on thirty male Wistar rats. The animals were segregated into two groups of fifteen rats. The rats of the first group weighed about 50 g and were about 3 weeks of age. The rats of the second group weighed about 150 g and were about 6 weeks of age. These two groups are referred to hereafter respectively as "younger rats" and "older rats".

The animals were anesthetized by intradermal injection of 0.1 ml of Thalamonal® (Janssen-Pharmaceutica) per 50 g of live weight. The skin was shaved and washed with 74° alcohol. The right leg was incised along its external posterolateral side, from the knee to the heel. The biceps femoris muscle was detached from its tibial insertion. The triceps surae and plantaris were entirely removed, except at the knee, where two short stumps about 1 mm long were left. It was placed into a sterile Petri dish. The soleus and the thick tendons were discarded. The remainder of the triceps surae and plantaris was minced into small pieces with scissors. The mince was grafted back into the leg.

The muscle biceps femoris and the skin were each sutured with separated stitches (Ethicon 6–0). No infections have been observed. The surgical instruments had been sterilized by heating at 150°C for 1 hr.

Animals were examined 15, 30, 60, 90 or 120 days after surgery. The regenerate was dissected free, great care being taken to avoid damaging nervous and vascular supply. The reference length $L_0$ was measured as the length of the muscle belly when the leg was flexed at 90° on the thigh, and the foot was flexed at 90° on the leg.

The leg was fastened vertically by two pairs of screws driven into the femoral condyles and the distal end of the tibia. The distal tendon of the regenerate was sectioned and tied to a strain gauge attached to an electromagnetic ergometer (described in Maréchal and Plaghki, 1979). The tension signals were recorded with a fast UV recorder (model 200 S.E.).

The sciatic nerve was isolated in the thigh, tied and cut. Its peripheral end was placed on two platinum electrodes. All its collaterals were sectioned, except the branch innervating the regenerate. In this way, only the regenerated muscle fibers that were functionally useful for the animal were stimulated. The nerve was stimulated by supramaximal square waves (0.2 ms; 3 to 6 V) at a frequency of 100 Hz for 0.25 s. A fused tetanus was thus obtained.

The regenerate was stretched from $0.90\,L_0$ to $1.22\,L_0$ by steps of $0.02\,L_0$, at intervals of 2 min. At each step the muscle was tetanized isometrically.

The surface temperature of the muscle was kept at 32°C ± 0.3. Drops of a Krebs solution were allowed to fall onto the muscle. The temperature of the drops was controlled just before falling. The rectal temperature was kept at 37.5 to 38°C. Control experiments showed that in these conditions muscles could be tetanized for 1 s every two minutes showing no decrease either of isometric force or of the rate of development of isometric force over a period of several hours.

After the experiments the regenerates were dissected and weighed.

## Results and Discussion

### 1. Functional Recovery

The rats are severely disabled immediately after surgery. Functional recovery occurs in two to three months in rats operated early, when they weighed about 50 g. In older rats (operated when they weighed about 150 g) functional recovery is often incomplete.

We have found it convenient to describe functional recovery by the following four clinical stages. They are schematically illustrated in Fig. 1.

*Stage I.* (Normal stage) The rat walks on the proximal tips of the metatarsals and on the distal tips of the toes. The calcaneum is above the ground. The foot well mobile can be extended until it is in the prolongation of the leg.

*Stage IV.* This stage is observed immediately after surgery. The foot is completely flexed on the leg. As a result the rat walks on the calcaneum when it tries to use the operated limb. A few days after surgery, the mobility of the foot decreases. It is not possible to extend it completely. The "extension deficit" is measured by the angle between the normal fully extended position of the foot and the actual position attained in the operated rat by a forced extension. The extension deficit is high (between 50 and 30°).

*Stage III.* This stage is observed three to four weeks after surgery. The foot seems to be at a normal angle relative to the leg, and the rat used its limb freely. However, the rat takes support on the proximal end of the calcaneum, the foot being arched. The extension deficit remains at the high value observed in stage IV (between 50 and 30°).

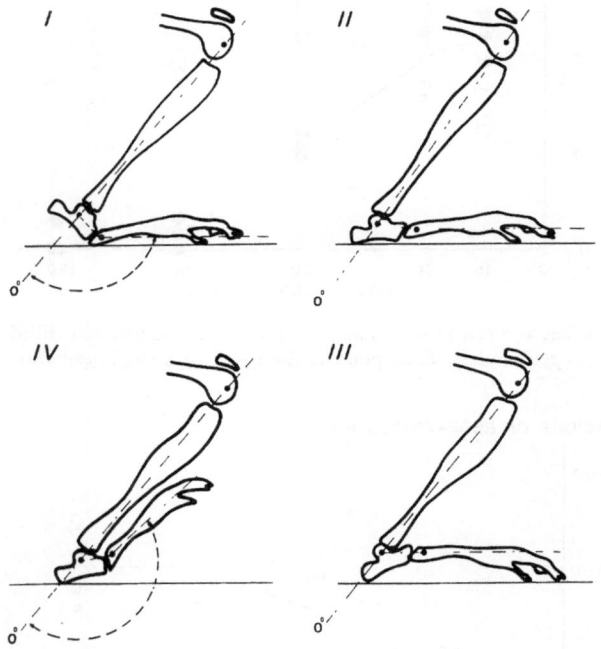

Fig. 1. Clinical stages of functional recovery during regeneration of minced triceps surae (see text)

*Stage II.* This stage is observed only when the functional recovery is good, 60 days or more after surgery. The arched shape characteristic of stage III has disappeared. The foot now lies flat on the ground, the main difference with the normal stage I being that the calcaneum still touches the ground. The extension deficit is moderate, never higher than 25°. The force with which the rat can extend the foot is however less than that observed in the normal unoperated side. Also palpation reveals that the regenerated muscle is appreciably thinner than the heterolateral muscle. At this stage, the rats seem to walk and to run quite normally.

## 2. The Effect of Age

The various stages of regeneration have been evaluated on 15 "younger" rats operated at three weeks of age (weight: 50 g) and 15 "older" rats operated at 6 weeks of age (weight: 150 g). The younger rats recovered well. Four months after surgery they were back to stage I or II. The older rats recovered to a lesser degree. Four months after surgery they were at stage III. As shown in Fig. 2, the extension deficit measured four months after surgery remains high in older rats, but has practically disappeared in younger rats. Thus the extension deficit provides an easy and rapid estimate of the degree of functional recovery in rats.

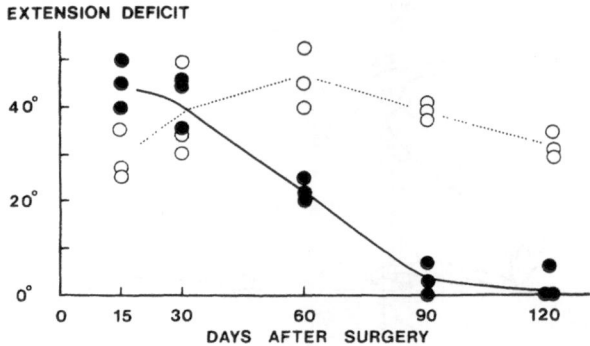

Fig. 2. Extension deficit as a function of time after surgery in younger rats (filled circles) and older rats (open circles). Each point is the result of a single experiment

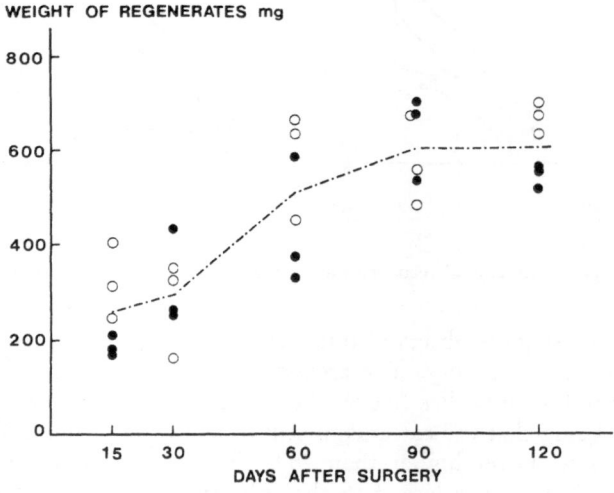

Fig. 3. Weight of the regenerates as a function of time after surgery in younger rats (filled circles) and older rats (open circles). Each point is the result of a single experiment

## 3. Weights of the Regenerates

Fig. 3 shows that the weights of the regenerates increase with time after surgery. It shows the important fact that younger and older rats do not show any differences in this respect, in spite of significant differences in their functional recovery. Three months after the surgery the weights of the heterolateral muscles were 2 to 3 times larger than those of the regenerates.

## 4. Passive Force-Length Relation

The muscle resting at its reference length $L_0$ develops very little force, not measurable with accuracy. If it is stretched to the maximal possible length in the animal (i.e. 1.18 $L_0$) it exerts a force of $3 \pm 0.5$ N. At intermediate lengths, the force is an exponential function of the difference $(L - L_0)$:

$$F = a \exp [(L - L_0)/b] \tag{1}$$

The length constant is $0.266 \pm 0.075$ (S.D., $n = 20$) in normal adult muscle. This value is similar to those reported by Schwartz (1961). In agreement with this author we found that this value does not depend on age or size of the animal. The force-length relation of regenerates is similar in shape to that of normal muscles. The maximal force at 1.18 $L_0$ is less ($0.7 \pm 0.03$ N) and the exponential increase of the passive force with $L - L_0$ is slower, the length constant b being nearly twice as large ($0.539 \pm 0.035$, $n = 24$).

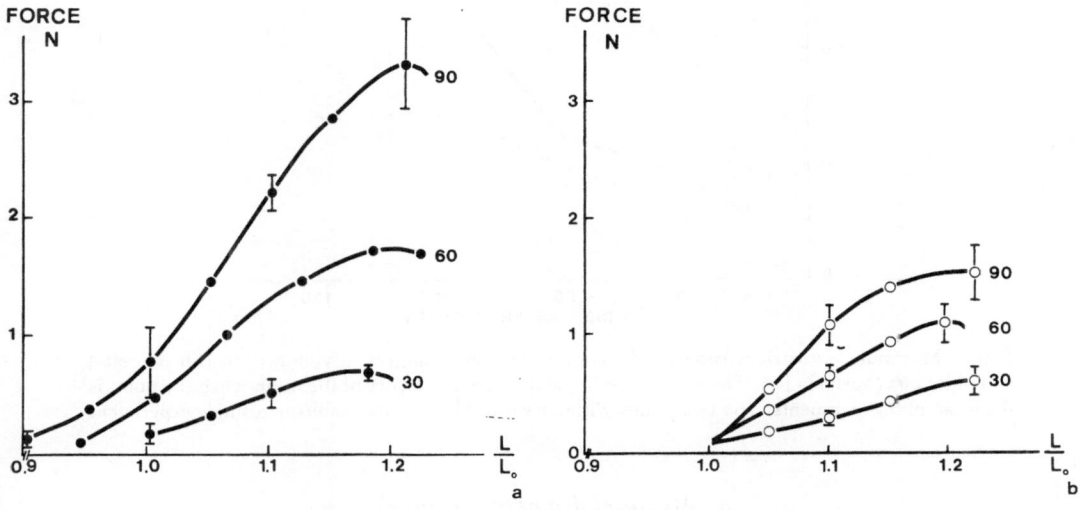

Fig. 4. Isometric tetanic force as a function of muscle length in younger rats (a) and older rats (b). The numbers in parameters refer to the time in days after the surgery. Each point is the main of 3 experiments. The standard errors of the mean are shown by the vertical bars for a few points

## 5. Active Force-Length Relation

The isometric force-length relation is plotted in Fig. 4 for the regenerates of muscles. Each curve is the mean of three experiments. The change in length corresponds to the physiological range. The shortest length 0.9 $L_0$ is obtained where the leg is fully flexed on the thigh, and the foot fully extended on the leg. The largest length 1.2 $L_0$ is obtained when the leg is fully extended on the thigh, and the foot is fully flexed on the leg.

Force-length relations are shown for regenerates 30, 60 and 90 days after surgery, in younger rats (4a) or older rats (4b). The maximum force is obtained near 1.2 $L_0$ in every case, as in normal muscle. It increases as regeneration proceeds: 90 days after surgery it is 3 to 4 times larger than after 30 days. However there is a large influence of age of the rat at the time of surgery. In younger rats, the post-surgery increase in maximal force is twice as fast. A second important difference concerns the shape of the force-length relation. At lengths smaller than $L_0$, younger rats show a conspicuous recovery of isometric force, whilst older rats are not able to develop any force at all. This fact has a serious effect on the functional recovery, because it means that older rats cannot forcibly extend their foot if their leg is completely flexed on their thigh, whilst younger rats can.

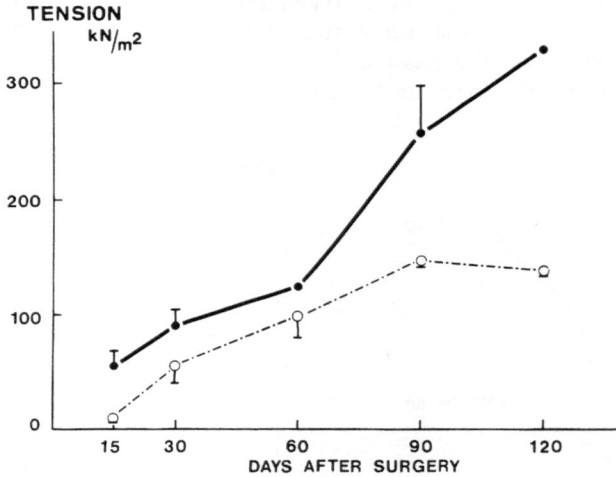

Fig. 5. Maximum isometric tension as a function of time after surgery in younger rats (filled circles) and older rats (open circles). The vertical bar show the standard errors of the mean when the point is the mean of 3 experiments. The two points without vertical bar are the results of a single experiment

## 6. Maximal Isometric Tension

The maximal isometric tension $P_0$ is the maximal force per unit cross-sectional muscle. Neglecting the density of muscle (set equal to 1), $P_0$ is equal to the force multiplied by length and divided by weight. The results are shown in Fig. 5. A further difference between younger and older rats emerges. Regenerates of younger rats are stronger, especially 90 to 120 days after surgery. Their tension at 120 days is 312 kN/m², a normal value. Regenerates of older rats are less powerful, their maximal isometric tension reaching only 40% of that of normal muscles.

Their actin content increases linearly with maximal isometric tension (Plaghki et al., 1980a). This fact indicates that the small tension produced by regenerates of older rats is mainly due to a poor regeneration of myofibrillar apparatus rather than to a disorderly arrangement of fibers or a poor reinnervation.

### References

1. Carlson, B. M.: The Regeneration of Minced Muscles (Monographs in Developmental Biology, Vol. 4). Basel: Karger. 1972.
2. Carlson, B. M., Gutmann, E.: Development of contractile properties of minced muscles regenerates in the rat. Exp. Neurol. *36*, 239–249 (1972).
3. Gallucci, V., Novello, F., Margreth, A., Aloisi, A.: Biochemical correlates of discontinuous muscle regeneration in the rat. Brit. J. Exp. Path. *47*, 215–226 (1966).
4. Maréchal, G., Plaghki, L.: The deficit of the isometric tetanic tension redeveloped after a release of frog muscle at a constant velocity. J. gen. Physiol. *73*, 453–467 (1979).
5. Plaghki, L., Maréchal, G.: Time course of regeneration of minced frog muscles estimated by the level of energetic substrates. Pflüg. Arch. *361*, 135–143 (1976).
6. Plaghki, L., Beckers-Bleukx, G., Bertrand, C., Maréchal, G.: Creatine and actin in regenerating rat gastrocnemius muscles, in: Energetics and Gas Exchange in Exercise Physiology (Cerretelli, P., Whipp, B. J., eds.). Amsterdam: Elsevier. 1980a.
7. Plaghki, L., Colson-Van Schoor, M., Beckers-Bleukx, G., Maréchal, G.: Creatine creatinekinase and glycolytic enzymes in regenerating muscles, in: Mechanism of Muscle Adaptation to Functional Requirement (Guba, F., Maréchal, G., Takacs, Ö., eds.). Acad. Sci. Hung. 1980b.
8. Rifenberick, D. H., Koski, C. L., Max, S. R.: Metabolic studies of skeletal muscle regeneration. Exptl. Neurology *45*, 527–540 (1974).
9. Salafsky, B.: Functional studies of regenerated muscle from normal and dystrophic mice. Nature (Lond.) *229*, 270–272 (1971).
10. Schwartz, N. B.: Changing size composition and contraction strength of gastrocnemius muscle. Am. J. Physiol. *201*, 164–170 (1961).
11. Snow, M. H.: Metabolic activity during the degenerative and early regenerated stages of minced skeletal muscle. Anat. Rec. *176*, 185–204 (1973).

Author's address: Dr. G. Maréchal, Laboratoire de Physiologie Générale, UCL-5540, Avenue Hippocrate, 55, B-1200 Bruxelles, Belgium.

# Skeletal Muscle Transplantation in Cats With and Without Nerve Repair

J. A. Faulkner, J. M. Markley jr., and T. P. White

Department of Physiology and Section of Plastic Surgery, Department of Surgery,
University of Michigan School of Medicine,
Ann Arbor, Michigan, U.S.A.

With 4 Figures

The regeneration of skeletal muscle fibers following free, whole muscle auto-transplantation has been well documented in rats (Carlson and Gutmann, 1975 a und b). Neither vascular nor nerve repair was made, so revascularization and reinnervation occurred spontaneously or not at all. The time course of regeneration and the degree to which control values are restored have been described (Carlson et al., 1979). A limited number of studies have focused on the regeneration of skeletal muscle fibers following transplantation of skeletal muscles in larger species. Successful transplantations have been reported in cats (Hakelius et al., 1975; Faulkner et al., 1976; Maxwell et al., 1978; Faulkner et al., 1980) and monkeys (Markley et al., 1978; Markley and Faulkner, 1980; Maxwell et al., 1979). In dogs, Thompson (1971) has reported successful grafts whereas Lavine and Cochran (1976) and Watson and Muir (1976) described unsuccessful transplantations.

In a series of experiments we transplanted 3 to 6 gram extensor digitorum longus (EDL) muscles of cats into the EDL site. Different experimental procedures were used to test the hypotheses that restoration of structure and function would be superior in predenervated grafts compared to grafts made without prior denervation; that orthotopic grafts would be superior to heterotopic grafts; and that grafts made with nerve repair would be superior to grafts dependent upon spontaneous reinnervation.

## Methods

Experiments were performed on male and female adult cats. All cats were healthy and free of disease. Operations were conducted under sterile conditions with the cats under pentobarbital anesthesia. Eight EDL muscles were denervated 2 to 4 weeks prior to transplantation. These muscles and four muscles denervated at the time of transplantation were removed from their site after all blood vessels were severed by electrocoagulation, and the proximal and distal tendons were cut. The grafts were then replaced in their original sites and the proximal and distal tendons of the graft were sutured to the tendon stumps. Since no attempt was made to repair the blood vessels or nerves, revascularization and reinnervation were left to occur spontaneously. These grafts were termed orthotopic standard grafts with or without predenervation. In a second series of experiments, four predenervated EDL muscles were removed and placed in the contralateral EDL site as heterotopic standard grafts. In a third series of experiments, eight EDL muscles were transplanted orthotopically without prior denervation. In addition to suturing the tendons of four grafts, the distal end of the cut peroneal nerve was anastomosed to the stump of the nerve pedicle remaining on the graft. Following each operative procedure, the fascia and skin were closed separately. The hypotheses regarding denervation and the influence of site were tested by comparisons of structure and function of stabilized grafts 140 to 520 days after transplantation. A stabilized graft was defined as a graft in which the mean fiber area in the central core was not significantly different from that in the peripheral areas (Faulkner *et al.*, 1980). The hypothesis on reinnervation was tested by comparisons of recovery 120 days after transplantation. We had no evidence that these grafts had stabilized.

At sacrifice, several functional and morphological variables were quantified. Measurements of contractile properties included time to peak twitch tension, half relaxation time, maximum isometric twitch and tetanic tension, twitch: tetanus tension ratio, maximum velocity of shortening; and fatigability (for details see Faulkner *et al.*, 1980). Muscle mass and fiber length were measured, and the percentage shortening was estimated. The succinate oxidase activities of whole muscle homogenates were assayed to provide an estimate of the oxidative capacity of the tissue (Maxwell *et al.*, 1980). Choline acetyltransferase activities of homogenates were assayed to provide an estimate of the mass of cholinergic nerve terminals in the tissue (Tuček, 1978). The maximum blood flow was measured using an arterial reference sample radioactive microsphere method (White *et al.*, 1980). Capillary density was determined by the p-hydroxy-mercurobenzoate technique (Maxwell *et al.*, 1980).

## Results

The maximum isometric tetanic tension correlates highly with the cross-sectional area of viable muscle fibers (Fig. 1) and is the single best measure of the degree of restoration of structure and function in an autograft (Faulkner *et al.*, 1980). The maximum tetanic tension was used to test the effect of predenervation on orthotopic grafts and the effect of orthotopic and heterotopic grafting (Fig. 2). The maximum tetanic tension of standard grafts without predenervation was not significantly different from that of predenervated grafts, nor were heterotopic grafts different from orthotopic grafts. Consequently, we rejected our hypotheses that predenervated grafts would be superior to standard grafts made without prior denervation, and that orthotopic grafts would be superior to heterotopic grafts.

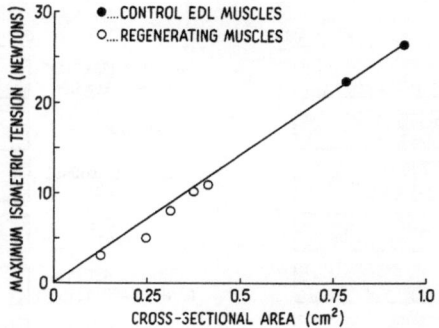

Fig. 1. The relationship between the cross-sectional area of skeletal muscle fibers and the maximum isometric tetanic tension (The solid line was drawn from the control data to the zero intercept)

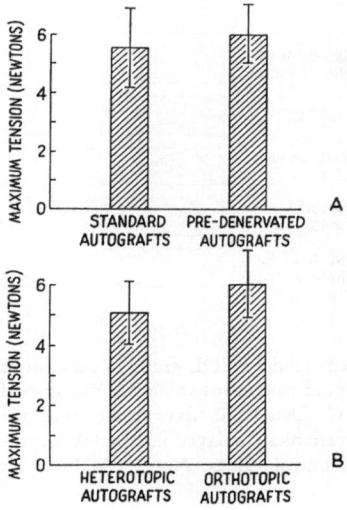

Fig. 2. The maximum isometric tetanic tension of standard EDL grafts in cats transplanted with and without prior denervation of the muscle (A) and transplanted heterotopically and orthotopically (B). Bars indicate ± 1 standard error of the mean

We then pooled the data for stabilized standard grafts of cat EDL muscles and found a number of variables in which there was complete restoration of the control values (Fig. 3A). Other variables showed an incomplete restoration with significant decreases in function (Fig. 3B).

The low choline acetyltransferase activity led us to hypothesize that the impairment in structure and function might result from defective reinnervation. Transplantation with nerve repair significantly improved maximum tetanic tension, muscle mass, and choline acetyltransferase activity, but fatigability and succinate oxidase activity remained at 60 percent of the control value (Fig. 3C).

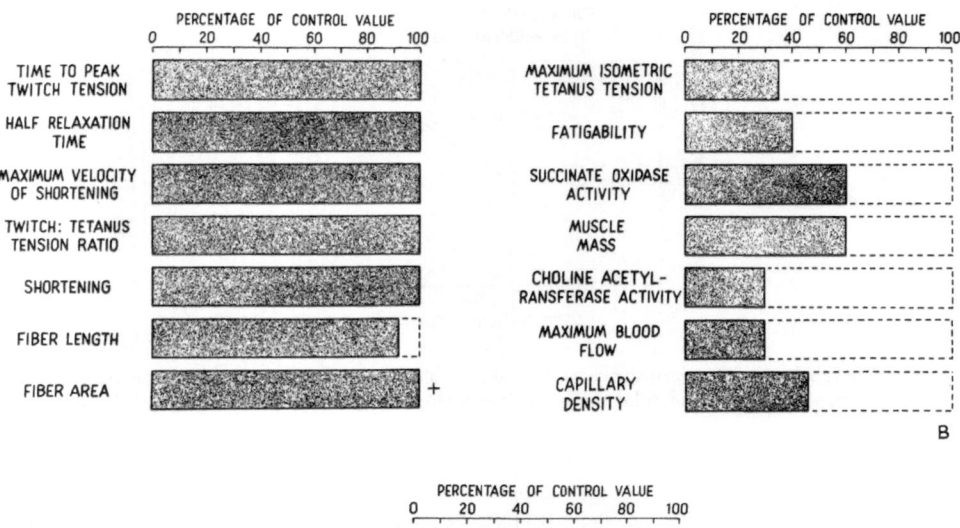

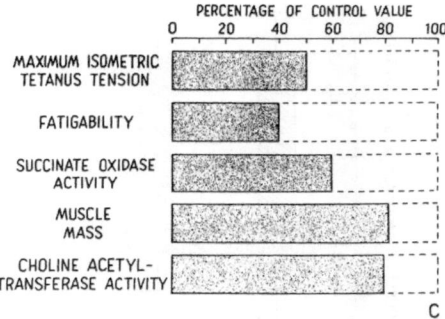

Fig. 3. Pooled data on stabilized standard EDL grafts in cats normalized as a percentage of control value. *A* Variables that are restored to control values. *B* Variables that show incomplete restoration of structure and function. *C* Data 120 days after transplantation on grafts made with nerve-anastomoses. Note: For variables displayed in Panel A, nerve-anastomosed grafts also attained 100 percent of the control values. Note: 3 A. Fiber area is of *single* fibers

## Discussion

Following transplantation of cat EDL muscles, skeletal muscle fibers degenerate and then regenerate (Mufti *et al.*, 1977). This sequence of degeneration and regeneration was shown previously in rat EDL muscles (Carlson and Gutmann, 1975a; Carlson *et al.*, 1979). The time course of events is slower in cats than in rats (Fig. 4). Grafts of EDL muscles in rats stabilize by 60–90 days (Carlson and Gutmann, 1975b) whereas cat EDL grafts require from 140 to 520 days (Faulkner *et al.*, 1980). The difference between cats and rats in the time of degenerative and regenerative events may be a function of the mass of the graft, the species involved, or an interaction between these two variables. In stabilized grafts in rats and cats, there are significant differences in the number of fibers that regenerate and in the mean cross-sectional areas of fibers.

Traditionally, the clinical applications of skeletal muscle transplantation to correct partial facial paralysis (Hakelius, 1974a; Thompson, 1971; Freilinger, 1975; Harii et al., 1976) or anal incontinence (Thompson, 1971; Hakelius, 1974b) have used predenervated muscles. Predenervation does not improve the function of stabilized grafts in cats or monkeys. Recently, grafts have been made successfully in humans without prior denervation of the muscle (Markley and Faulkner, 1980). Since predenervation requires an additional operative procedure, we recommend the practice be discontinued. Predenervation does decrease the mass of the muscle due to denervation atrophy. This smaller mass could be obtained equally well by selection of a smaller muscle or by surgical removal of part of a larger muscle.

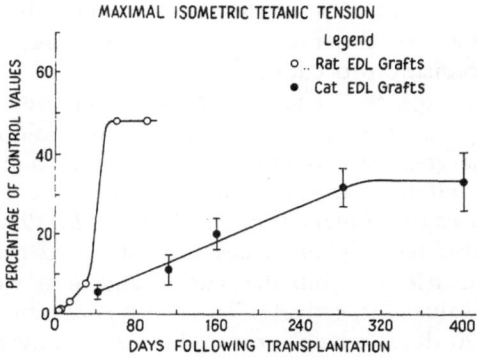

Fig. 4. The relationship between maximum isometric tetanic tension and time after transplantation for free, whole, standard grafts of 100 mg rat EDL muscles (from Carlson and Gutmann, 1975b), and 3 g cat EDL muscles (from Faulkner et al., 1980). Bars indicate ±1 standard error of the mean

In humans, surgeons have used palmaris longus, gracilis, extensor digitorum brevis, and pectoralis major for grafting purposes (Markley and Faulkner, 1980). We have previously reported (Markley et al., 1978; Maxwell et al., 1979) successful transplantation of palmaris longus and sartorius muscles to correct experimentally induced facial paralysis in monkeys. The observation that there were no significant differences in maximum tetanic tension between heterotopic and orthotopic grafts is consistent with the premise that the fiber length, fiber typing, and fascial sheaths present in the donor muscle are not critical variables. Upon regeneration, the fibers in the heterotopic graft develop the structural and functional characteristics of the muscle normally present in the recipient site. These observations allow plastic and reconstructive surgeons considerable choice in their selection of appropriate donor skeletal muscles for autologous transplantations.

After pooling the data on standard EDL grafts, it was apparent that some variables returned to control values. The concept that emerged was that skeletal muscle fibers that were revascularized and reinnervated developed normal structure and contractile properties, but that not all fibers would become revascularized and reinnervated. In cats, approximately 13,000 muscle fibers regenerated, compared to the 45,000 fibers present in the control EDL muscles. The fibers that do regenerate and become reinnervated tend to have slightly larger cross-sectional areas than fibers in control EDL muscles. The lower maximum tetanic tension of the grafts is consistent with the concept of normal function in a smaller number of fibers providing a reduced functional cross-sectional area (Fig. 5). The normalized maximum tetanic tension of grafts at any given stage of regeneration is not significantly different from the control value of 28.5 Newtons/cm² (Faulkner et al., 1980).

Compared to control EDL muscles, the lower succinate oxidase activity, maximum blood flow, and resistance to fatigue of grafts indicate an impaired functional capacity. Our major goal was to devise an operative procedure that would restore these variables closer to the control values. Since the choline acetyltransferase activity was 30% of the control value, the impaired function might be attributable to denervated fibers, therefore, nerve-anastomosis appeared to be a promising procedure.

The significantly greater choline acetyltransferase activity of the nerve-anastomosed grafts suggests a successful reinnervation of more skeletal muscle fibers in the nerve-anastomosed grafts than in the standard grafts (Carlson et al., 1980). The choline acetyltransferase activity correlates well with morphological measures of reinnervation (Carlson et al., 1980). The grafts with nerve anastomoses also had higher values than standard grafts for maximum tetanic tension and muscle mass but the tension and mass were still only 50% and 82% of control values respectively. The nerve-anastomosed grafts may not have stabilized by 120 days, which means additional recovery is still possible. However, the low succinate oxidase activity and blood flow associated with a rapid onset of fatigue suggest additional operative or post-operative procedures may be necessary before these grafts regain full function.

## Summary

Three to six gram EDL muscles were transplanted in adult cats with and without predenervation, orthotopically and heterotopically, and with and without nerve repair. In stabilized grafts, no significant differences were observed between autografts made with or without predenervation or between grafts transplanted heterotopically and those transplanted orthotopically. Regeneration of skeletal muscle fibers in cat EDL grafts was slower than in 100 mg rat EDL grafts but the degree of restoration of approximately 35 to 50 percent of the control value for maximum tetanic tension is similar. Compared to standard grafts, grafts with nerves anastomosed show better innervation, larger mass, and greater tension but oxidative capacity and fatigability were still impaired. The degree of restoration of structure and function through regeneration observed in large grafts in cats, particularly following nerve repair, provide experimental support for the continued use of free whole muscle transplantation in appropriate clinical cases.

### Acknowledgements

The authors thank Carol Brangwyn for her assistance in the collection and reduction of the histochemical and biochemical data. The current address of Timothy P. White is Department of

Physical Education, University of Michigan. The research was supported by grants from the Muscular Dystrophy Association and National Institutes of Health AM-18727.

## References

Carlson, B. M., Gutmann, E.: Regeneration in free grafts of normal and denervated muscles in the rat: morphology and histochemistry. Anat. Rec. *183*, 47–62 (1975 a).

Carlson, B. M., Gutmann, E.: Regeneration in grafts of normal and denervated rat muscles. Contractile properties. Pflüg. Arch. *353*, 215–225 (1975 b).

Carlson, B. M., Hansen-Smith, F. M., Magon, D. K.: The life history of a free muscle graft, in: Muscle Regeneration (Mauro, A., et al., eds.), p. 501. New York: Raven Press. 1979.

Carlson, B. M., Hník, P., Tuček, S., Vejsada, R., Bader, D. M., Faulkner, J. A.: Improvement of size and strength of rat muscle grafts possessing an intact nerve. (Submitted for publication, 1980.)

Faulkner, J. A., Maxwell, L. C., Mufti, S. A., Carlson, B. M.: Skeletal muscle fiber regeneration following heterotopic autotransplantation in cats. Life Sci. *19*, 289–296 (1976).

Faulkner, J. A., Maxwell, L. C., White, T. P., Niemeyer, J. H.: Characteristics of autografted mammalian skeletal muscles, in: Muscle Regeneration (Mauro, A., et al., eds.), p 493. New York: Raven Press. 1979.

Faulkner, J. A., Niemeyer, J. H., Maxwell, L. C., White, T. P.: Contractile properties of transplanted extensor digitorum longus muscles in cats. Am. J. Physiol. *238* (Cell Physiol. *7*), C120–C126 (1980).

Freilinger, G.: A new technique to correct facial paralysis. Plast. Reconstr. Surg. *56*, 44–48 (1975).

Hakelius, L.: Transplantation of free autogenous muscle in the treatment of facial paralysis. Scand. J. Plast. Reconstr. Surg. *8*, 220–230 (1974 a).

Hakelius, L.: Free autogenous muscle transplantation in two cases of total anal incontinence. Acta Chir. Scand. *141*, 69–75 (1974 b).

Hakelius, L., Nyström, B., Stålberg, E.: Histochemical and neurophysiological studies of autotransplanted cat muscle. Scand. J. Plast. Reconstr. Surg. *9*, 11–27 (1975).

Harii, K., Ohmori, K., Torii, S.: Free gracilis muscle transplantation, with microneurovascular anastomosis for the treatment of facial paralysis. Plast. Reconstr. Surg. *57*, 133–143 (1976).

Lavine, D. M., Cochran, T. A.: The failure to survive of autogenous free grafts of whole *gracilis* muscles in dogs. Plast. Reconstr. Surg. *58*, 221–227 (1976).

Markley, jr., J. M., Faulkner, J. A., Carlson, B. M.: Regeneration following transplantation of skeletal muscles in monkeys. Plast. Reconstr. Surg. *62*, 415–422 (1978).

Markley, jr., J. M., Faulkner, J. A.: Transplanted skeletal muscle regeneration in primates with clinical correlation. New York: Raven Press. In Press (1980).

Maxwell, L. C., Faulkner, J. A., Markley, jr., J. M., Winborn, D. R.: Neuroanastomosis of orthotopically transplanted palmaris longus muscles. Muscle & Nerve *2*, 44–52 (1979).

Maxwell, L. C., Faulkner, J. A., Mufti, S. A., Turowski, A. M.: Free autografting of entire limb muscles in the cat: histochemistry and biochemistry. J. Appl. Physiol. *44*, 431–437 (1978).

Maxwell, L. C., White, T. P., Faulkner, J. A.: Oxidative capacity, blood flow, and capillarity of skeletal muscles. J. Appl. Physiol.: Respirat. Environ. Exercise Physiol. *49*, 627–633 (1980).

Mufti, S. A., Carlson, B. M., Maxwell, L. C., Faulkner, J. A.: The free autografting of entire limb muscles in the cat. Anat. Rec. *188*, 417–429 (1977).

Thompson, N.: Autogenous free grafts of skeletal muscle. Plast. Reconstr. Surg. *48*, 11–27 (1971).

Tuček, S.: Acetylcholine in Neurons. London: Chapman and Hall. 1978.

Watson, A. C. H., Muir, A. R.: Failure of free muscle grafts in dogs. Brit. J. Plast. Surg. *29*, 27–33 (1976).

White, T. P., Sosin, D. M., Maxwell, L. C., Faulkner, J. A.: Capillarity and blood flow of transplanted muscles in cats. Am. J. Physiol.: Heart and Circ. (Accepted with revision for publication, September 1980.)

Author's address: Dr. J. A. Faulkner, Department of Physiology and Section of Plastic Surgery, Department of Surgery, University of Michigan School of Medicine, Ann Arbor, MI 48109, U.S.A.

## Discussion

*Tolhurst:* Would not Dr. Faulkner agree, that a 30% recovery of function is not good enough for reconstruction facial palsy. 30% recovery in a facial palsy is not adequate, so therefore shouldn't we use revascularized and reinnervated muscle grafts?

*Faulkner:* There are several things that make the possibility of using a muscle transplantation without vascular anastomose quite feasable in the face: first 30% function of the transplanted palmaris longus muscle in place of the zygomaticus major muscle is almost more than the normal function of the zygomaticus muscle–that means that it is enough for this purpose and secondly in a normal smile or in normal animation of the face the zygomaticus muscle does not contract 100%, only much less. In reality, when we do palmaris longus muscle transplants into the face, measurements made of the function in monkeys has been, such that at least up to 120 or 150 days there is more tension than there was previously in the zygomaticus major muscle. Thus you may even get more function than you had with the original facial muscles.

*Thompson:* I have done two series in facial palsy patients: one series received microsurgical anastomosis only and the other series recieved microvascular and neural anastomosis. The results fall very much into the pattern that Dr. Faulkner has described.

*Faulkner:* We have used, because of the connective tissue in the graft, measurement of the absolute force of an autograft and comparing it in grams. This does not work because of the connective tissue. We therefore attempt to estimate the true muscle fibre cross-sectional area of the autograft and the control muscle. It is 28 Newtons per cm square of muscle fibres 40 days after transplantation in every single case. Our conclusion is that the fibres are consistent in the force of regenerating, but that the number of fibres is changed.

# Summary

*Carlson:* As far as regenerating muscle is concerned, there is no doubt that regenerating muscles function, and there seem to be certain characteristics which are true across the various lines of laboratory animals which have been studied. We now have to find out if these characteristics are, in fact, also found in human beings. The question of pre-denervation, I think, is still open. There should be more time to discuss that; we have already seen some of the experimental results today.

# Muscle Transplantation in Experimental Surgery

# Experimental Basis for Free Muscle Transplantation*

## L. Hakelius

Department of Plastic Surgery,
University Hospital, Uppsala, Sweden

In our experimental research on free muscle transplantation in Uppsala we have systematically tried to follow the different steps of a graft's course from a free muscle transplant to a functioning muscle. We have studied the transplanted muscle fibres, the revascularization and reinnervation of the transplants with histological, histochemical, electronmicroscopic and neurophysiological techniques. I will give you a short survey of our research with the emphasis on the reinnervation and the end-plate formation in the grafts.

As research animals we used adult cats, in which the peroneus longus and tertius muscles were used as grafts after they had been denervated two weeks before transplantation. The muscles were transplanted to the cats' intercostal spaces with the muscles placed under the intercostal fascia in direct contact with the fibres of the intercostal muscles. They were positioned at right angles to the intercostal fibres. Both ends of the transplanted muscle were sutured to the intercostal fibres, with the transplants in slight tension. We studied six different enzymes and substrates of the muscle fibres of the grafts in serial sections in transplants from five days to 44 weeks after grafting.

In a normal peroneus longus muscle stained for succinic dehydrogenase there is a checkerboard pattern of red and white muscle fibres and there is a polygonal configuration of the fibres in cross sections.

In transplants 5 to 8 days old we found with histochemical methods that three zones could be distinguished. In the outer zone the red and white fibres could be distinguished quite easily by staining for oxidative enzymes. In the middle zone no normal muscle fibres were observed. The constituents appeared to be necrotic remnants of muscle fibres but it stained well for oxidative

* This paper is built on the following papers:
Hakelius, L., Nyström, B., Stålberg, E.: Histochemical and neurophysiological studies of autotransplanted cat muscle. Scand. J. Plast. Reconstr. Surg. 9, 15 (1975); Hakelius, L., Nyström, B.: Histochemical studies of end-plate formation in free autologous muscle transplants in cats. Scand. J. Plast. Reconstr. Surg. 9, 9 (1975); Hakelius, L., Nyström, B.: Blood vessels and connective tissue in autotransplanted free muscle grafts of the cat. Scand. J. Plast. Reconstr. Surg. 9, 87 (1975); Schaiaffino, S., Sjöström, M., Thornell, L. E., Nyström, B., Hakelius, L.: The process of survival of denervated and freely autotransplanted skeletal muscle. Experientia 31, 1328 (1975).

enzymes. The inner zone occupying more than half of the cross-section area consisted of structurally intact muscle fibres. Here it was not possible to stain for oxidative enzymes. We could not clearly establish the nature of these changes by light microscopy. Because of that we made a separate electron microscopic investigation of transplants from this early period in order to define more precisely the process of survival of the graft. This study showed that the outer zone consisted of surviving atrophic fibres and there was no evidence of necrosis or muscle regeneration in this zone. In the middle zone the cell composition was markedly heterogenous and in conclusion this zone was characterized both by extreme muscle atrophy and by fiber regeneration and there was an increasing number of satellite cells and thus of the population of myoblasts participating in the regenerative process. In the inner zone muscle fibres were all necrotic and macrophages often appeared in these fibres. The study showed that two distinct processes occur in the autografts in the early critical phase of the transplantation. A survival of transplanted fibers at the periphery of the graft and a regeneration of new muscle fibres following breakdown of the originally transplanted fibres in the central area. This process of regeneration seems to occur as a progressive concentric wave, penetrating deeper into the grafts. In sections made from 8 week old grafts there is beginning of redifferentiation in red and white fibres as a sign of reinnervation. The reinnervated fibres have started to increase in size and there is a tendency towards type grouping which means that there is no checker-board pattern of red and white fibres any more but there are clusters of red and white fibres, each cluster innervated through sprouting from a single motor neuron. This tendency towards grouping can be expected when the reinnervation is accomplished through direct sprouting. In other parts of the sections there are small atrophic fibres still uninnervated. In sections from a 40 week-old graft stained in the same manner as the previous ones almost all of the muscle fibres are redifferentiated and type grouping is quite evident.

In a second series of transplants the end-plates of the grafts have been visualized by means of staining the cholinesterase in the subsynaptic clefts. A longitudinal section of a normal peroneus longus muscle shows the normal fan-shaped arrangement of the muscle fibres and the narrow zone of end-plates placed at the middle of the fibres. The normal mature end-plates are ramified with unbroken ramifications. Sections of a 5 week-old transplant reveals a striking difference in comparison with the normal muscle. Here relatively few end-plates are located in small narrow zones, which did not extend over all the fibres to form a complete innervation band as in the normal muscle. These limited zones were seen in sections from both deep and superficial parts of the muscle. These end-plates have ramifications although some parts are heavily stained and others don't stain at all; they are apparently old disintegrating end-plates. In transplants 12 weeks old, no old fragmented end-plates were found but an exceptional number of small rounded cholinesterase positive plaques through out the muscle. These plaques were rounded without ramifications and their internal structure was irregular. This is the picture of immature end-plates. In 12 week-old transplants the end-plates were found along the entire muscle fibres and quite often there were more than one end-plate on each muscle fibre. In the oldest transplants 40–44 weeks old the normal narrow band of end-plates was lacking, instead there were short innervation zones at different sites in the muscle and also some scattered end-plates through out it. They showed further differentiation than the immature end-plates seen at earlier stages but they were still immature with broken ramifications giving the end-plates an appearance of a cluster of islands.

We have also made electromyographic recordings of the transplanted muscles at the time of extirpation. This was possible because the intercostal muscles were working even during general anesthesia. Voluntary activity, defined as activity synchronous to the EMG of the underlying intercostal muscle, was seen as early as 4 weeks after grafting.

Finally I will discuss the interesting appearance of muscle spindles, the tension feeling organs of the muscle. In the normal cat muscle you find them easily, but during the early stages of muscle transplantation we could not see a single muscle spindle in our material. This is in marked contrast to the situation after simple denervation when there is little effect on the spindles. In normal muscle the spindles have a very high oxidative activity and therefore the scanty vascular supply during early transplantation may be inadequate for their large oxygen demands and they can not survive. In the later transplants we found two newly formed muscle spindles, one in a 12 weeks old transplant and one in a 40 weeks old transplant. They were quite normal and reacted very strongly when stained for oxidative enzymes.

Author's address: Prof. Dr. L. Hakelius, Department of Plastic Surgery, University Hospital, S-750 14 Uppsala 14, Sweden.

## Discussion

*Thompson:* Have you had the opportunity to get human material and how did you find does it correlate with your animal findings?

*Hakelius:* I have not had human material enough to correlate. I think it is practically quite different to reoperate the patient and take specimens from a well-functioning muscle. I have not done that.

*Freilinger:* I agree, there are many differences between different animals, and especially between animals and human beings, in findings relating to free muscle transplantation.

*Hakelius:* I agree very much with you, Dr. Freilinger. For instance, there is a much more intensive power for muscle regeneration in cats than in other animals and especially than in human beings. In experiments on cats it is very difficult to keep a muscle denervated for a longer period, the tendency for reinnervation is always very high.

*Harii:* It is quite difficult to estimate the functional recovery of a transplanted muscle in animals and I may ask you about the variety of the muscle survival in a histological section and the functional recovery. Can you tell us anything about the variety of these parameters?

*Hakelius:* I cannot tell anything about the contractile power of these muscles, because we have not done any experiments with measurements.

*Faulkner:* It is difficult to compare the functional properties of a grafted muscle in different areas of the body; for instance in your model, when you put the muscle onto the intercostal space, the muscle fibres were contrary to the normal direction. Therefore there must be a great variation in the muscle function. Can you comment on this, Dr. Hakelius?

*Hakelius:* Of course, this model was used to examine the early stages of muscle transplantation and these muscles have no function. To get an information about the contractile power of transplanted muscles, other models should be used.

# Experimental Studies on Factors Influencing Muscle Transplantation*

M. Frey, H. Gruber, J. Holle, G. Kleinpeter, and G. Freilinger

Department for Plastic and Reconstructive Surgery
of the Second Surgical University Clinic of Vienna and
Institute for Anatomy
of the University of Vienna, Austria

With 9 Figures

Since the development of microsurgical techniques enables the immediate reestablishment of blood circulation in a transplanted muscle by microvascular anastomoses, a number of problems of free muscle transplantation may possibly be overcome.

1. The muscle graft is independent from capillary ingrowth.

2. One has not to expect central ischemic necrosis.

3. Larger muscles can be used for grafting without fear of losing the greater part of the muscle for lack of revascularization.

4. There is no need for predenervation as postulated by Studitsky *et al.*, 1963 (9) and Thompson, 1971 (12, 13). The reduction of the muscle to a plastic state and the reduction of the metabolic requirements of the muscle are no longer necessary because of the absence of temporary devascularization after transplantation.

The first free muscle transplants with microneurovascular anastomoses were performed in dogs by Tamai and coworkers (10). The rectus femoris muscle was used for orthotopic and heterotopic transplantation. The results published in 1970 consist of a microsurgical success rate of 70 percent and an almost normal histological structure 5 months after transplantation as seen in light and electron microscopes. Evoked potentials, regularly similar to normal tracings more than 5 months after the operation are used as an argument for perfect recovery of function.

* This study was supported by the "Fonds zur Förderung der Wissenschaftlichen Forschung in Österreich" (Project 2618) and by the Jubiläumsfonds der Oesterreichischen Nationalbank (Project 1691).

Similar results were reported in 1976 by Kubo *et al.* (7). In this experimental study the biceps brachii and the rectus femoris of the dog were used for ortho- and heterotopic transplantation with micro-neurovascular anastomoses. After about 5 months the macroscopic, histological, electron-microscopic, histochemical and electromyographic findings had returned to normal.

In the following years several clinical cases of muscle transplantation using microsurgical procedures have been reported. Harii (4, 5) began the clinical application for reanimation of facial paralysis in 1973 and published the first case in 1976. According to Harii transferred muscle undergoes some degenerative atrophy and its bulk is reduced during the period of reinnervation. In addition the acquired contraction of the transferred muscle is weaker than its original excursion.

Assessing recovery of muscle function is very difficult in clinical cases. Therefore physiological assessment of transplanted muscles with micro-neurovascular anastomoses in experimental series is of special interest.

Terzis *et al.* (11) studied the functional capabilities of the rectus femoris muscle of the rabbit after tenotomy, simple neurovascular repair, and orthotopic and heterotopic transplantation. She showed that tenotomy alone altered the function more than did neurovascular repair, and although a muscle survived after replantation, maximum working capacity achieved only one fourth of the normal.

In spite of different results of survival and regeneration rates on the one hand, and of functional recovery on the other hand, it is a common opinion that muscle transplantation with microneurovascular anastomoses seems to be the best way to substitute muscles with greater volume and powerful contraction.

With our experimental series we intended to analyse the effect of ischemia, of nerve-suture and the combination of both on the muscle function, using the rectus femoris of the rabbit as an experimental model.


## Material and Method

### Anatomy

The rectus femoris of the rabbit is a good model for studying muscle transplantation, because it is a defined unit, spindle-shaped, with a circumscript origin and insertion. The muscle is supplied by a single artery as a branch of the femoral artery. This artery with a diameter of 0.5 to 0.8 mm enters the muscle mediodorsally together with a smaller comitant vein, which drains directly or sometimes indirectly into the femoral vein. Another vein with a diameter of about 1 mm runs close to the ventral surface of the muscle and drains over a larger transverse vein, crossing the muscle near and parallel to the inguinal ligament, into the femoral vein. The nerve supply enters the muscle as branches of the femoral nerve. A thicker bifascicular nerve accompanies the artery and the comitant vein, usually two small and short branches entering the muscle slightly proximal to its hilus (Fig. 1).

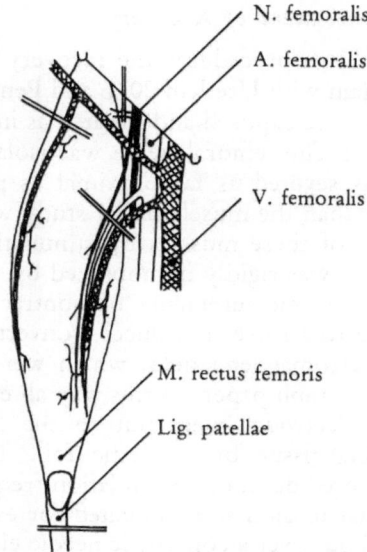

N. femoralis

A. femoralis

V. femoralis

M. rectus femoris

Lig. patellae

Fig. 1. *Topographic scheme* of the rectus femoris muscle of the rabbit and its vascular and nervous supply (// = level of clamping the vessels and of the division and suture of the nerve)

## Operative Procedures

In 21 male rabbits (3–3.5 kilograms each), divided into three groups of 7 each, the following microsurgical procedures were performed: In the first group the rectus femoris muscle was denervated by division of the muscle nerve near its entrance into the muscle. Immediately afterwards the bifascicular main branch was sutured and further small, unimportant branches to the muscle were resected. In the second group the blood supply was interrupted by clamping the artery and the two veins for three hours. In the third group both, the division and suture of the nerve and the clamping of the vessels were performed. For all experiments the combination of Urethan 20% and Pentothal® was used for anaesthesia.

Starting from the anterior superior spine, the skin of the ventromedial thigh was incised onto the tibial tuberosity. After dissecting a thin layer of covering muscle tissue and cutting the patellar tendon, the rectus femoris muscle was easily freed; by pulling the muscle laterally a clear inspection of the femoral vessels and nerve with their branches to the muscle became possible. In some cases the muscle origin was severed too, but the reinsertion of the origin is difficult. In the results there is no difference between severing the origin or not. In this way we imitated the orthotopic transplantation but eliminated the effect of postoperatively reduced blood flow in the case of microvascular anastomoses with different patency rates. When the microsurgical part was finished, the patellar tendon and its connections to the insertion of the other parts of the quadriceps femoris were sutured and the skin was closed.

The operations were performed on the muscle on one side, with the muscle of the other side as a comparable control in the same animal.

## Assessment of Recovery

Six months after the operative procedures the recovery was assessed. The animals were anaesthesized again with Urethan 20 % and Pentothal®. The rectus femoris muscles of both sides were exposed and isolated as in the first operation by cutting the patellar tendon. The femoral nerve was isolated by cutting the inguinal ligament, and it was severed as far proximal as possible. All nerve branches to the muscles other than the muscle under study were also severed in order to exclude contractions of these muscles by stimulation of the femoral nerve. The origin of the muscle was rigidly immobilized by transfixation of the iliac bones and the femur. For measurements of contractile properties the patellar tendon was connected to a force transducer, converting the mechanical forces into changes of an electromagnetic field, which were transformed into contraction curves recorded on graph paper. In this way all evoked contractions were isometric. Stimulating electrodes were put to the femoral nerve and isolated from the surrounding tissue by a plastic foil. The suprathreshold electrical stimuli were of 0.2 msec duration. Stimulation frequency was 100 Hz for tetanus. The optimal initial tension was evaluated for every tested muscle. EMG recordings were carried out over a concentric needle electrode, which was always inserted at the middle of the muscle. Macroscopic observations were documented.

At the end of the functional assessment each muscle was dissected free from its origin and was weighed. Afterwards a standard middle segment of the muscle was quick-frozen in isopentane, cooled by dry ice, for histochemical procedures. 30 $\mu$m thick cross sections were cut from the frozen blocks in a cryostat at −20 °C. Sections of operated and control muscles were incubated for NADH-diaphorase and myofibrillar ATPase at pH 9.4. Hematoxylin-Eosin and Sudan III stainings were performed (1, 3). ATPase stained sections were evaluated quantitatively. Photographic samples with a standard distribution over total cross-sections were projected on a planimetric board. The fiber area, the perimeter, the diameter of the equal area circle (D-circle) and the correlation of area and perimeter were determined and distribution histograms were plotted out by an Videoplan® apparatus (Fa. Kontron).

## Results

### Macroscopic Findings

About 6 months postoperatively the treated muscles were reexplored and compared with the control muscles. It was astonishing that there were only small macroscopic alterations. The muscles were of normal volume, the only imposing fact being the augmentation of connective and fat tissue especially in the nerve-suture and the ischemia group. Only in one ischemia-case was the reinsertion of the muscle distracted, and the absence of resting tension caused serious alterations of the muscle. The muscle size was significantly reduced, and scar tissue replaced a large part of the muscle tissue.

### Measurements of Muscle Force

At the beginning of the electric, indirect stimulation of each muscle the *optimal initial tension* was estimated. Although there is no significant difference between the three groups and the control (Table 1), a distinct increase was found in the ischemia and the nerve suture group.

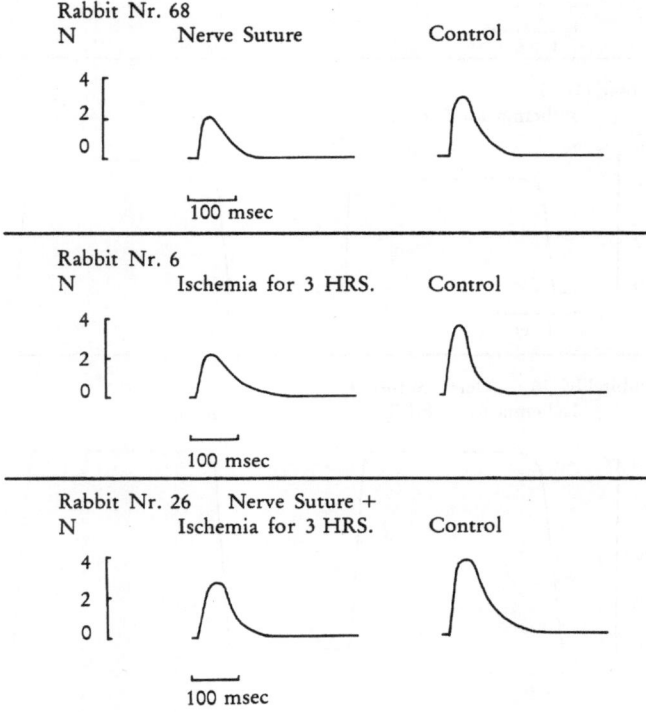

Fig. 2. *Isometric twitch contractions* of the rectus femoris muscle of the rabbit six months after operation – one example of each group, compared with the untreated, contralateral side

Comparing the *twitch-tensions*, the muscles of the nerve-suture group reached 74.6 (± 17.8) % of the control side (= 100 %), the ischemia group 78 (± 18.3) % and the group after ischemia and nerve-suture 95.3 (± 23.2) % (Table 1, Fig. 2).

Time parameters of single twitch, as *total twitch time, contraction time* and *one half relaxation time* showed no significant differences (Table 2). On the average, *maximal tetanic tension* at a stimulation frequency of 100 Hz reached 84.3 (± 13.1) % of the control in the nerve-suture group, 80.5 (± 7.8) % in the ischemia group and 96.5 (± 2.9) % in the group after ischemia and nerve-suture (Table 1, Fig. 3).

After functional testing the muscles were taken out and weighed. In all groups *muscle weight* of the treated muscles was somewhat higher than in the control. This increase is caused by a greater amount of connective and adipose

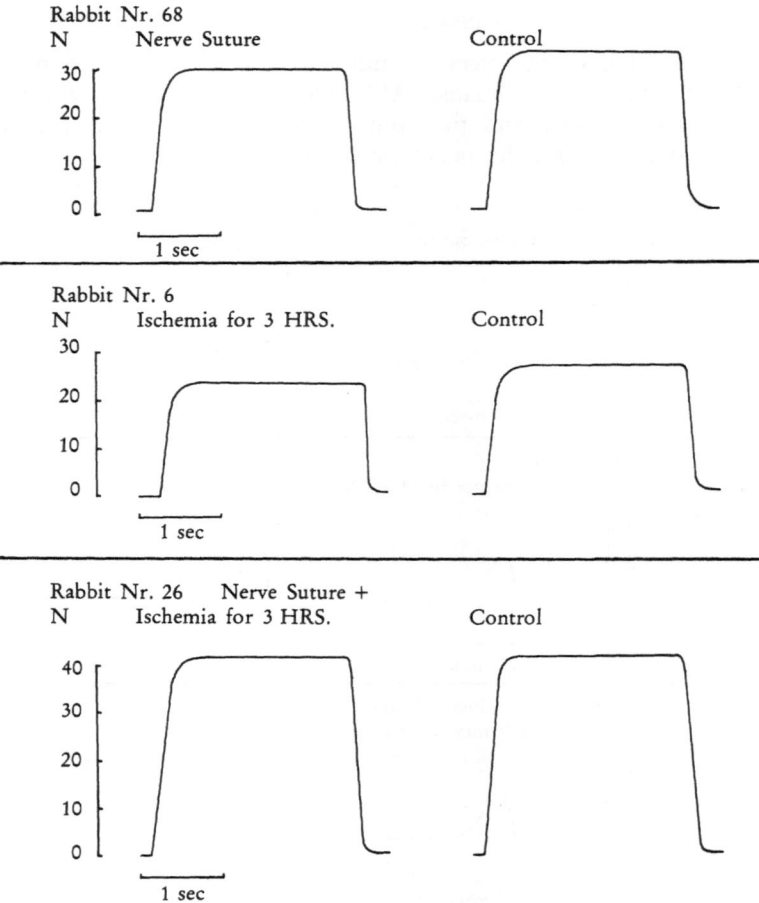

Fig. 3. *Isometric tetanic contractions* of the rectus femoris muscle of the rabbit six months after operation—one example of each group, compared with the untreated, contralateral side

tissue in the operated muscles as was verified both macroscopically and histologically. The incomplete recovery of muscle force speaks against an increase of muscle tissue (Table 3).

Therefore this fact has to be mentioned, when force data are normalized by expressing them as *force per gram of muscle weight*. This parameter does not exactly represent muscle function. Prior to normalizing, it would be necessary to subtract the increased amount of connective and fat tissue from muscle weight. Since it excludes the great variability of muscle weights, the parameter is very useful. Comparing the different groups, a knowledge of the contents of tissues other than muscle tissue is important. Expressed as a percentage relation to the control muscle, the force per gram of muscle weight reached 75.8 ($\pm$ 23.8) % for the twitch and 75.7 ($\pm$ 9.7) % for the tetanus in the nerve-suture group, 72.5 ($\pm$ 17.8) % in the ischemia group for the twitch and 76.2 ($\pm$ 2.8) %

Table 1. *Force parameters of contractions six months after the microsurgical procedures in the rectus femoris muscle of the rabbit (compared with the contralateral, untreated muscle)*

|  | Operated | Control |
|---|---|---|
| *Optimal initial tension* (Newton = N) | | |
| Nerve suture | 5.30  (± 1.78)  N | 4.90  (± 1.38)  N |
| Ischemia for 3 hrs. | 4.51  (± 0.80)  N | 4.12  (± 0.43)  N |
| Nerve suture and ischemia for 3 hrs. | 5.89  (± 2.68)  N | 7.06  (± 1.27)  N |
| *Total twitch tension* (Newton = N) | | |
| Nerve suture | 2.433 (± 0.952) N | 2.943 (± 1.04)  N |
| Ischemia for 3 hrs. | 2.757 (± 1.128) N | 3.522 (± 1.05)  N |
| Nerve suture and ischemia for 3 hrs. | 3.443 (± 0.746) N | 3.728 (± 0.873) N |
| *Maximal tetanic tension* (Newton = N) | | |
| Nerve suture | 19.424 (± 7.26)  N | 22.975 (± 7.05)  N |
| Ischemia for 3 hrs. | 27.615 (± 4.02)  N | 32.648 (± 8.59)  N |
| Nerve suture and ischemia for 3 hrs. | 39.142 (± 6.632) N | 40.420 (± 5.81)  N |

Table 2. *Time parameters of contractions six months after the microsurgical procedures in the rectus femoris muscle of the rabbit (compared with the contralateral, untreated muscle)*

|  | Operated | Control |
|---|---|---|
| *Total twitch time* (msec) | | |
| Nerve suture | 164 (± 27) msec | 142 (± 47) msec |
| Ischemia for 3 hrs. | 206 (± 48) msec | 198 (± 23) msec |
| Nerve suture and ischemia for 3 hrs. | 204 (± 56) msec | 220 (± 43) msec |
| *Contraction time* (msec) | | |
| Nerve suture | 23 (±  4) msec | 23 (±  3) msec |
| Ischemia for 3 hrs. | 24 (±  4) msec | 26 (±  2) msec |
| Nerve suture and ischemia for 3 hrs. | 28 (±  2) msec | 26 (±  4) msec |
| *One half relaxation time* (msec) | | |
| Nerve suture | 37 (± 15) msec | 40 (± 21) msec |
| Ischemia for 3 hrs. | 50 (± 37) msec | 38 (±  7) msec |
| Nerve suture and ischemia for 3 hrs. | 34 (±  6) msec | 34 (± 11) msec |

for the tetanus, and in the group after ischemia and nerve suture 89.7 (± 13.3) % for the twitch and 99.3 (± 22.0) % for the tetanus (Table 3). It was surprising that the loss of resting tension by rupture of the tendon suture in that one case mentioned above caused a rather poor functional result, in sharp contrast to the good recovery in all the other animals.

## EMG-Recordings

Together with the twitch contraction curves, needle EMG's were registered. Even in the two groups in which a nerve-suture had been performed, normal multiphasic EMG's were observed and interpreted as a sign of restored innervation.

Table 3. *Muscle weight and force per gram of muscle weight six months after the microsurgical procedures in the rectus femoris muscle of the rabbit (compared with the contralateral, untreated muscle)*

|  | Operated | Control |
|---|---|---|
| *Muscle weight* (grams = g) | | |
| Nerve suture | 13.1 (±2.5) g (112%) | 11.7 (±1.6) g |
| Ischemia for 3 hrs. | 9.3 (±2.5) g (108%) | 8.6 (±2.3) g |
| Nerve suture and ischemia for 3 hrs. | 10.9 (±3.2) g (106%) | 10.3 (±2.5) g |
| *Twitch contraction:* | | |
| *Force per gram of muscle weight* (Newton/gram = N/g) | | |
| Nerve suture | 0.186 (±0.069) N/g [75.8 (±23.8) %] | 0.249 (±0.076) N/g |
| Ischemia for 3 hrs. | 0.358 (±0.300) N/g [72.5 (±17.8) %] | 0.461 (±0.281) N/g |
| Nerve suture and ischemia for 3 hrs. | 0.315 (±0.101) N/g [89.7 (±13.3) %] | 0.347 (±0.071) N/g |
| *Tetanic contraction:* | | |
| *Force per gram of muscle weight* (Newton/gram = N/g) | | |
| Nerve suture | 1.49 (±0.45) N/g [75.7 (±9.5) %] | 1.97 (±0.53) N/g |
| Ischemia for 3 hrs. | 2.49 (±0.40) N/g [76.2 (±2.8) %] | 2.99 (±0.49) N/g |
| Nerve suture and ischemia for 3 hrs. | 3.76 (±1.36) N/g [99.3 (±22.0) %] | 3.77 (±1.04) N/g |

## Histological Findings

Histological examination of the cross-sections had the following results: The cross-sections of all treated muscles seem to be larger than the cross-sections of the controls because of an augmentation of connective and adipose tissue.

In the nerve-suture group complete denervation and almost complete reinnervation was ascertained by typical type grouping all over the cross-sections (Fig. 4). The myonuclei were often found in the center of the cell (Fig. 5). In all cases of this group areas of atrophic fibers were found, but they were limited to a small percentage of the cross-section. Both adipose tissue and augmented connective tissue were situated near the central aponeurosis which divides the rectus femoris muscle into two, almost equal parts. The muscle nerves showed excellent regeneration.

Isolated injury of the muscle by transient ischemia alone seems to be attested by healthy nerves and missing signs of denervation and reinnervation (Fig. 4). In contrast to untreated muscle we found central myonuclei, but not so diffuse as after nerve suture (Fig. 5). Only single bundles of muscle fibers were involved. There was more fat than in normal muscle but less than after nerve-suture. The

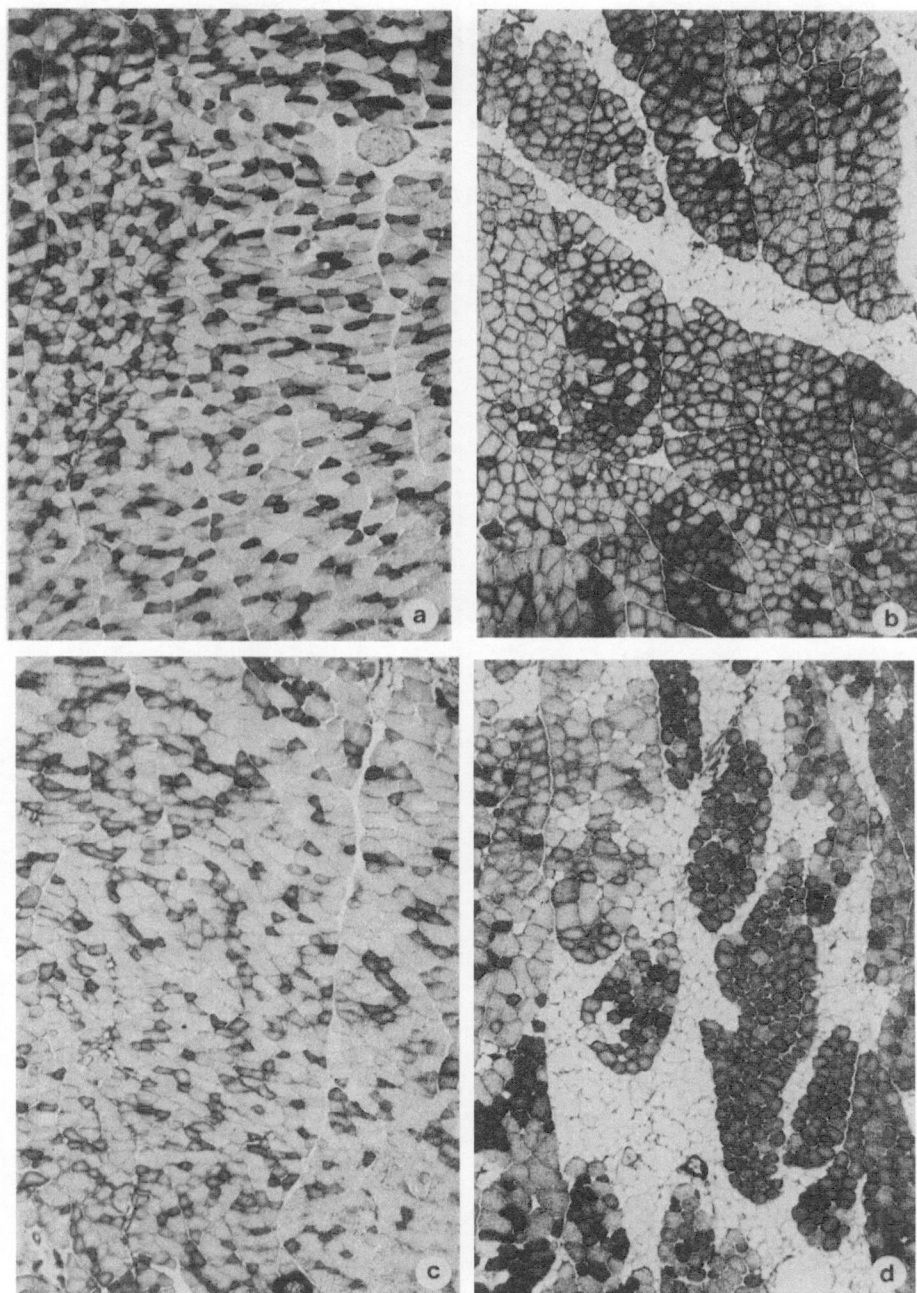

Fig. 4. NADH-diaphorase stained cross-sections of the rectus femoris muscle: *a* Untreated control, *b* 6 months after division and suture of the muscle nerve, *c* 6 months after ischemia for 3 hrs., *d* 6 months after nerve suture and ischemia for 3 hrs. Magnification: 25 ×

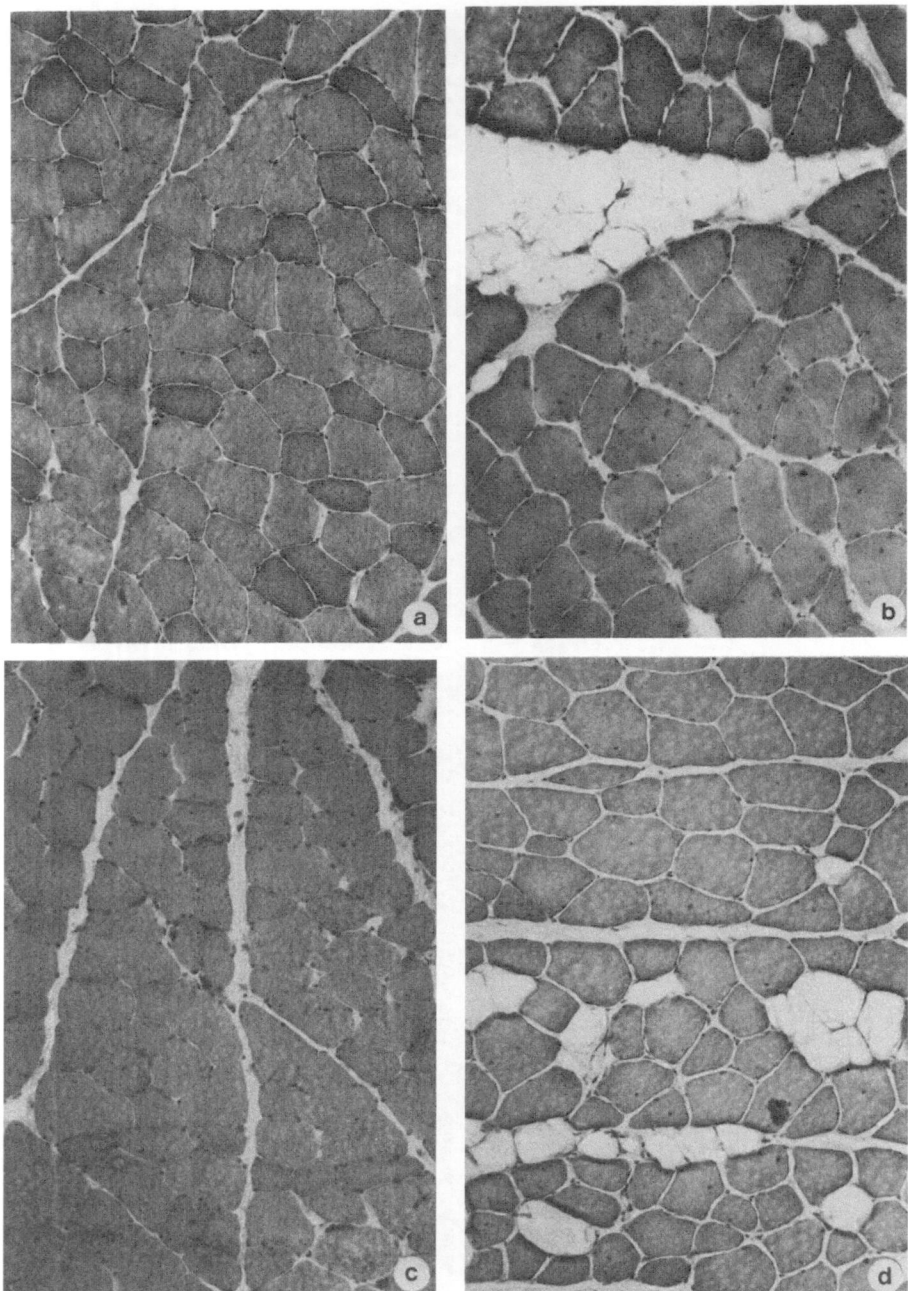

Fig. 5. Hematoxylin-Eosin stained cross-sections of the rectus femoris muscle: *a* Untreated control, *b* 6 months after division and suture of the muscle nerve, *c* 6 months after ischemia for 3 hrs., *d* 6 months after nerve suture and ischemia for 3 hrs. Magnification: 100 ×

morphology of the muscle fibers and the distribution of fiber-types were not altered.

The group after nerve-suture and ischemia for 3 hours showed signs of reinnervation to the same extent as the group with nerve suture alone (Fig. 4). Small differences consisted in further progressed regeneration. Groups of atrophic fibers were seldom seen. The myonuclei seemed to lie more at the periphery, but central myonuclei were still found all over the cross-section (Fig. 5). The extent of fat tissue was similar to that in the ischemia group.

All these histological findings correlated very well with the functional results.

## Planimetry

For the planimetric analysis an example of each group should be demonstrated (Figs. 6, 7, 8). 1700 to 2700 fibers were evaluated in the cross-section of each muscle. In a comparison of the mean values and the distribution curves for area, perimeter and diameter of the circle with the same area (D-circle), and of the correlation between area and perimeter no difference could be found between the treated and the control side. Even in the groups with reinnervation there was no significant alteration of these morphologic parameters.

## Discussion

In concluding and comparing all these results of macroscopic observation of functional assessment, and of histological examination including planimetry, some facts in muscle transplantation with microneurovascular anastomoses can be pointed out:

The suture of the muscle nerve near its entrance into the muscle results in practically full reinnervation. The regeneration rate leads to muscle fibers of normal dimensions and to functional recovery of 75 % for maximal twitch and 84 % for maximal tetanic tension (Fig. 9). A small part of the muscle tissue is replaced by fat and connective tissue. Transient ischemia for 3 hours was used as an imitation of the clinical situation of ischemia during muscle transplantation. Several authors (Terzis, Schenk, Harii; lit. 11, 8, 6) report that it takes 60 to 100 minutes for the reestablishment of blood circulation in the muscle. Gordon, Buncke and Townsend (2) investigated the histological changes in the quadriceps muscle of the rat after temporary independent occlusion of arterial and venous supply. Their results indicate that the period of warm ischemia should be limited to about one hour, because a longer period of arterial ischemia produces severe histological changes in the muscle. The limiting factor seems to be the arterial rather than the venous supply. They did not investigate the possibility of muscle regeneration after such ischemic insults. According to our own clinical experience about half an hour is needed from the division of the neurovascular pedicle of the muscle until the opening of the clamps at the arterial anastomosis, and about another 20 minutes to complete the venous anastomosis. From this point of view it seems to be better to anastomose the artery before the vein. In our experimental model we used an ischemia for 3 hours and found

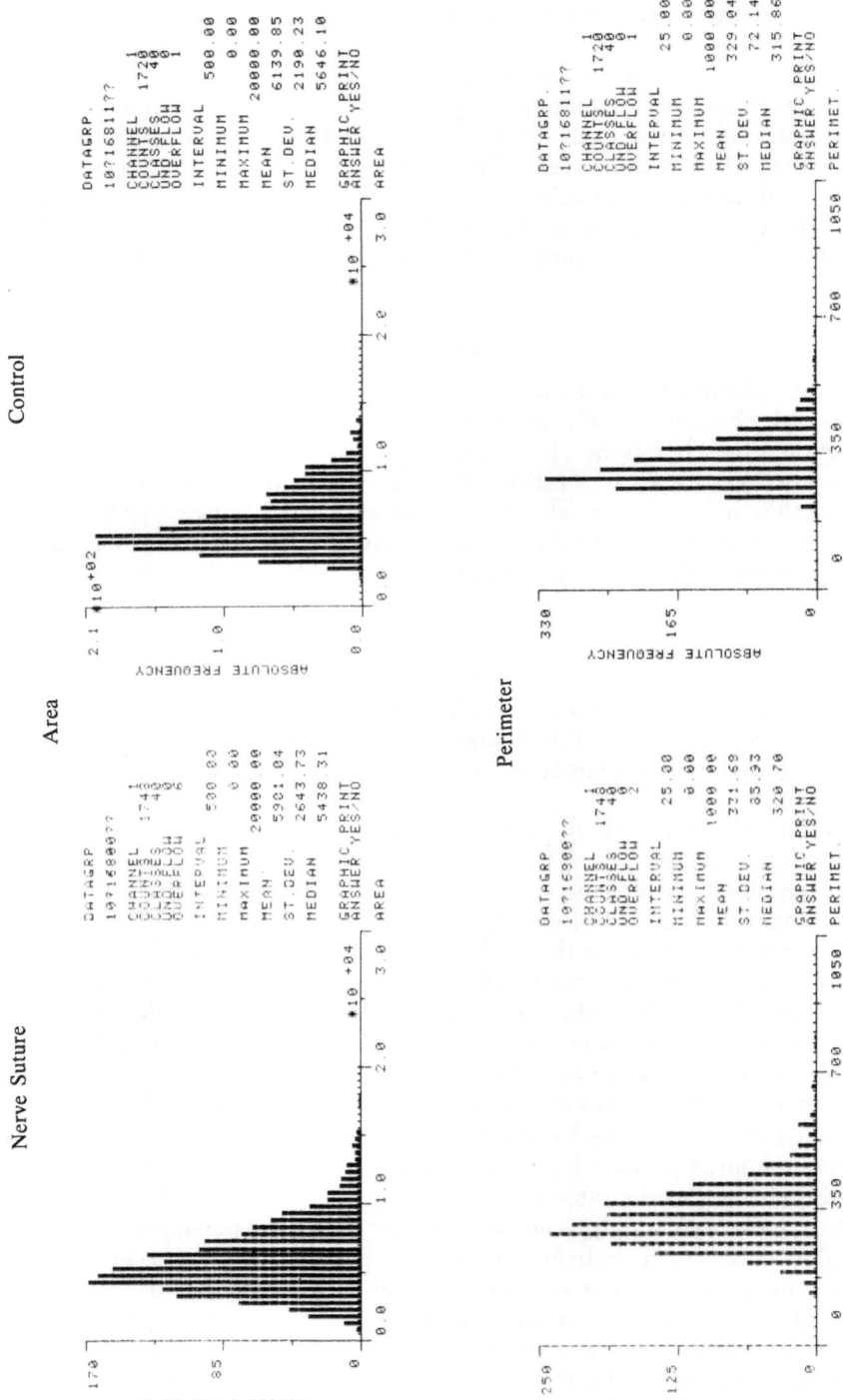

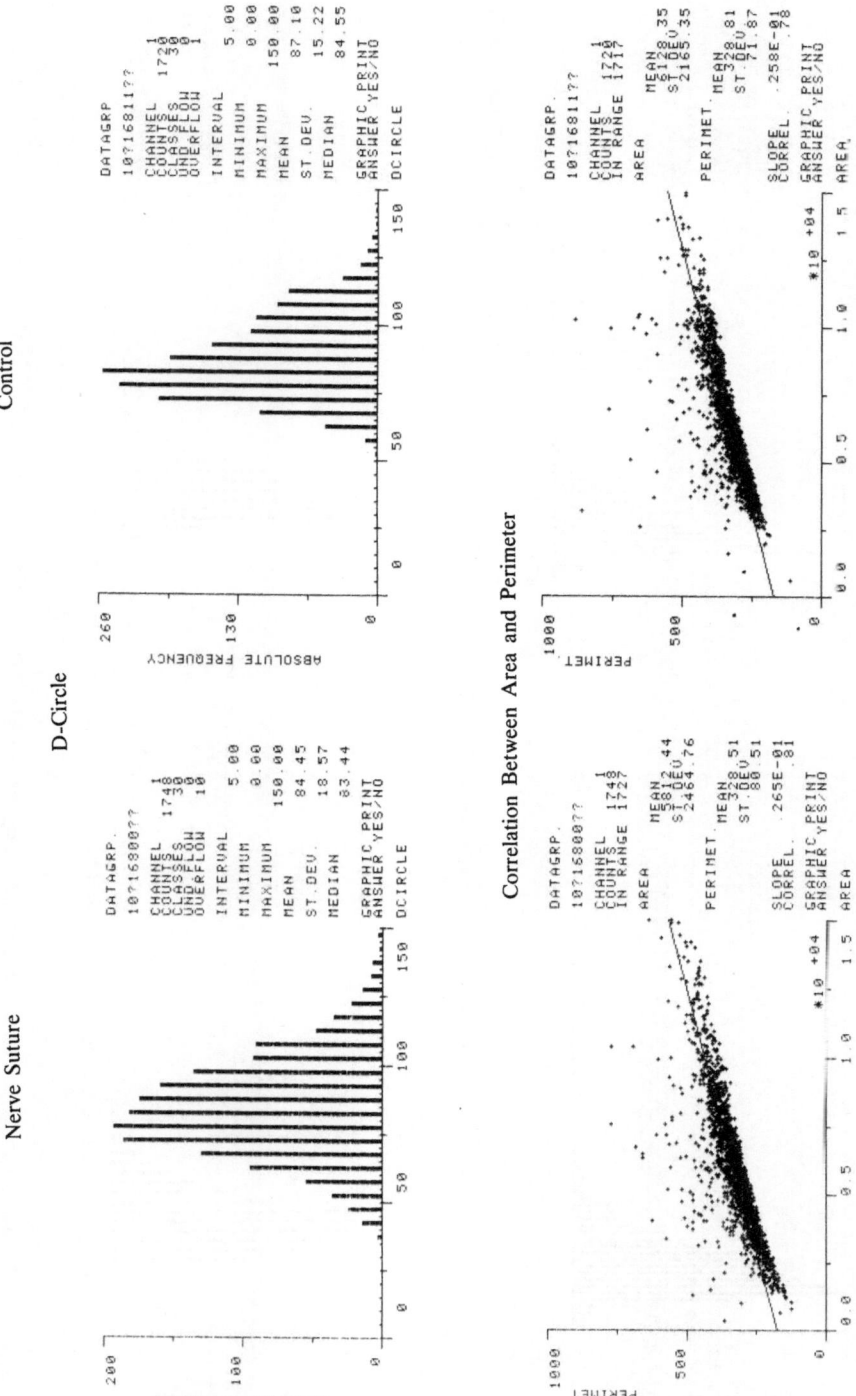

Fig. 6. Rabbit Nr. 68. Distribution curves for area, perimeter and D-circle, correlation between area and perimeter of the muscle fibers 6 months *after division and suture of the muscle nerve.* ATPase stained cross-sections were used for the evaluation

M. Frey, H. Gruber, J. Holle, G. Kleinpeter, and G. Freilinger:

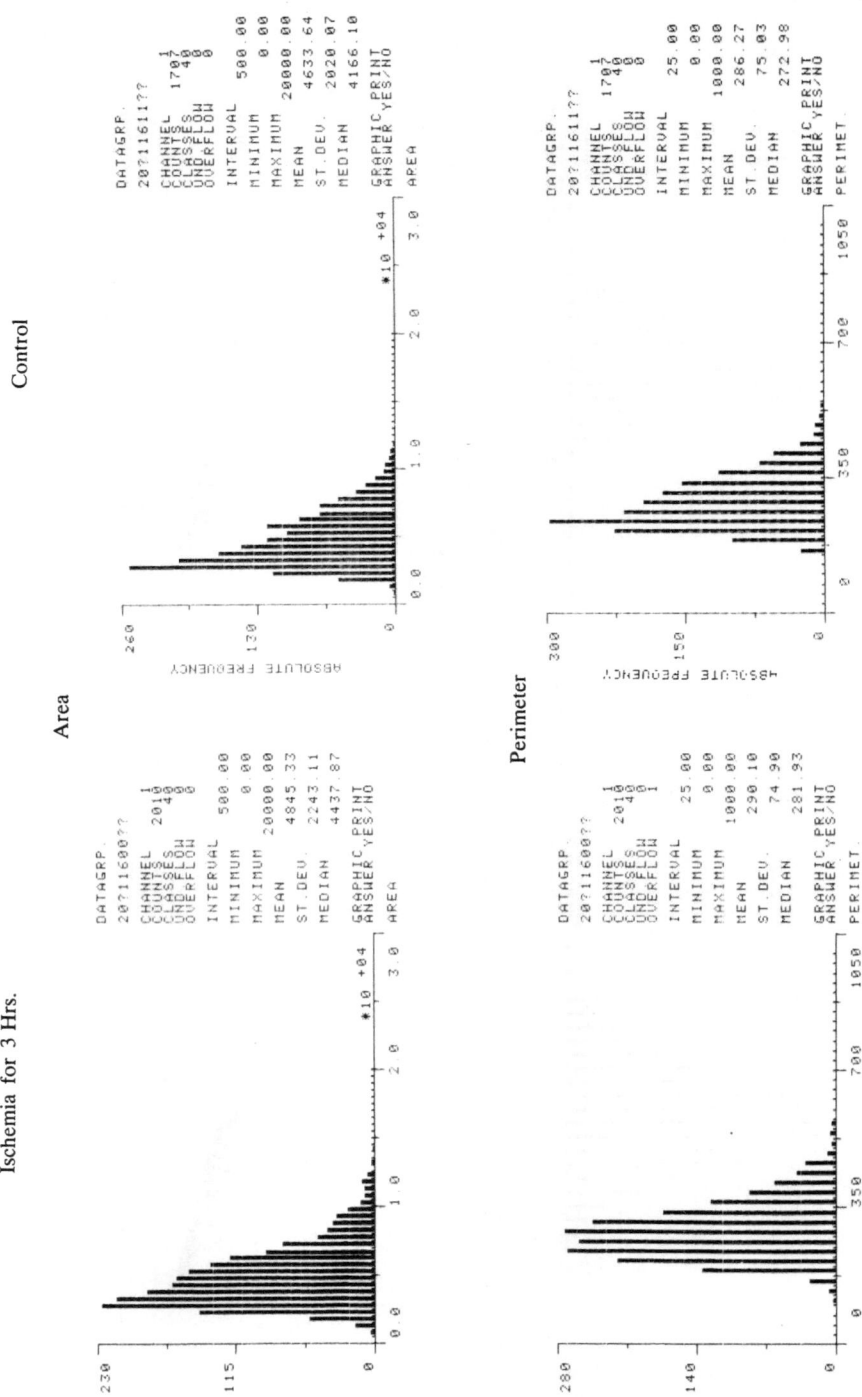

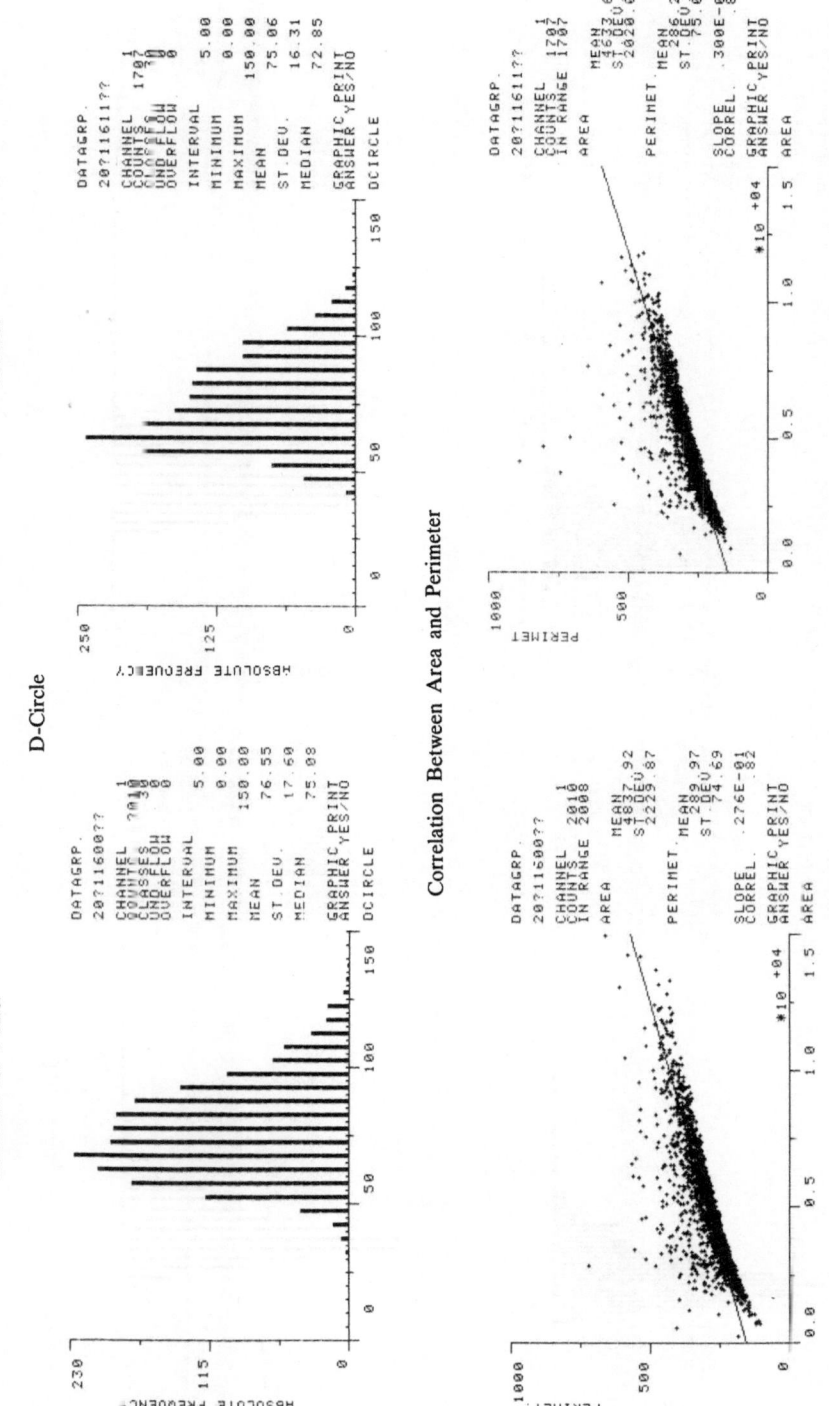

Fig. 7. Rabbit Nr. 16. Distribution curves for area, perimeter and D-circle, correlation between area and perimeter of the muscle fibers 6 months *after ischemia for 3 hrs*. ATPase stained cross-sections were used for the evaluation

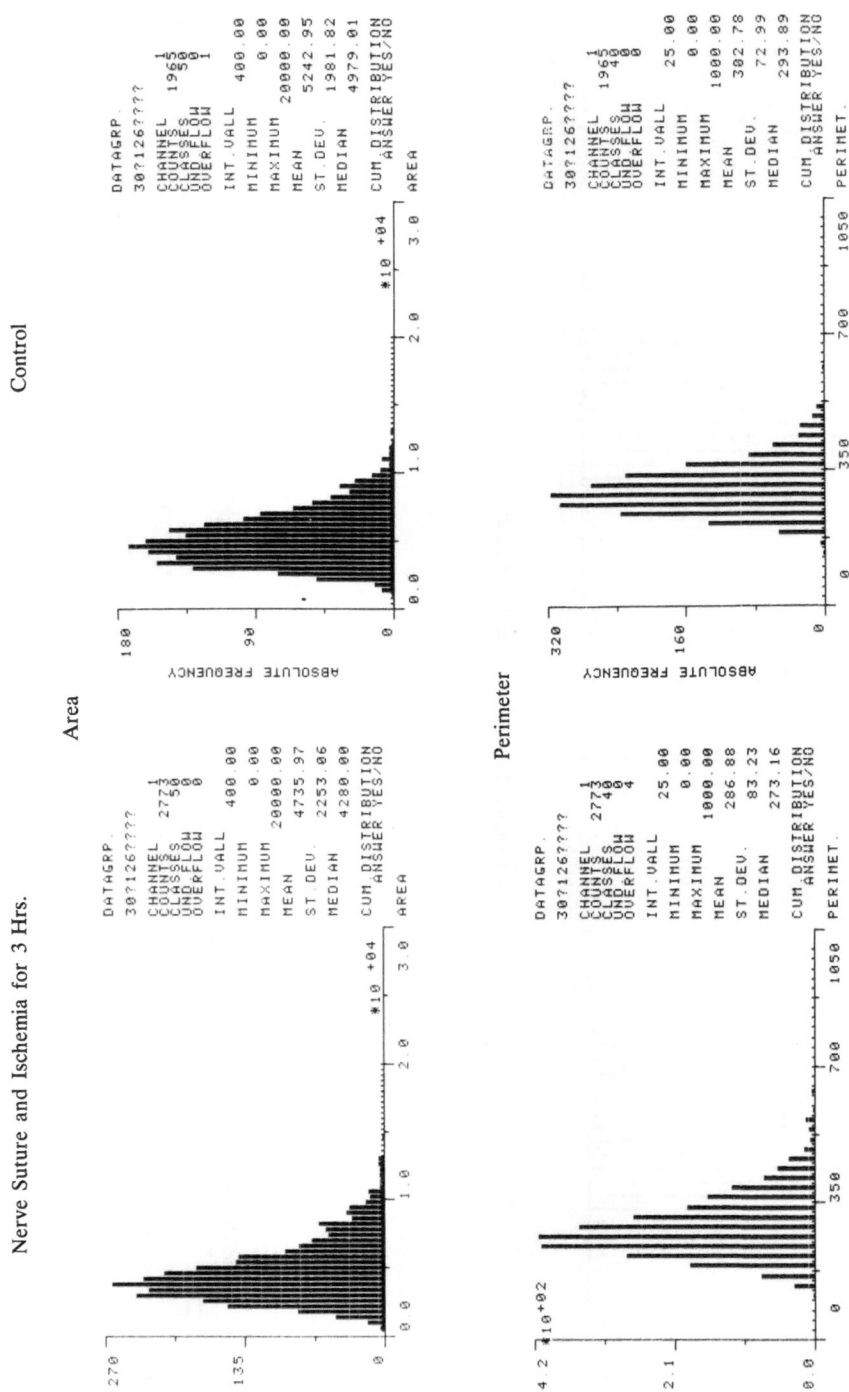

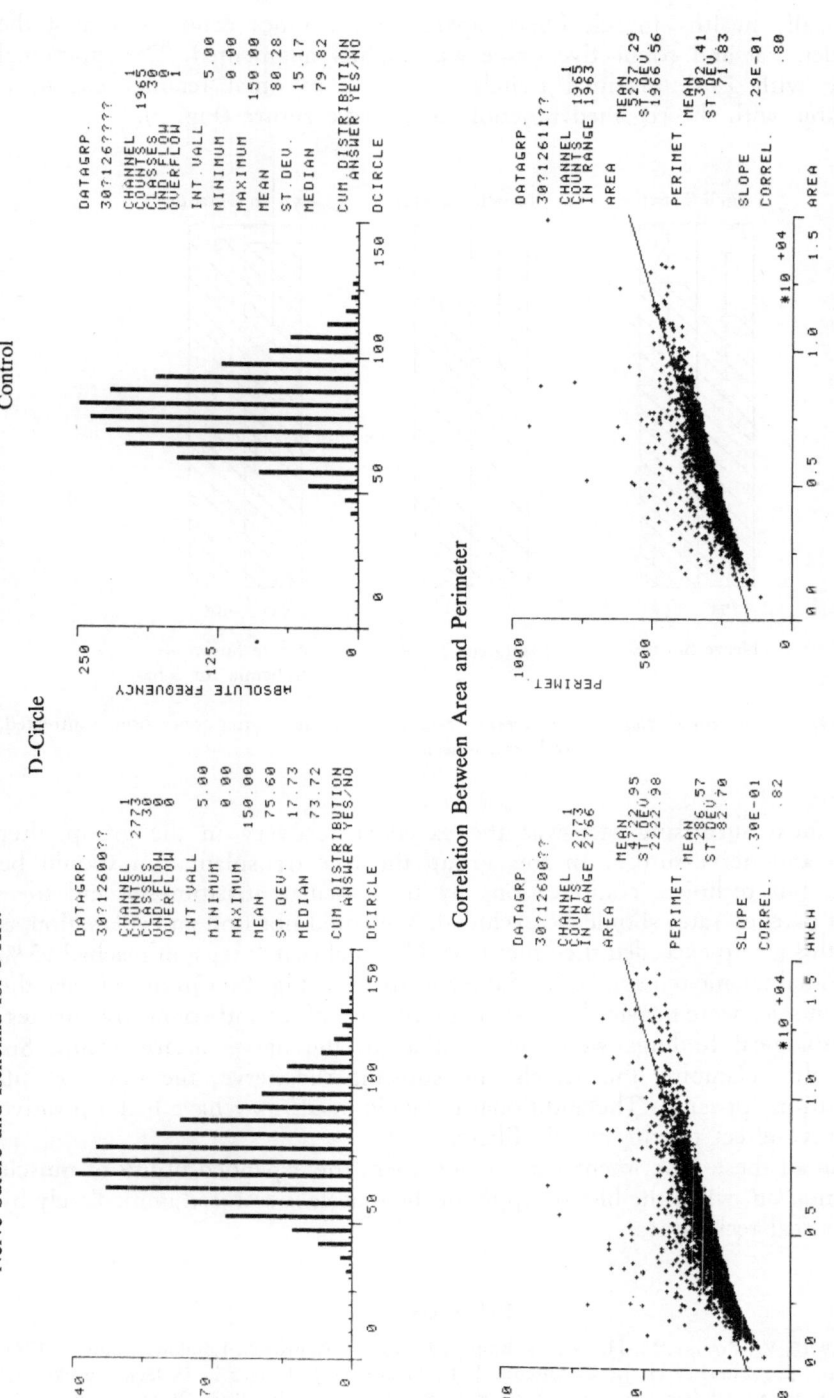

Fig. 8. Rabbit Nr. 26. Distribution curves for area, perimeter and D-circle, correlation between area and perimeter of the muscle fibers 6 months *after ischemia for 3 hrs. and division and suture of the muscle nerve.* ATPase stained cross-sections were used for the evaluation

histologically healthy muscle fibers, apart from a minor centralisation of the myonuclei. Fat and connective tissue was slightly augmented. The functional recovery with 78 % maximal twitch and 81 % maximal tetanic tension is comparable with the regained function after nerve suture (Fig. 9).

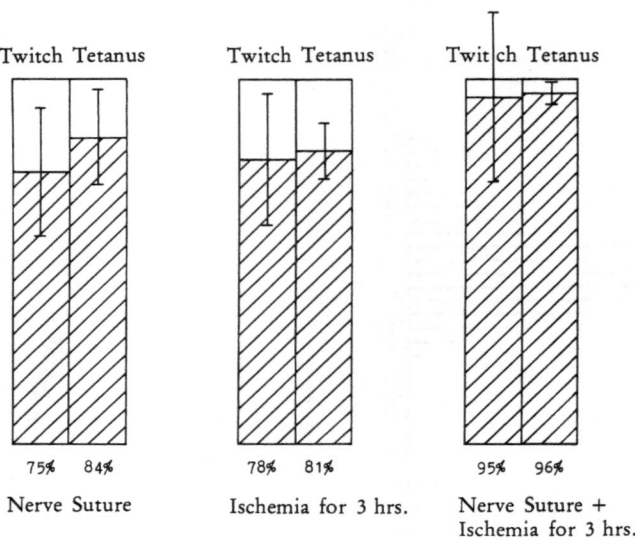

| Twitch Tetanus | Twitch Tetanus | Twitch Tetanus |
|:---:|:---:|:---:|
| 75%   84% | 78%   81% | 95%   96% |
| Nerve Suture | Ischemia for 3 hrs. | Nerve Suture + Ischemia for 3 hrs. |

Fig. 9. *Regained maximal twitch and tetanic tension* 6 months after operation (untreated, contralateral muscle = 100 %)

The most surprising fact was the excellent recovery in the group after ischemia and nerve-suture. In this group the free transplantation should be imitated, but technical complications by the vascular anastomoses and their different patency rates should be excluded. We could not find an explanation as to why this group exceeded the other two. Maximal twitch tension reached 95 % and maximal tetanic tension 96 % of the control side (Fig. 9). On the average the treated muscles were heavier because of an increase of fat and connective tissues. The histological findings were very similar to the nerve suture group. Six months after clamping the vessels and suturing the nerve, the signs of full reinnervation appeared. The additional ischemic insult may have had a positive regenerative effect on the muscle fibers.

All in all these experimental series document the expanded utility of muscle transplantation, when the blood supply of the muscle is restored immediately by microsurgical techniques.

### References

1. Dubowitz, V., Brooke, M. H.: Muscle Biopsy: A Modern Approach. London: Saunders. 1973.
2. Gordon, L., Buncke, H. J., Townsend, J. J.: Histological changes in skeletal muscle after temporary independent occlusion of arterial and venous supply. Plast. Reconstr. Surg. *61*, 576–580 (1978).

3. Guth, L., Samaha, F. J.: Procedure for the histochemical demonstration of actomyosin ATP-ase. Exp. Neurol. *28*, 365–367 (1970).
4. Harii, K., Ohmori, K., Torii, S.: Free gracilis muscle transplantation with microneurovascular anastomoses for the treatment of facial paralysis. Plast. Reconstr. Surg. *57*, 133–143 (1976).
5. Harii, K.: Microneurovascular free muscle transplantation for reanimation of facial paralysis. Clin. Plast. Surg. *6*, 361–375 (1979).
6. Harii, K.: Free muscle transplantation with microneurovascular anastomoses. Symposium on Microsurg. *14*, 177–185 (1977).
7. Kubo, T., Ikuta, Y., Tsuge, K.: Free muscle transplantation in dogs by neurovascular anastomoses. Plast. Reconstr. Surg. *57*, 495–501 (1976).
8. Schenck, R. R.: Rectus femoris muscle and composite skin transplantation by microneurovascular anastomoses for avulsion of forearm muscles: A case report. Hand Surg. *3*, 60–69 (1978).
9. Studitsky, A. N., Zhenevskaya, R. P., Rumyantseva, O.: The role of neurotrophic influences upon the restitution of structure and function of regenerating muscles. In: The Effect of Use and Disuse in Neuromuscular Functions (Gutmann, E., Hník, P., eds.), p. 71. Prague: Publ. Czech. Acad. Sci. 1963.
10. Tamai, S., Komatsu, S., Sakamoto, H., Sano, S., Sasauchi, N., Hori, Y., Tatsumi, Y., Okuda, H.: Free muscle transplants in dogs, with microsurgical neurovascular anastomoses. Plast. Reconst. Surg. *46*, 219–225 (1970).
11. Terzis, J. K., Sweet, R. C., Dykes, R. W., Williams, H. B.: Recovery of function in free muscle transplants using microneurovascular anastomoses. Hand Surg. *3*, 37–59 (1978).
12. Thompson, N.: Investigation of autogenous skeletal muscle free grafts in the dog. Transplantation *12*, 353 (1971).
13. Thompson, N.: Autogenous free grafts of skeletal muscle. Plast. Reconst. Surg. *48*, 11 (1971).

Author's address: Dr. M. Frey, Abteilung für Plastische und Wiederherstellungschirurgie, II. Chirurgische Universitätsklinik, Spitalgasse 23, A-1090 Wien, Austria.

## Discussion

Question: Dr. Frey, do you see fibrillation potentials or poly-morph reinnervation potentials by EMG-recordings during your experiments and for how long can they be found?

*Frey:* We have no exact data on this point.

*Benetar:* We all have the experience that in replantations of extremities, where the ischemia time is longer than 3 hours. In spite of this we gain very useful functional recovery. One of the questions that arrived, is—what is the amount of functional recovery that human being need after replantation, because from clinical experience we know, that human muscles can sustain more time ischemia than 3 hours.

*Frey:* We have chosen the time of 3 hours ischemia, because this should be the longest ischemia time during free muscle transplantation. But it is possible, that after 5 hours we have the same results.

# An Early Report of Free Muscle Grafts in Rabbits

## T. A. Miller and S. K. Das

Plastic Surgery Section, Plastic Surgery Research Laboratory,
Veterans Administration, Wadsworth Medical Center, Los Angeles, California,
and Division of Plastic Surgery, UCLA Medical Center,
Los Angeles, California, U.S.A.

With 4 Figures

The first successful free muscle graft was performed in the rat by Studitsky and Bosova in 1960. In the following two decades an increasing number of successful free muscle grafts, particularly in small animals, have been reported from laboratory experiments (Studitsky and Bosova, 1960; Carlson, 1968; Studitsky, 1964; Allbrook, 1975; Carlson and Gutmann, 1976; and Maxwell, 1964), and clinical situations (Thompson, 1971; Hakelius and Stålberg, 1974; Freilinger, 1975; Hakelius, 1974; and Holle et al., 1974).

The first successful clinical grafts utilized predenervated extensor digitorum brevis and palmaris longus muscles to reconstruct facial palsy (Thompson, 1971). Success was attributed to two factors: preoperative denervation and transplantation of the entire muscle. However, utilizing the same technique, other investigators were unsuccessful (Roy, 1966; Lavine and Cochran, 1976; Watson and Muir, 1976, and Harii et al., 1976, and Miller, 1978).

The recent laboratory experiments strongly suggest that viable muscle seen following grafting is the result of *regeneration* rather than survival of original graft fibers (Zhenevskaya et al., 1965; Carlson and Gutmann, 1976; Allbrook, 1975). This phenomenon has also been observed following injections of bupivacaine (Marcaine) (Carlson and Gutmann, 1976; Benoit, 1970; Hall-Craggs, 1974).

Because of variations in the experimental animals, their age, the type of muscle used and the site of grafting, it is difficult to make comparisons or to draw general conclusions from these investigations. Important technical considerations (whether or not muscle fascia was removed; whether or not physiological tension was reestablished; size of graft) are often not provided.

As an example, the concept of preoperative denervation is illustrative of some of the contradictions and complexities involved in muscle grafting. From the earliest reports it was emphasized that preoperative denervation was absolutely essential for muscle graft survival (Thompson, 1971; Studitsky and Bosova, 1960), but recently it has been demonstrated that comparable numbers of muscle fibers were seen in grafts regardless of whether they were pre-denervated or not (Carlson and Gutmann, 1976).

The purpose of our studies is to attempt to clarify some of these unanswered questions.

## Laboratory Model

The rabbit forelimb model was used because of our previous experience with laboratory investigations of muscular neurotization (Miller, 1978), and its anatomical similarity to the human flexor muscles. The muscle used as a graft

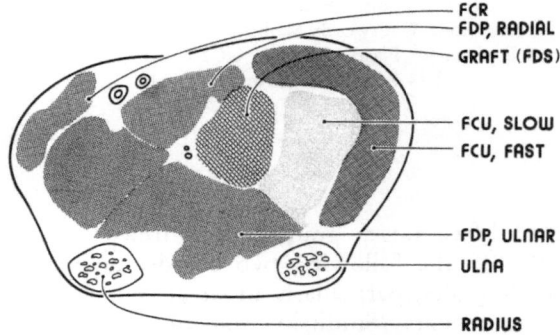

Fig. 1. Schematic diagram of the flexor compartment of the forearm, used as a model. *FCR* Flexor Carpi Radialis; *FDP* Flexor Digitorum Profundus–predominantly a fast muscle, the graft; *FDS* Flexor Digitorum Superficialis–a predominantly fast muscle; *FCU* Flexor Carpi Ulnaris–medial head–predominantly slow muscle and lateral head predominantly fast muscle

was the flexor digitorum superficialis (FDS). The relation of flexor digitorum superficialis muscle to flexor carpi ulnaris and flexor digitorum profundus is shown in Fig. 1. The FDS has a mean total muscle fiber count 5532 ± 730; in young (<1 mo.) rabbits it is 9367 ± 500. With ATPase histochemical stains, it was found that 79% of these fibers were fast staining in mature animals and 81% in young rabbits. The weight of this muscle ranges from 0.2 grams to 1.2 grams, depending on the age of the animals. This size was nearly ten times larger than the extensor digitorum longus muscle in rats of comparable age (Carlson, 1975).

## Method and Materials

### Group I. Young Rabbits

Twenty white New Zealand rabbits, one month old (1 kg in weight) were studied. Anesthesia was induced by ketamine hydrochloride 50 mg per kg and xylazine 10 mg per kg, intramuscularly (White and Holmes, 1976). On one side, the flexor digitorum superficialis was orthotopically grafted as a whole graft, and on the other side, the FDS graft was minced into 1 mm cubes and replaced orthotopically. The fascia of the graft was not removed.

## Group II. Mature Rabbits

There were 30 mature, white New Zealand rabbits in this group (weighing approximately 2.5 kg each and 12 weeks in age). The flexor digitorum superficialis was grafted in the following three groups:

1. *Whole Graft Group:* (25 limbs) orthotopic whole muscle grafts.
2. *Minced Graft Group:* (20 limbs) orthotopic minced grafts.
3. *Marcaine Treated Group:* (15 limbs) the FDS graft was removed and injected with 1 cc of 0.5% Marcaine and 30 IU of Hyaluronidase and then dipped in 0.5% of Marcaine solution for 10 minutes. It was replaced orthotopically.

In all grafts, the distal tendon was resutured and the proximal end was reattached to the area of muscle origin.

All rabbits were inspected daily for signs of local infection or graft detachment from its proximal or its distal sites of attachment. The animals were sacrificed at time intervals of six days, two weeks, three weeks, one month and three months postoperatively; the whole flexor muscle group of the forelimb was removed and examined histologically. No clamps were used when the grafts were harvested because of previous experience which showed significant histological distortion of the muscle. After removing the flexor muscle group, transverse sections were taken at the upper one-third of the muscle and stained with hematoxylin and eosin, and histochemically for alpha glucose phosphate dehydrogenase, succinic-dehydrogenase, and myosin ATPase.

The results of the grafts were evaluated and expressed in terms of percentage of the total fiber count and fiber type in the surviving graft at the various time periods compared to normal controls. Counts were performed by utilizing the Bausch and Lomb microprojector and Zeiss photomicroscope Mark 3.

## Results

### Group I. Young Rabbits

Six days after grafting, no viable muscle fibers were seen (Fig. 2). However, after two weeks a mean of 5,700 fibers were found (Fig. 3), larger numbers of fibers were seen in minced grafts at two weeks compared to whole grafts. Fiber counts at three weeks were comparable (see Table). At one month, the total fiber count decreased in both groups. This decrease, which consistently followed the initial appearance of fibers, seemed to be greater in minced grafts (compared to whole grafts).

At three months, a significant increase in the number of viable muscle fibers was seen in the recipient area in both mature and young animal groups (Fig. 4). Again, there were consistently more fibers seen in the whole grafts compared to the minced (6,045 vs. 1,850 fibers respectively). Histologically, the grafts appeared to be well organized into fascicles at two weeks and at three months. However, one month postoperatively, the fibers were more poorly organized.

All the fibers seen until the three week period demonstrated fast staining characteristics. At that time a few slow staining fibers appeared. After one month, approximately 7.5% of the total fibers were slow staining.

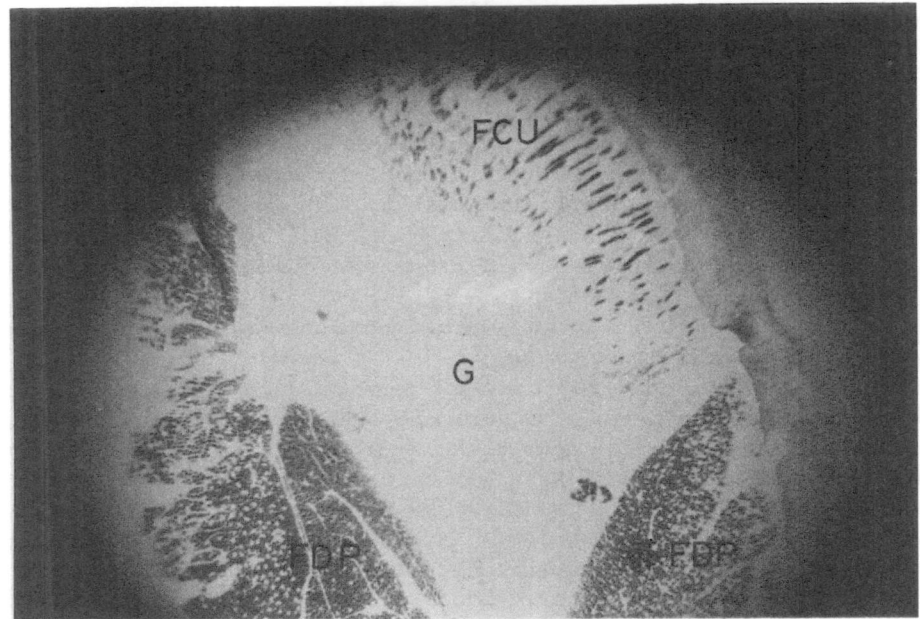

Fig. 2. Nearly total degeneration of Marcaine graft at six days. *G* graft; *FCU* flexor carpi ulnaris; *FDP* flexor digitorum profundus

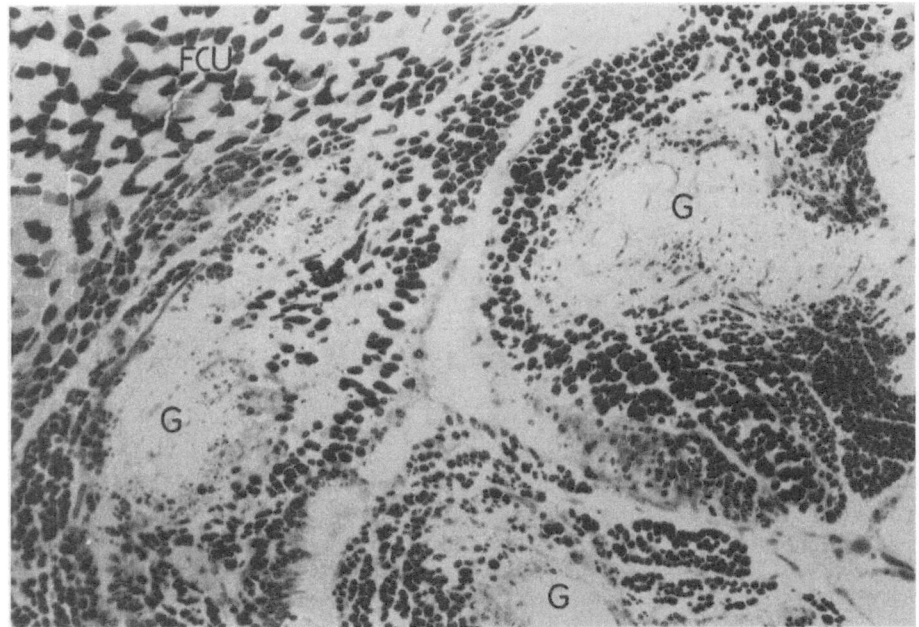

Fig. 3. Survival of graft at two weeks. *G* graft; *FCU* flexor carpi ulnaris

## Group II. Mature Rabbits

Six days postoperatively, there was almost total degeneration of the muscle fibers within the graft. A thin ring of viable muscle fibers was observed along the periphery of the graft. There was a mean of 285 of these peripheral fibers and it was noted that 30% of these fibers were slow staining.

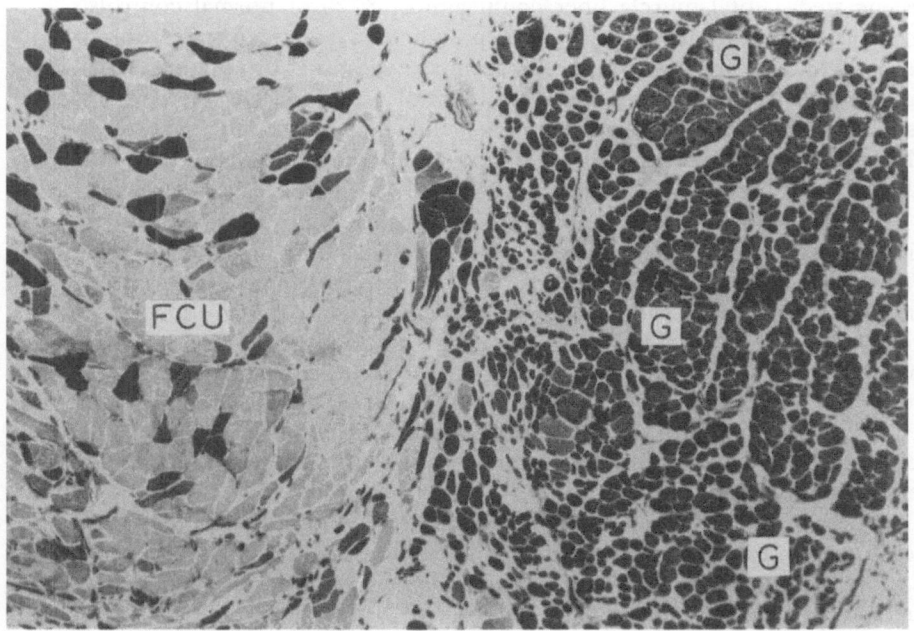

Fig. 4. Survival of the whole graft at three months in young rabbits. *FCU* flexor carpi ulnaris

Table 1. Survival of free muscle graft in rabbits

|  | 6 days | 2 weeks | 3 weeks | 1 month | 3 months |
|---|---|---|---|---|---|
| Young–Whole | 0 | 5075 | 6495 | 3185 | 6045 |
| Young–Minced | 0 | 6360 | 1100 | 775 | 1850 |
| Mature–Whole | 102 | 1029 | 680 | 583 | 1550 |
| Mature–Minced | 200 | 2900 | 900 | 2440 | 2550 |
| Mature–Marcaine | 350 | 2475 | 1000 | 1500 | 1240 |

The number of muscle fibers in the graft increased significantly two weeks post grafting (mean 2,700) but appeared to fall one week later in all groups (mean 1,000).

The numbers of each group are relatively small. The differences in total fiber counts are reflected in Table 1.

## Discussion

The early results of our study confirms the observation of others that viable muscle seen following grafting is the result of regeneration rather than persistence of the original fibers. At six days, almost all of the fibers of the original graft appeared to have undergone ischemic necrosis, yet two weeks later a substantial amount of viable muscle was consistently present. And even at this early stage of investigation, it seems clear that the regenerative potential of younger rabbits is significantly greater than mature animals, both quantitatively and qualitatively. Three months post-grafting, whole grafts in young rabbits regenerated a total muscle fiber count almost 80% of normal controls.

At this time, we have not studied enough animals in each sub-group to make general conclusions. However, early trends suggest that in young animals whole grafts result in significantly larger amounts of viable muscle fibers than minced grafts. In contrast, the reverse relationship appeared in the mature animals. More accurate statements can be made after greater numbers of animals are studied.

Another much more definite trend appears in this study: a consistent biphasic variation in the numbers of fibers seen following grafting (Table 1). There appears to be an initial burst of muscle regeneration sometime between one and two weeks, followed by a decrease around the third week. This is followed by a second burst of regenerative activity between one and three months. This pattern was observed in all of the experimental groups. At this time, we can only speculate on the significance of this pattern. The time sequence suggests that it is conceivable that the first increase in muscle fibers is related to the acquisition of a new blood supply and the second burst related to reinnervation.

Whether reinnervation is by a direct neural-muscular route or muscular neurotization is unclear. The histochemical fiber patterns suggest that the former is more significant. In the young animals fiber-type grouping is rarely seen. In the adult group this phenomenon appears to be limited to peripheral areas. It should be pointed out that the graft (which is composed of predominantly fast fibers) is replaced into its orthotopic site between a fast and slow number (Fig. 1). From our previous experience with muscular neurotization (Miller, 1978) we would expect the appearance of more slow staining fibers within the graft adjacent to the slow portion of the FCU if, indeed, muscular neurotization was taking place to any significant extent. Careful attention is being focused on the source of reinnervation in our current investigations.

### References

Allbrook, D.: Transplantation and regeneration of striated muscle. Ann. Royal Coll. Surg. Eng. *56*, 312 (1975).

Benoit, R. W., Belt, W. D.: Destruction and regeneration of skeletal muscle after treatment with a local anesthetic, bipuvacaine (Marcaine). J. Anat. *107*, 547 (1970).

Carlson, B. M.: Regeneration of the completely excised gastrocnemius muscle in the frog and rat from minced muscle fragments. J. Morph. *125*, 447 (1968).

Carlson, B. M.: A quantitative study of muscle fiber survival and regeneration in normal, predenervated and Marcaine-treated free muscle grafts in the rat. Exp. Neurol. *52*, 421 (1976).

Carlson, B. M., Gutmann, E.: Regeneration in grafts of normal and denervated rat muscles: Contractile properties. Pflügers Arch. *353*, 215 (1975).

Carlson, B. M., Gutmann, E.: Free grafting of the extensor digitorum longus muscle in the rat after Marcaine pretreatment. Exp. Neurol. *53*, 82 (1976).

Freilinger, G.: A new technique to correct facial paralysis. Plast. Reconstr. Surg. *56*, 44 (1975).

Hakelius, L.: Transplantation of free autogenous muscle in the treatment of facial paralysis. Scand. J. Plast. Reconstr. Surg. *8*, 220 (1974).

Hakelius, L., Stålberg, E.: Electromyographical studies of free autogenous muscle transplants in man. Scand. J. Plast. Reconstr. Surg. *8*, 211 (1974).

Hall-Craggs, E. C. B.: Rapid degeneration and regeneration of a whole skeletal muscle following treatment with bupivacaine (Marcaine). Exp. Neurol. *43*, 349 (1974).

Harii, K., Ohmori, K., Tarii, S.: Free gracilis muscle transplantation with microneurovascular anastomoses for the treatment of facial paralysis. Plast. Reconstr. Surg. *57*, 133 (1976).

Holle, J., Freilinger, G., Gruber, H., et al.: Tierexperimentelle Untersuchungen zur freien autologen Muskeltransplantation. Langenbecks Arch. Chir. Suppl. Chir. Forum *235* (1974).

Lavine, D. M., Cochran, T. A.: The failure of autogenous free grafts of whole gracilis muscle in dogs. Plast. Reconstr. Surg. *58*, 221 (1976).

Mauro, A.: Regeneration of skeletal muscle fibers. J. Biophys. Biochem. Cytol. *9*, 493 (1961).

Maxwell, L. C., et al.: Free autografting of entire limb muscles in the cat: Histochemistry and biochemistry. J. Appl. Physiol. *44*, 432 (1978).

Miller, T. A., Korn, H. N., Wheeler, E. S., Eldridge, L.: Can one muscle reinnervate another? A preliminary study of muscular neurotization in the rabbit. Plast. Reconstr. Surg. *61*, 50 (1978).

Miller, T. A.: Are free muscle grafts a reliable reconstructive method? Plast. Reconstr. Surg. *62*, 597 (1978).

Roy, R. P.: Behavior of a free autogenous muscle graft into the skeletal muscles of the dog. J. Exp. Med. Sci. *9*, 78 (1966).

Studitsky, A. N.: Free auto- and homografts of muscle tissue in experiments on animals. Ann. New York Acad. Sci. *120*, 789 (1964).

Studitsky, A. N., Bosova, N. N.: Development of atrophic muscular tissue in conditions of transplantation in place of mechanically damaged muscles. (Russian.) Arch. Anat. Gist. Embriol. *39*, 18 (1960).

Thompson, N.: Autogenous free grafts of skeletal muscle. Plast. Reconstr. Surg. *48*, 11 (1971).

Watson, A. C. H., Muir, A. R.: Failure of free muscle grafts in dogs. Brit. J. Plast. Surg. *29*, 27 (1976).

White, G. L., Holmes, D. D.: A comparison of ketamine and the combination ketamine-xylazine for effective surgical anesthesia in the rabbit. Lab Animal Sci. *26*, 804 (1976).

Zhevevskaya, R. P., Rumyantseva, O. N., Navaselona, F. L., et al.: Regenerative processes in the transplantation of unprepared muscle of young rats. (Russian.) Zhur Obshch. Biol. *26*, 569 (1965).

Authors' address: Dr. T. A. Miller, Chief, Plastic Surgery Section (691/112F), Wadsworth Medical Center, Los Angeles, CA 90073, U.S.A.

## Discussion

*Gruber:* You missed any differentiation of fibre types in your graft in the last two pictures. How can you explain this? I would suggest, that the stage after the transplantation was too short and the fibres were rather thin and still in regeneration. And I think, two months later there would be differentiation between type 1 and type 2 fibres.

*Miller:* I think, you are right. One thing, we are seeing at the two months level, that we are now following up, is the presence of intermediate staining of fibres. This is something that does not occur in the rabbit normally, and the explanation of this is totally unclear.

# The Relevance of Preliminary Denervation in Muscle Transplantation

D. Benatar, J. Terzis, and B. Williams

Department of Plastic Surgery,
McGill University, Quebec, Canada

With 6 Figures

It has long been recognized that the transfer of autogenous skeletal muscle has been associated with an inability to obtain complete functional recovery (Neuhof, 1923; Peer, 1955). Its ability to survive as an anatomical entity has been observed for a long time. More recent investigations using electrophysiological recordings have shown that the capacity of a transferred muscle to perform useful work is significantly impaired, Terzis (1978). Striated muscle survival and function following its transfer depends on our ability to maintain both adequate vascularization and innervation, to respect its original tension and to induce a "Plastic State" prior to transplantation (Hakelius, 1974–1975 a, b; Thompson, 1971 a, b, c).

"The Plastic State" concept has been introduced in 1959 by Studitsky and Zhenevskaya (1964). They described it as a condition during which a high regenerative capacity is present, making the muscle therefore more suitable for reparative surgery.

This state (during which proliferation of protoplasm, amitotic division of the nuclei, emergence of myoblasts and development of typical muscle fibers have been observed) is obtained when the muscle is minced, tenotomized, traumatized or *denervated*.

The last technique has been popularized by Thompson (1971) and Hakelius (1974). Denervation two to three weeks before transplantation has been recommended in order to create a more efficient metabolism in the transplanted muscle.

White muscle that has been denervated undergoes a shift of its anaerobic glycolytic metabolism toward a more efficient aerobic lipolytic metabolism (Romanul and Hogan, 1965; Romanul and Meulen, 1967). Changes in the energy production system, causing more efficiency, would increase the survival of transplanted skeletal muscle.

Following denervation of the muscle, a marked shift in enzyme activity was associated with a change in the vascular network of the same muscle (Hakelius, 1975). Clinical application of denervation prior to transplantation has been motivated by the satisfactory results obtained, using histology, chemical staining or E. M. G. as investigative tools. However, these techniques of evaluation do not reflect .the real working capacity of a transplanted muscle that has been previously denervated.

This project was designed to evaluate on a functional basis the effects of preliminary denervation to the free transplantation of skeletal muscle and to determine the optimal time interval between denervation and transplantation.

The findings that are described here are related to transplantation done without repair of the neurovascular pedicle. Results on transplantation done with vascularized and neurotized muscle will be presented in a companion paper.

## A. Materials and Methods

Twenty-seven white male rabbits (2.5–3.0 kg each) had the medial portion of their right and left rectus femoris muscles investigated. Each group was composed of three animals or 6 muscles, treated as follows: Group N: normal rabbit–normal muscle, not transplanted; group O: muscles transplanted without preliminary denervation; group 1 to 7: muscles denervated respectively from 1 to 7 weeks before orthotopic transplantation.

## B. Surgical Procedures

General anaesthesia was induced with a facial mask containing ether; then blind peroral endotracheal intubation was performed. A stainless steel tubing connected to a small container, where a 50% air-ether mixture was present, was used in order to control the long-standing anaesthesia Mersereau (1976). Then the animals were shaved from the knees to the mid-abdomen and the surgical field was prepared with proviodine solution.

*First operation*

All twenty-seven animals had a first operation. Using a ventro-medial incision, the right and left rectus femoris were exposed. The nerves were identified and 0.8 to 1 cm. of nerve was resected. Denervation of the rectus femoris was confirmed by stimulation of the femoral nerve at a more proximal level. The vascular pedicle was left intact.

*Second operation* (0 to 7 weeks after first operation for each respective group)

The entire muscle belly was mobilized from its origin and its insertion as a free graft using blunt dissection. The fascia was left intact. The vascular pedicle was severed. Each muscle was replanted reconstituting original tension. No neurovascular anastomoses was performed.

Skin closure was achieved with interrupted 5–0 nylon and antibiotic ointment was used on the wound without dressing. The average time of muscle ischemia was 15 to 20 minutes. Before replantation, the muscle was measured and weighed. Details of the color, ischemia time, duration of anaesthesia and any complications were carefully recorded.

## C. Method of Assessing Recovery

1. Measurement of muscle weight
2. Physiological assessment
   a) Measurement of the threshold to elicit
      a visual contraction
   b) Measurements of the threshold to elicit
      a recorded contraction
   c) Measurement of the muscle force
      twitch contraction strength
      rise time
      tetanic tension
      fusion frequency
      fatigue rate
   d) Needle E. M. G. recording
3. Histology

This method of assessing the recovery of muscle replantation is an attempt to evaluate objectively the functional ability of the muscle unit. This technique of electrophysiological recording has been described in a previous paper Terzis (1978) and was meticulously duplicated.

However, we added data to complement this study; a) Measurement of the threshold to elicit a visual contraction; b) Measurement of the threshold to elicit a recorded contraction. The first threshold is equal to a stimulus capable of eliciting a muscle response that could be seen by at least two observers while the second threshold was equal to a stimulus capable of eliciting a measurable muscle response that could be displayed on a Grass Polygraph (Model 7P15). These measurements were done in order to stress the importance of having objective measurement, since the first threshold is too often used by authors who claimed success when they can visualize their muscle contracting. Unfortunately, this contraction does not always correlate with significant work capacity.

*Histology:* When all physiological testing was done, the muscle was fixed on a cork backing and left in a 10 % formaldehyde solution. Transverse sections of proximal and distal muscle, and longitudinal sections of the middle part were taken and stained with hematoxylin-eosin. Representative areas of each slide were photographed and were compared histologically using the following criteria.
   fatty infiltration
   fibre atrophy
   hyaline degeneration
   focus of necroses and of floccular change
   relative increase of nuclei
   hyperchromatic and pyknotic nuclei
   loss of fiber contour
   basophilic fibres

## D. Results

### a) Muscle Weight

In Fig. 1 we observe that muscle weight of rabbits of the same age and weight and performing the same activity is smaller when the denervation period is longer. This progressive atrophy of denervated muscle is not surprising and reconfirms previous work on this subject. However when we compare the weight of these same muscles 18 to 20 weeks after transplantation (Fig. 1) we observe that muscle weight is higher when the denervation period is longer—which is the contrary to what has been observed before transplantation.

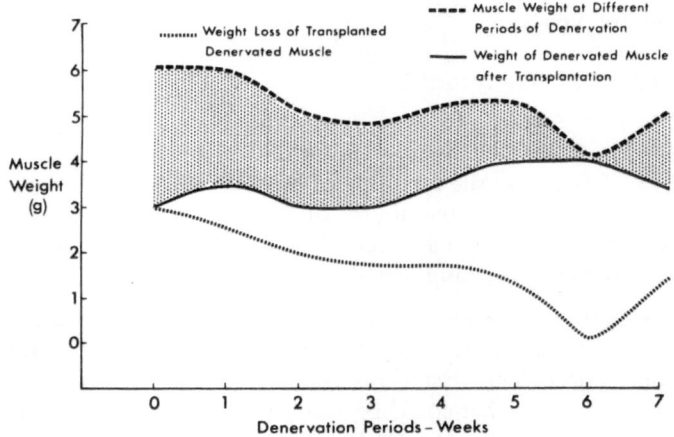

Fig. 1. Weight loss *vs* denervation periods in transplanted muscles

Considering that all muscles lose weight when they are transplanted, but since this average weight loss is less in muscles that have been denervated, we might be tempted to conclude that preliminary denervation before transplantation minimizes the muscle atrophy, mainly when muscles are denervated for 6 weeks.

### b) Threshold for Contraction

In order to assess the sensitivity of a transplanted muscle that has been denervated for various periods before transplantation, we measured the minimum amount of electrical stimulation applied directly to the muscle to elicit a contraction. This amount of electric current is called threshold. So as to have a basis for further discussion, we compared the threshold necessary to elicit a visual contraction with the threshold necessary to obtain a measurable contraction as depicted with a Grass Polygraph 7P15. No correlation was found between these two thresholds.

The threshold for eliciting a measurable contraction being more objective, we have chosen this one for comparative purposes. Fig. 2 shows that supramaximal electrical stimulation was necessary to record a muscle contraction in the groups of muscles denervated for 0, 1, 2, 3 and 4 weeks; while the muscles denervated for 5, 6 and 7 weeks needed a stimulation that varied from 30 to 40 volts in order to elicit a contraction.

From this observation we can conclude that: a transplanted muscle is more sensitive to electrical stimulation when it has been denervated 5, 6 and 7 weeks before transplantation.

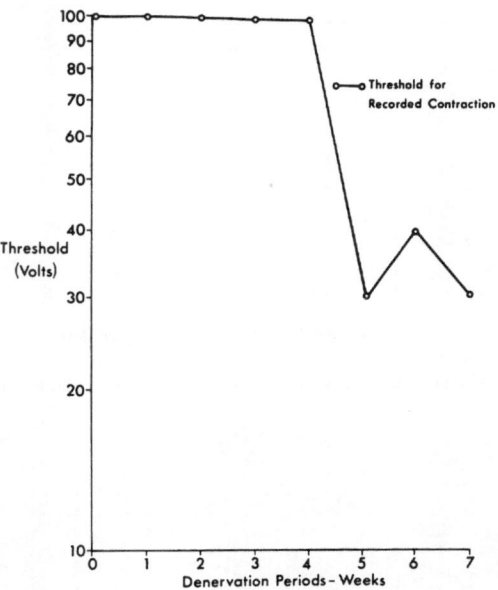

Fig. 2. Threshold for contraction *vs* denervation periods in transplanted muscles

One should notice that if the threshold for eliciting a visual contraction is to be considered, it will bring about a different conclusion, the most sensitive muscle being at 2 and 6 weeks. However, the contraction of only a few fibers could be seen without producing a contraction capable of reducing the length of the muscle and being recorded by the graph transducer. This type of focal contraction is useless considering that in order to achieve normal function, a muscle should reduce its total length when the muscle fibers are stimulated. We can conclude that: the necessary threshold for eliciting a visual contraction of a muscle should not be considered as a criterion for assessment of the functional capabilities of a muscle.

### c) Measurement of the Muscle Force

Fig. 3 shows that in the muscle transplanted without previous denervation at a threshold stimulation, at 2 times the threshold or with a supramaximal stimulation the muscle force recorded was nil. The same result was obtained when muscles were denervated for 1 to 4 weeks before transplantation. However, a preliminary denervation of 5, 6 or 7 weeks increased the muscle force of the transplanted muscle. This increase is not significant if we compare it with the force of a normal muscle.

The normal rectus femoris of the rabbit will produce an average twitch contraction of 500 gm. at supramaximal stimulation (100 volts) while Fig. 3

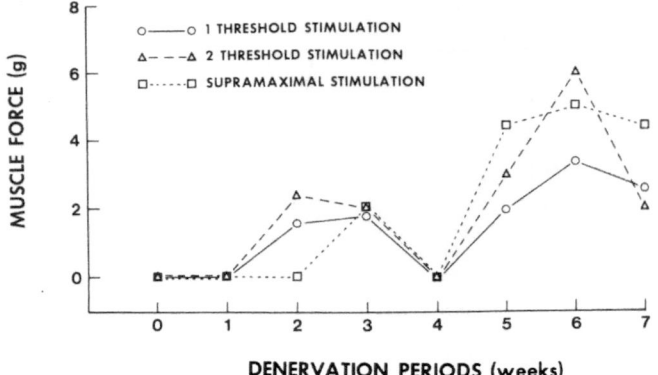

Fig. 3. Muscle force *vs* stimulus intensity in transplanted muscles

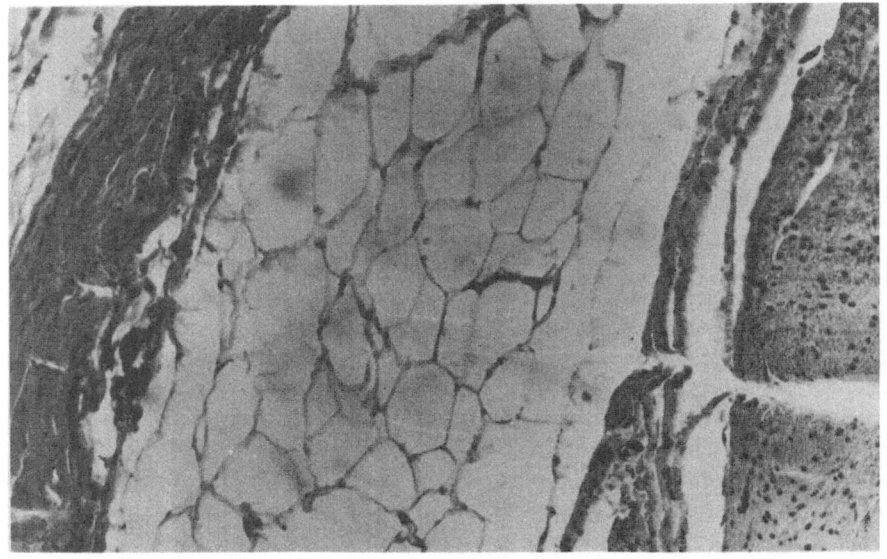

Fig. 4. Fatty infiltration in a 3 week denervated muscle

shows that the denervated transplanted muscle could only produce twitch contraction varying from 0 to 2 gms. This muscle force being so low, we were unable to obtain sufficient numbers of rise times, and fusion frequency values for discussion.

From these observations we can conclude that: preliminary denervation of a transplanted muscle increased slightly the force of the graft.

### d) *Histology*

We found a close correlation between our electrophysiological results and histologic observation.

In the muscles where poor contraction was obtained histological sections showed large amounts of necroses, fatty infiltration and severe atrophy (Fig. 4).

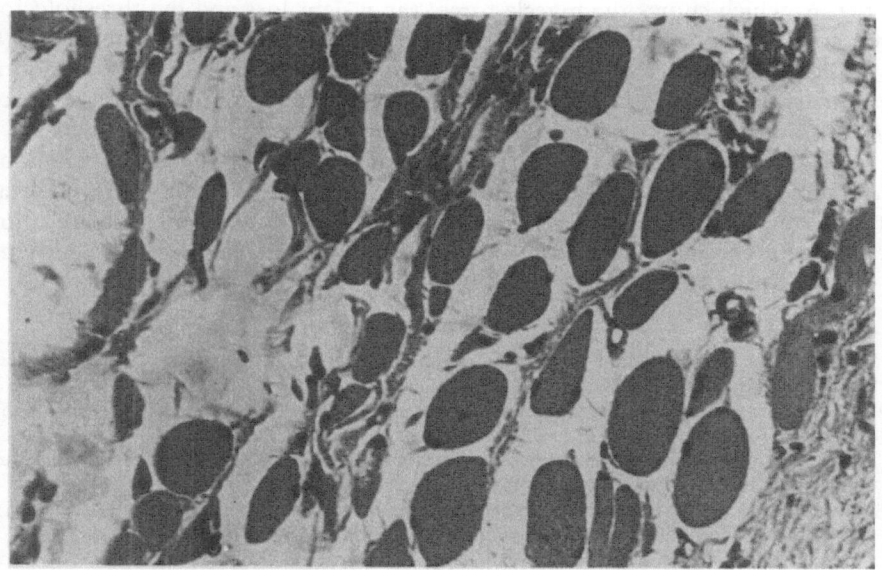

Fig. 5. Muscle fiber atrophy in a 4 week denervated muscle

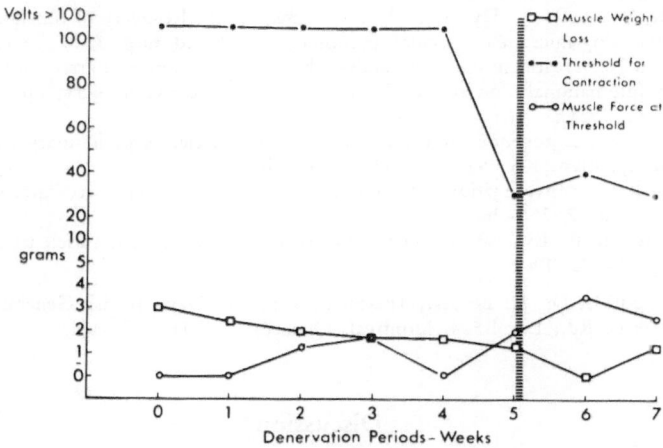

Fig. 6. Diagrammatic depiction of the functional data obtained from transplanted muscles denervated at various time intervals

In more responsive muscles, corresponding to 5, 6 and 7 weeks of denervation, a greater percentage of normal muscle cells was observed (Fig. 5).

Common to all muscles was the presence of larger numbers of normal cells at the periphery with more necroses and fat in the center.

## Conclusion

Fig. 6, which shows the muscle force, the weight loss and the threshold for contraction of the muscles after different periods of preliminary denervation (0 to 7 weeks), allowed us to conclude that: it is only after 5, 6 or 7 weeks of preliminary denervation that transplanted muscle shows an increase force associated with a low threshold of contraction and a minimal weight loss.

One should consider this period of 5 to 7 weeks as the ideal period of denervation that should precede muscle transplantation. However in skeletal muscle transplantation where microneurovascular anastomoses are not performed, preliminary denervation does not significantly improve the ability of the muscle to perform work.

### References

1. Hakelius, L.: Transplantation of free autogenous muscle in the treatment of facial paralysis. Scand. J. Plast. Rec. Surg. *8*, 22–230 (1974).
2. Hakelius, L.: Blood vessels and connective tissue in autotransplanted free muscle grafts of the cat. Scand. J. Plast. Rec. Surg. *9*, 87–91 (1975 a).
3. Hakelius, L., Nyström, B.: Histochemical studies of end plate formation in free autologous muscle transplants in cats. Scand. J. Plast. Surg. *9*, 9–14 (1975 b).
4. Mersereau, W. A.: Endotracheal ether anesthesia in the rabbit. J. Surg. Res. *21*, 63–66 (1976).
5. Neuhof, H.: The transplantation of tissue. New York: Appleton. 1923.
6. Peer, L. A.: Transplantation of tissues, Chapt. V. Baltimore: Williams & Wilkins Co. 1955.
7. Romanul, F. C., Hogan, E.: Enzymatic change in denervated muscle. I. Histochemical Studies. Arch. Neurol. *13*, 263–274 (1965). II. Biochemical Studies. Arch. Neurol. *13*, 274–280 (1965).
8. Romanul, F. C. A., Meulen, J. P.: Slow and fast muscles after cross innervation. Enzymatic and physiological changes. Arch. Neurol. *17*, 387 (1967).
9. Studitsky, A. N.: Free auto and homografts of muscle tissue in experiments on animals. Annals N. Y. Acad. of Sci. *120*, 789–800 (1964).
10. Terzis, J., Sweet, R. C., Dykes, R. W., Williams, H. B.: Recovery of function in free muscle transplants using microneurovascular anastomoses. J. Hand Surg. *3*, 37–59 (1978).
11. Thompson, N.: Treatment of facial paralysis by free skeletal muscle grafts. In: Transactions of the Fifth International Congress of Plastic and Reconstructive Surgery, pp. 66–82. Sydney: Butterworth. 1971 a.
12. Thompson, N.: Autogenous free grafts of skeletal muscle. A preliminary experimental and clinical study. Plast. Rec. Surg. *48*, 11–27 (1971 b).
13. Thompson, N.: Investigation of autogenous skeletal muscle free grafts in the dog. Transplantation *12*, 353–363 (1971 c).
14. Zhenevskaya, R. P.: Experimental histologic investigation of striated muscle tissue. Rev. Canad. Biol. *21*, 457–470 (1962).

Author's address: Dr. D. Benatar, The Sir Mortimer B. Davis Jewish General Hospital, 3755 Cote St. Catherine Rd., Local 524, Montreal, Quebec, H3T 1E2, Canada.

## Discussion

*Schenk:* What is the mechanism of the improvement by this denervation? What is your explanation of that?

*Benatar:* At the time when Dr. Thompson started the denervation before the transplantation, I understood it because of the change of the metabolism. It has been proved by the histochemical stainings of Romanul, showing that there is a change in the enzyme profile of the muscle and there is a shift from a more anaerobic metabolism to a more efficient aerobic metabolism. So we thought by changing this metabolism of the muscle by time of the transposition, we may increase the ITT and we may get better results. This is number one. Number two it is suggested, that denervation increases the vascularity and the capillary network of the muscle. Unfortunately we don't know exactly when it starts and when it is finished and when we follow the curve, the vascularity increase follows the metabolic change of the muscle. This is the reason, why we are measuring the functional recovery to see if, in fact, it was later that it was more efficient or sooner. But I want to say that it is important to realize, we only gain—if we gain anything—by denervation 10 grams of muscle power how efficient is that in clinical efficiency? If we deal with facial paralysis, where we are dealing with very small muscles and only a minimal force of contraction required to mobilize the lid, it might be efficient. But if we work on a Volkmann-contracture, I would personally not do denervation before muscle transplantation, unless my further studies on denervation of muscle transplants will show some significant difference.

*Holle:* The results of your experiments concerning the functional force of the transplanted muscles differ greatly from the results of our experiments. My question is: do you have any explanations for these differences? I think there can be two facts to be taken into account. The first is, that the vascular anastomosis in the experiments were not patent in every case and in the second, you did reanastomose only one vein and this muscle, which you and we transplanted in our experiments, has at least two big veins, which should be reanastomosed. So please, what is your opinion about that?

*Benatar:* The patency rate of our vascular anastomosis was about 95 %, so we don't think that this could be a reason for the different results. But on the other hand I must leave the question open, if the anastomoses of both veins would have given better functional results of the transplanted muscle.

*Tolhurst:* Dr. Benatar, do you think we should denervate a muscle graft prior to transplantation, even if it is a revascularized muscle graft?

*Benatar:* At this stage I cannot answer this question exactly. It seems to be no great difference between denervated and non-denervated grafts.

# Experimental Investigations Concerning Muscle Function

## G. Meissl

Ludwig Boltzmann-Institute for Experimental Plastic Surgery, Vienna,
and the Department for Plastic and Reconstructive Surgery
of the First Surgical University Clinic of Vienna, Austria

With 4 Figures

Several studies were undertaken to gain some information e. g. on how to determine muscle tendon unit properties during tendon transfer, and also on kinesiological studies of the human body under normal and pathological conditions. In the first period of the time these investigations were performed on cadavers. Since 1965 some articles were published, at first by Omer and Vogel, who investigated muscle tendon units during tendon transfer by muscle stimulation. They used the muscle stimulation to determine the physiological length of reconstructed muscle tendon units. Freehafer, Percham and Keith (1979) described theire techniques, accomplishing by electrical stimulation the muscle and monitoring of its strength.

Our purpose was to find the relationship between muscle function and nerve repair, using a technique similar to that described by Freehafer and co-workers. Up to now no real comparative data exist in the clinic on effective muscle function after nerve repair. Only Highet's scheme gives some information in humans as well as in experiments.

## Experiment

An experiment was carried out, using rabbits with a body weight from 23 to 35 Newton. All animals were anaesthesized intravenously with Nembutal. The test organ was the tibial nerve and the triceps surae muscle with the Achilles tendon. Two transducers, one for the force and one for the shortening of the muscle, coupled with an electronic unit, which consists of peak value detectors, digital displays for the distance in millimeters, force in newton and time, and at last a stimulator was applied. This equipment was necessary for stimulating the nerve, and recording length-tension data and force data of the measured muscle.

We have established three groups:

Group I: In eight animals the right leg was dissected, the tibial nerve prepared and a piece of 5 mm resected.

After this, a nerve suture under tension was carried out. After two months at first the unoperated leg was prepared in general anaesthesia, the triceps surae muscle was carefully dissected until the muscle bellies were hanging on their neuromuscular bundle and their origin. The knee joint was fixed on the table and the Achilles tendon transfixed by a suture. The suture was connected with both transducers. Two platinum electrodes were wrapped around the tibial nerve for stimulating them. In the same way we tested the operated side on which we had performed a nerve suture under tension.

Group II: Eight rabbits. On the right side the tibial nerve was transected and re-established with nerve suture without tension. The succeeding test of both legs was performed in the same fashion as described above.

Group III: Eight rabbits. The right tibial nerve was transected, 5 mm were excised and a defect created of about 10 mm. This defect was bridged by nerve grafts. The succeeding test, two months later, was performed in the same manner as described above. Stimulating electrodes were applied centrally of the proximal nerve suture.

No. 865. Triceps surae muscle–operated (Nerve suture under tension) and unoperated side. Pretension and peak value in mm and N

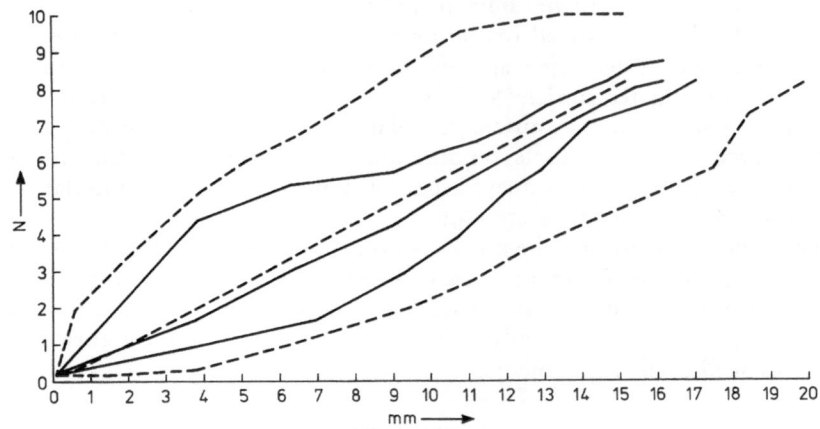

Fig. 1. The solid line represents the measurement of the operated leg after repeated tetanic stimulation. The dashed line represent the data for the unoperated leg. There is a significant difference in the function of muscle

## Results

For each nerve-muscle unit we obtained 24 measurements for the distance in millimeters and 24 for Newton.

The measurements start from the slack length, i.e., the length to which the muscle had retracted previously, following transection of its tendon.

Group I: In Fig. 1 the difference between the operated leg–the solid line represents the measurement of the operated leg in which we had performed a nerve suture under tension and the un-operated leg–dashed line–could be seen. Both lines in the middle show the data of the passive lengthening and the passive tension, respectively.

No. 865. Intact tibial nerve–transected tibial nerve and immediate nerve suture under tension

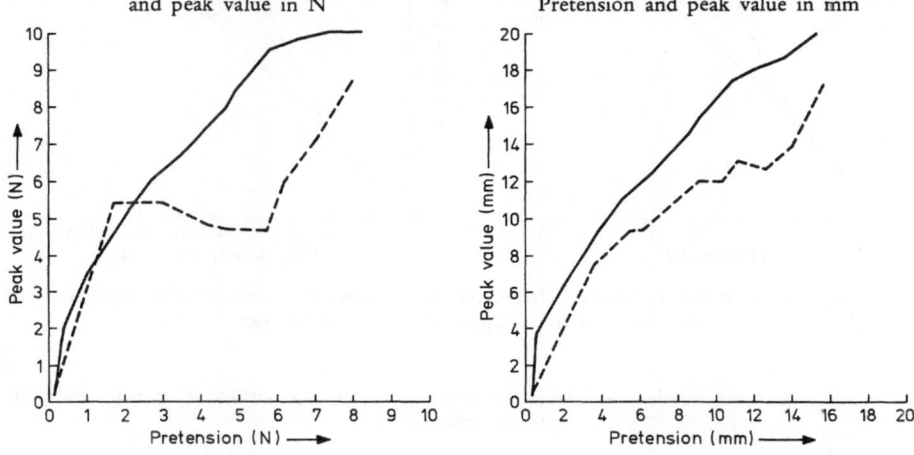

Muscle force in unop.–and op. side. Pretension and peak value in N    Muscle contraction in unop.–and op. side. Pretension and peak value in mm

Fig. 2. On the left side the peak value of muscle power in Newton. On the right side the peak value of muscle contraction. The dashed line represents the muscle-tendon unit of which the nerve was sutured under tension

For example, two actual measurements of the operated leg compared with the healthy side: passive lengthening to 3.8 mm, after stimulation 7.8 mm; at the undamaged leg 3.9 mm and actual shortening about 9.5 mm. Similar data could be observed by measuring the force.

In Fig. 2 the characteristics of muscle power are demonstrated. The solid line represents the healthy muscle, the dashed line the re-innervated muscle. It shows an active muscle, but of course if power is necessary, a significant decrease can be observed. Similar curves can be seen in active shortening of the triceps muscle.

Group II: In this group we investigated muscle function after immediate direct tensionless nerve suture. The ranges of actual measured data are, e.g. 16.71 mm passive lengthening, active shortening 17.06 mm at the re-innervated muscle, in the same muscle 16.71 mm passive tension and active shortening after nerve stimulation was 16.91 mm. The curves in muscle power, as well as in active contraction at the same muscle and re-innervated muscle, are nearly identical (Fig. 3).

Group III: In Group III we are comparing the undamaged muscle and the re-innervated muscle after nerve grafting. In force as well as in active shortening no difference can be found in both muscles (Fig. 4).

No. 807. Intact tibial nerve–transected tibial nerve and immediate nerve suture without tension

Muscle force in unop.–and op. side. Pretension and peak value in N · Muscle contraction in unop.–and op. side. Pretension and peak value in mm

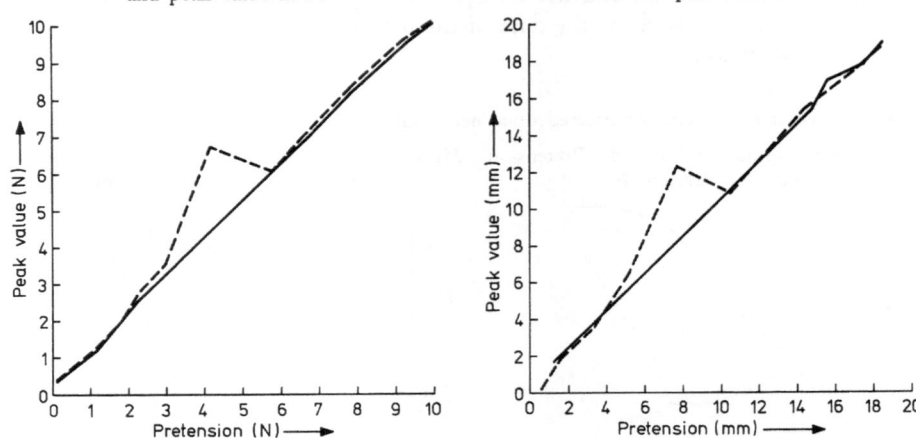

Fig. 3. An example of muscle function after nerve suture without tension. No difference between the operated and unoperated side could be seen

No. 917. Triceps surae muscle–operated (nerve grafting) and unoperated side. Pretension and peak value in mm and N

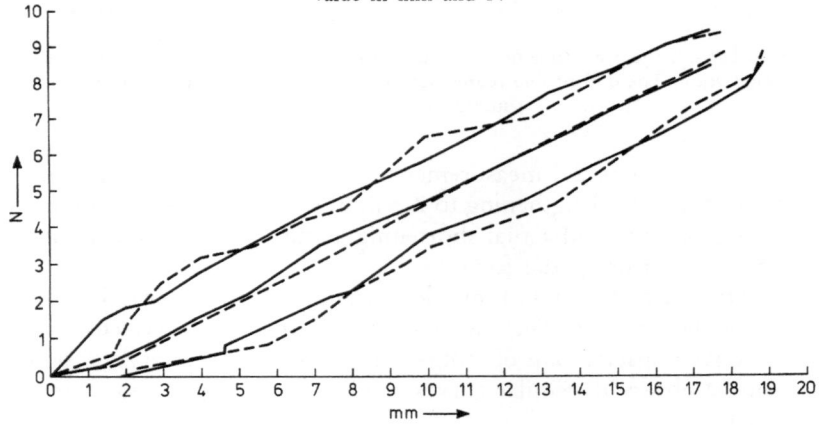

Fig. 4. After nerve grafting there is no difference in muscle function. Operated and unoperated nerves seem nearly identical

We may conclude that muscle function expressed in force and active shortening, achieves normal values after nerve suture without tension, even so after nerve grafting. By a nerve suture under tension we could observe normal values of the muscle function by a slight passive muscle tension. By increasing passive tension up to normal levels, a significant decrease occurred, because more muscle units are needed. But if by increasing passive tension more muscle units are necessary to gain normal function, the recruitment of more units is not possible, therefore, the force and the length of contraction decreases significantly. That means by a nerve suture under tension fewer nerve fibres are regenerating and re-innervating the innervated muscle. Furthermore we can say this is an objective test concerning muscle function in experimental conditions as well as in humans, as confirmed by Freehafer.

### References

Omer, G. E., Vogel, J. A.: Determination of physiological length of a reconstructed muscle-tendon unit through muscle-stimulation. J. Bone Joint Surg. (AM) *47*, 304–312 (1965).

Freehafer, A. A., Peckham, P. H., Keith, M. W.: Determination of muscle-tendon unit properties during tendon transfer. J. Hand Surg. *4*, 331–339 (1979).

Author's address: Doz. Dr. G. Meissl, Abteilung für Plastische und Wiederherstellungschirurgie, I. Chirurgische Universitätsklinik, Alser Strasse 4, A-1090 Wien, Austria.

### Discussion

*Frey:* Dr. Meissl, you measured the contracting forces of one muscle during different elongations of the muscle. Do you mean, this can give exact parameters, because we know that the contracting force differs greatly when the muscle is investigated during different periods of tensions? And my second question is about the time of your investigations after surgery. You measured the functional parameters 8 weeks after surgery. Don't you think that in a later stage of recovery different results could be gained?

*Meissl:* We have measured the tension *and* the amplitude of the muscle contractions together and not only the tension force. According to the time of our investigations we know that *nerve* regeneration occurs within 2 months after surgery is completed.

# Tissue Tolerance and Muscular Degeneration and Regeneration After Ischemia

## G. Brunelli

Department of Orthopaedics,
E.U.L.O. University School of Medicine,
Brescia, Italy

With 10 Figures

The aim of this study was to obtain precise data on muscular degeneration and regeneration after ischemia, with reference to reimplantation in human beings. Ischemia was induced in 386 rabbits in order to study the tolerance of muscle to various types of ischemic conditions and the capacity of muscle to regenerate in these conditions.

After having performed several initial amputations and reimplantations, we adapted another method because of the difficulty in obtaining exact times of the duration of ischemia; therefore ischemia was induced by means of a tourniquet applied to the base of the left hind limb (while the right limb was used for physiological controls).

The ischemic limb was kept at room temperature in all "normothermic ischemia" experiments, and wrapped in a plastic bag filled with ice and water in "hypothermic ischemia" experiments.

Normothermic ischemia was induced for periods which varied from 2 hours up to 8 hours, hypothermic ischemia was induced for periods which varied from 2 hours up to 18.

Modifications in muscle tissue were studied by means of optical and electron microscopy at the end of the ischemic period and at varying times after revascularisation (1 day, 3, 5, 10, 15–30).

Electrophysiological analysis of nerve and muscle and physiopathological analysis of muscle and blood were used to obtain values for the following:

conduction velocity at threshold and at maximal stimulation,
maximal stimulation of the nerve and muscle response,
deep temperature (as compared to rectal and control limb temperatures),
muscle weight (depending on the levels of oedema and atrophy),
plasmatic creatine-kinase and lactic dehydrogenase,

blood potassium, calcium and lactic acid,

protein content of muscle, C.P.K. and L.D.H.,

muscles, nerves, arteries, veins and capillaries were also examined by light and electron microscopy.

The deep muscle temperature (measured by means of thermistors) showed: 1) a faster rise in temperature of the cooled off limb (in hypothermic ischemia) which may be interpreted as indicating an obstructed blood flow caused by endothelial lesion in cases of ischemia at room temperature.

2) a rise in the limb temperature lasting at least 10 days after revascularisation which may be explained: a) by an increase of capillaries, b) by heat production in muscles due either to inflammation or to the separating of phosphorylation from oxidation and c) by a decrease in thermical dispersion.

This rise in temperature was reduced in cooled limbs.

As regards the functional analysis of nerve and muscle the outstanding finding is that there was no difference in response depending on recovery days.

This means that when recovery occurs it occurs after a short time.

Even after only 2 hours of ischemia half the rabbits did not respond, and the effects were much more dramatic than might be expected: conduction velocity was reduced by more than half and fulness of response reduced to a tenth of normal levels.

After both 4 and 6 hour ischemia the cooling off gave an improvement in physiological responses. Additional experiments seem to show a later minor recovery which might be correlated with histological regeneration. The variations of muscle mass after ischemia were positive (oedema) for 7 days and major for longer ischemias and room temperature ischemias, reaching a maximum value on the 3rd day (30–50 %). Then they became negative (atrophy up to 10–20 %).

As regards levels of C.P.K. and L.D.H. there was an increase proportional to the duration of the ischemia, which continued for 3 days with a decrease to their normal values on the seventh day.

The cooling-off process limited this increase more for C.P.K. values (one eighth normothermic limb values) than for L.D.H. values which it only halved.

Blood potassium rose after 4 and 6 hour warm ischemia but diminished over 24 hours.

This indicates a membrane alteration at the level of the Na-K ATP-dependent pumps because of an energy deficit.

Cooling off the blood potassium diminished probably due to the hypothermic itself.

Blood calcium decreased more after warm ischemia but it returned to normal within 3 days, probably due to larger absorption by the sarcoplasmic reticulum or to precipitation at mitochondrial level.

The amount of lactic acid present shows the metabolic behaviour of ischemic tissue.

There was a rapid increase during the first 24 hours after revascularisation (without significant cooling-off modification) which lasted for the whole observation period and this can be interpreted either as: 1) an increase in the

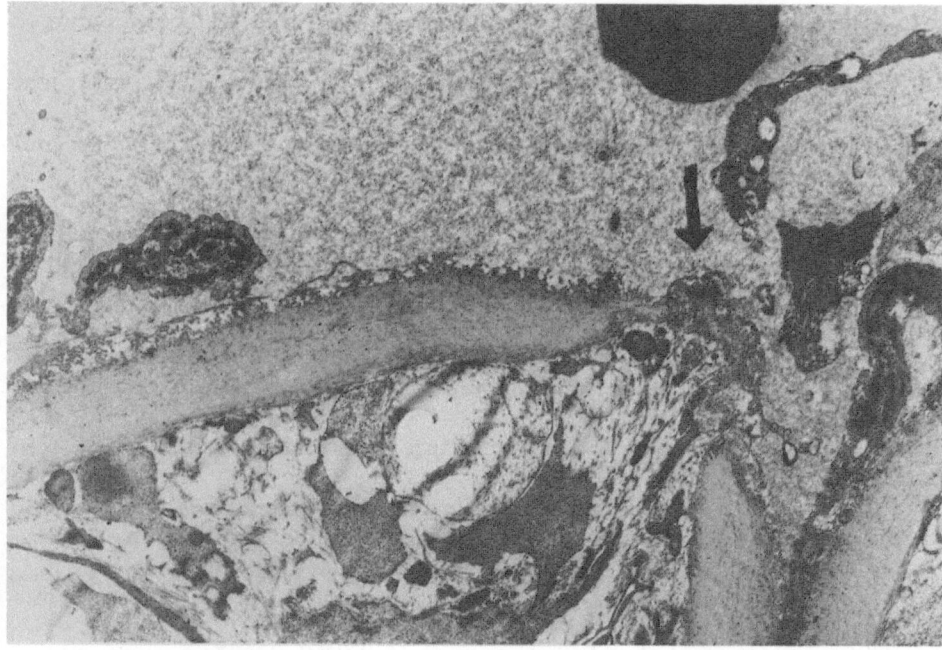

Fig. 1. Small vessel after 4 hours room temperature ischemia. The endothelium fell, the internal elastic membrane thickened and in places broke with media protrusion (arrow)

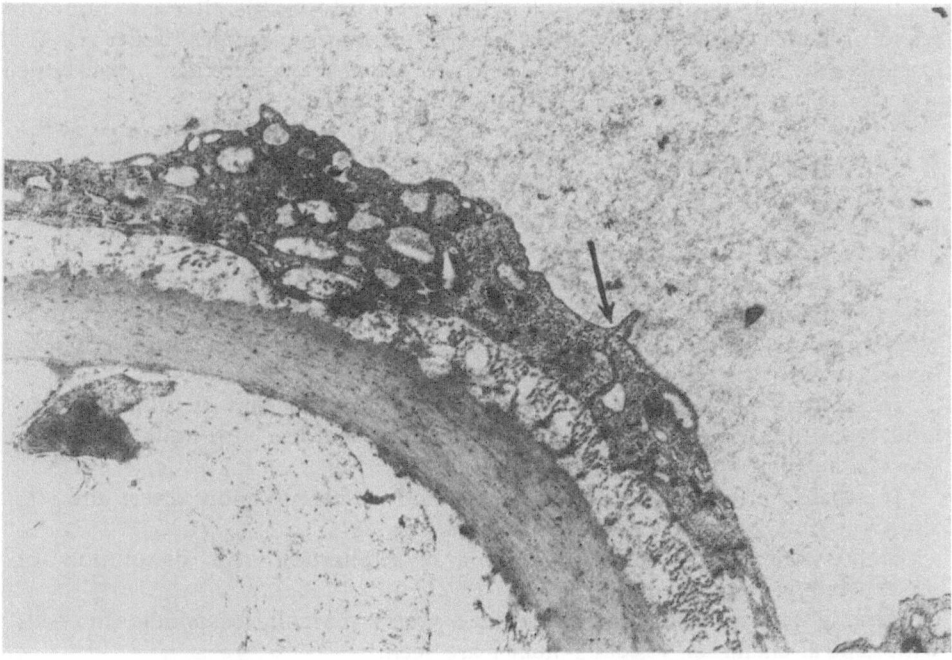

Fig. 2. Normal appearance of endothelium within 5 days of revascularisation after 2 h. of warm ischemia. Normal cell junction (arrow)

damaged tissues' energy needs with prevalent anaerobic metabolism due to repair or 2) an alteration of the micro-circulation with decreased oxygen.

The protein content of muscle decreased for 3 days because of enzymatic protein loss and dilution due to oedema.

The situation returned to normal after 7 days except for long term ischemia in which there was a fall in protein content due to atrophy. In cooled-off limbs there was no protein alteration.

Under the microscope the vessels showed degenerative changes after only 3 hours. The endothelium fell, the internal elastic membrane thickened and in places broke, over a period of 2 hours beginning presumably from the second hour (Fig. 1).

The vessels that underwent ischemia for 2 to 4 hours returned to normal within 24 hours, while in those having undergone 6 hours' ischemia the changes were visible after 15 days.

A normal cell junction is a sign of return to normality which can be seen after 5 days (Fig. 2).

Nerves, especially small and unmyelinated fibers tolerated ischemia better; in large axons myelin showed a quick vacuolization until complete layer separation took place after 4 to 6 hours of ischemia.

After 5 days the myelin seemed to be re-established (in normothermic ischemias).

With 4–6 hours of ischemia there was a typical Wallerian degeneration above all in the large nerve fibers.

If there was no necrosis, regeneration was rapid. After 10 or 15 days, medium-sized and weakly myelinated fibres were observed (Fig. 3).

In the muscle the first effect of ischemia, already visible after one hour of warm ischemia, was the disappearance of glycogen granules under E. M. examination. After only 2 hours of ischemia, oedema, nuclear chains, fish-bone appearance and disappearance of striation were found.

Under the electron microscope fiber separation, oedema and breakage of the Z lines were observed.

After 3 hours cross-striations disappeared, the mitochondria were swollen and longitudinally disposed and the Z lines were even more altered: after 4 hours the fibers were fragmented.

At 6 hours there was a partial disappearance of nuclei, initial hyalinosis, phagocytosis and eventually a total disappearance of muscular fibers with a waxy appearance (Fig. 4). After revascularisation a rapid normalisation was seen in ischemias which lasted less than 3 hours.

In ischemias lasting 4 hours macrophages appeared and an inflammatory infiltration (more precocious in 4-hour ischemias and less in 6-hour ischemias) was visible (Fig. 5).

If ischemia lasted longer, the damage to the muscle was more severe and was already visible 24 hours after revascularisation.

Under the E.M., megamitocondria, vacuolisation and dissolution of myofibers were observed (Fig. 6).

Among necrotic fibers and inflammatory cells muscular basophilic thin cells with central chains of vesicular nuclei are seen.

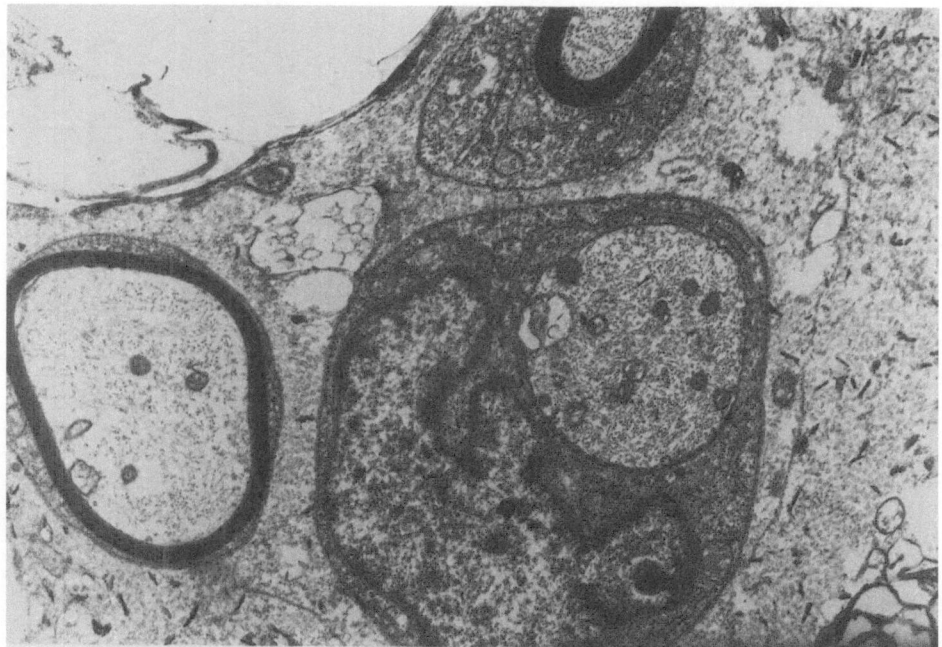

Fig. 3. Nerve regeneration and remyeliation within 10 days after 4 h. warm ischemia

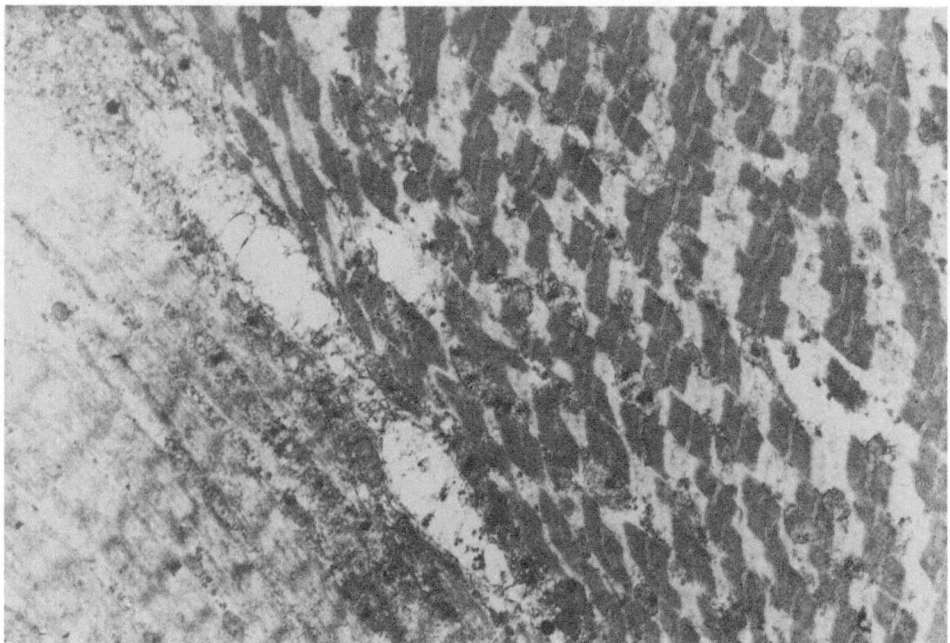

Fig. 4. Muscle. 6 h. warm ischemia. Mixed appearance: a zone with almost total disappearance of muscular fibers and waxy appearance in contact with another zone of less severe degeneration (fish bone aspect)

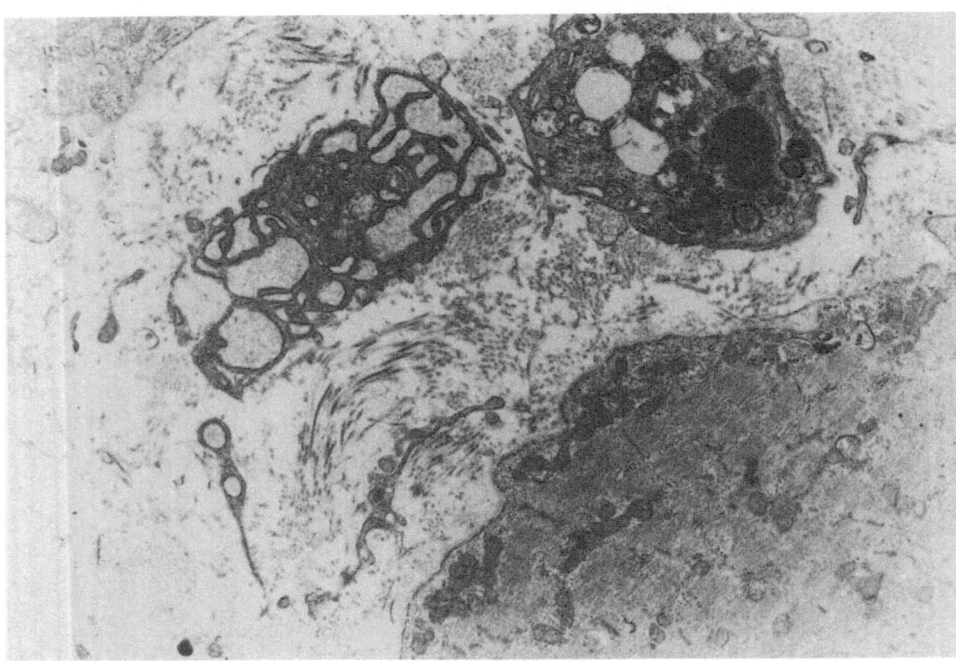

Fig. 5. Severe muscular degeneration and macrophage infiltration. 4 h. warm ischemia, 24 h. Revascularisation

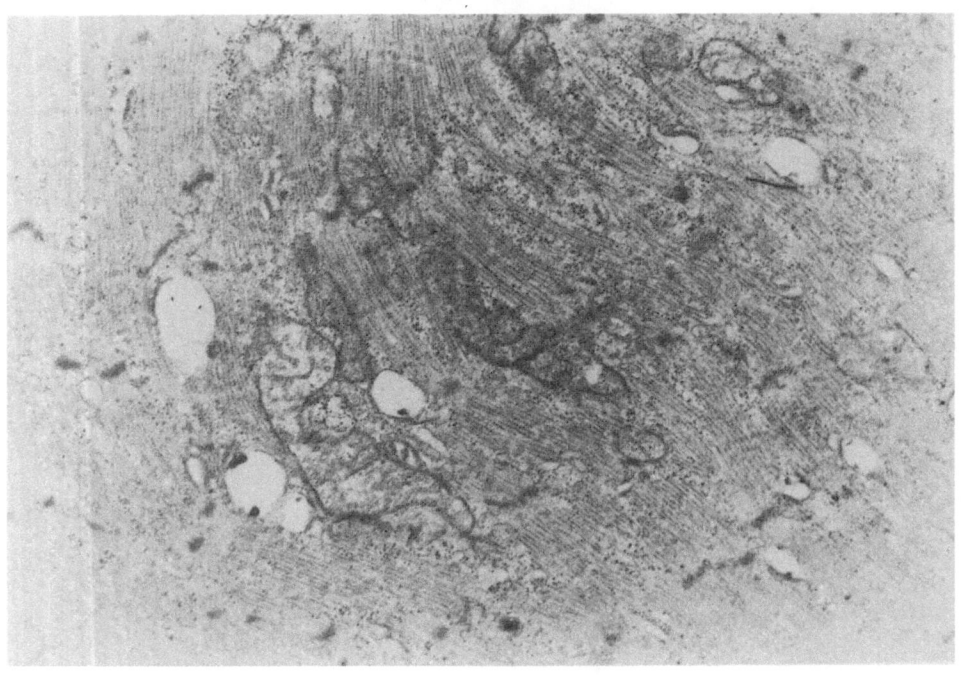

Fig. 6. 6 h. warm ischemia, 24 h. after revascularisation: Megamitochondria, vacuolisation and dissolution of myofibers

We also observed clumps of cytoplasmic material containing living nuclei that could be the starters of muscular regeneration.

10 days after revascularisation there was a consistent increasing of basophilic regenerating multinucleated myotubes with myofibrils and Z band formation (Fig. 7, 8).

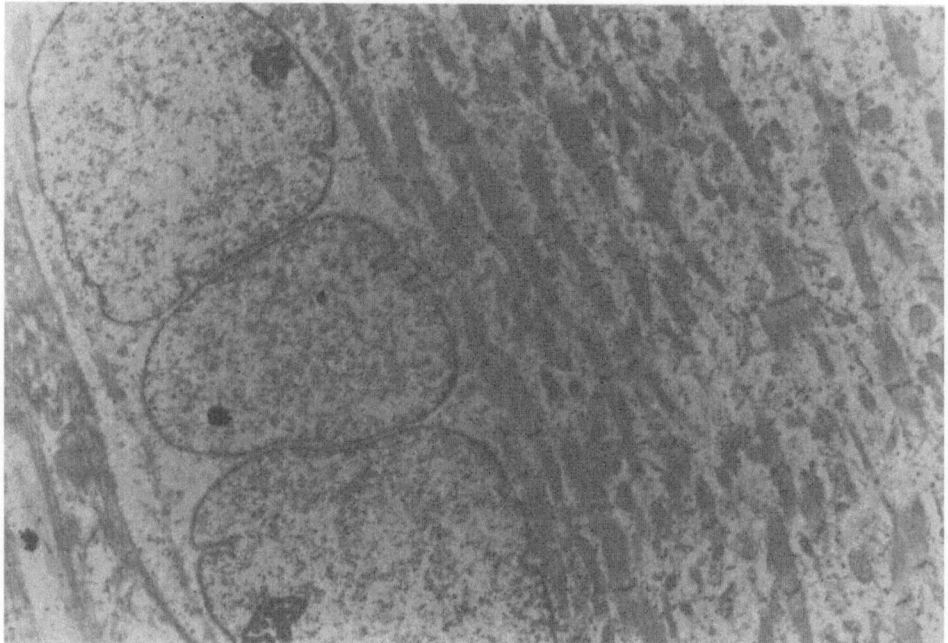

Fig. 7. 6 h. warm ischemia after 10 days of revascularisation: regenerating myotube with nuclear chain myofibrils appearance and Z band formation

Satellite cells increased in number and size, their nucleoli becoming prominent, their rough ergastoplasmic reticulum was activated (Fig. 9), myofibrils appeared (Fig. 10) and in some zones it seems possible to see the formation of Z lines.

From this anatomical, physiological and pathological research, it can be said that at room temperature there is a possibility of good conservation of tissues and of their function for up to a maximum of 3 hours without evident enzymatic alterations.

It has also been shown that longer ischemia, from 3 to 5 hours, causes progressively more severe damage which is still repairable. The damage becomes irrepairable when ischemia lasts 5−6 or more hours, and repair, when it occurs, is made by scarring.

The cooling-off process seems to have the capacity of slowing down the degenerative process although more evident for certain parameters than for

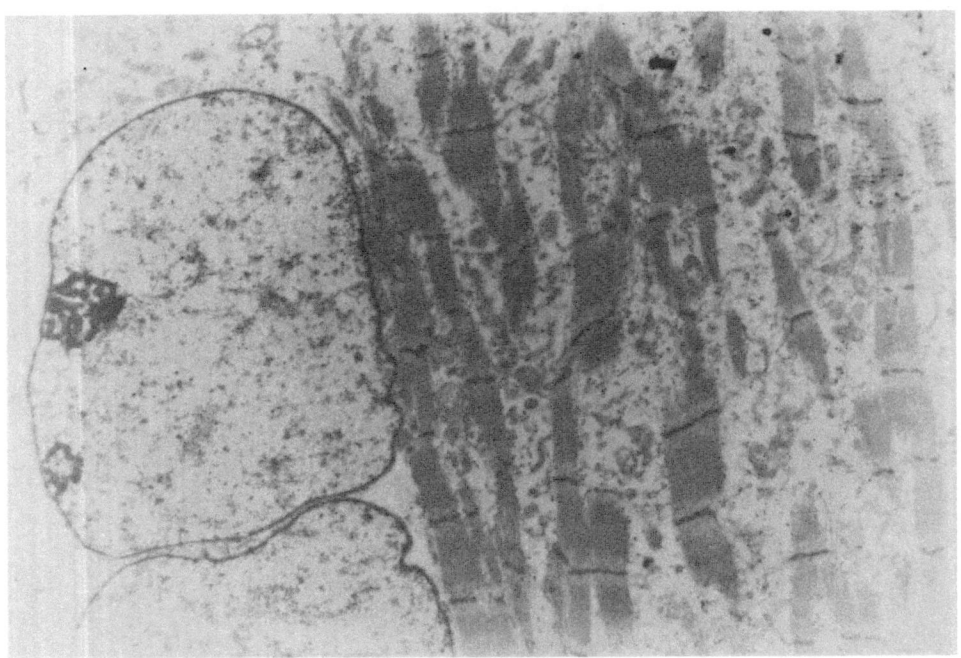

Fig. 8. 6 h. ischemia, 10 days recovery: Polynucleated myotube advanced myofibrils and Z bans formation

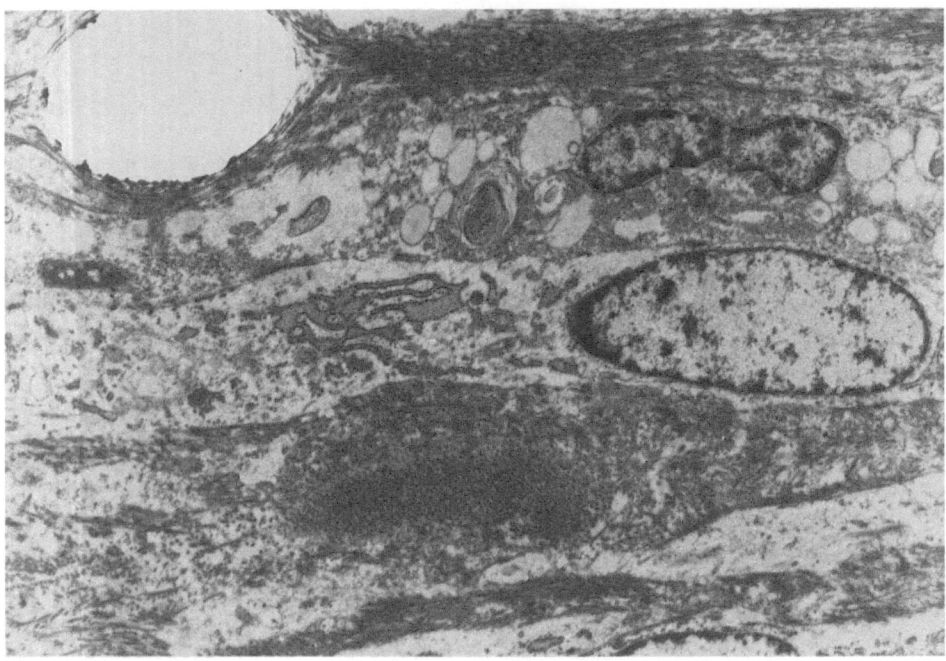

Fig. 9. 6 h. ischemia, 10 days recovery: Activation of a satellite cell with rough ergastoplasmic reticular enlargement and myofibrilar appearance

others. 12 hour cold ischemias showed appearances that were very similar to those of 2–3 hour warm ischemias, and even after 16 hours of cold ischemia fibers were not too severely damaged.

It can thus be said that if the cooling is begun immediately after the onset of ischemia and is correctly done, the cooling can increase the tolerance of muscle to ischemia by a factor of 3, if not 4 or 5 times. Regeneration of muscle has been proved and it seems to occur by means of 3 mechanisms: proliferation of vital clumps, continuous myotube prolongation and activation of satellite cells and their transformation into myoblasts.

These findings may be useful in the evaluation of indications of limb replantation.

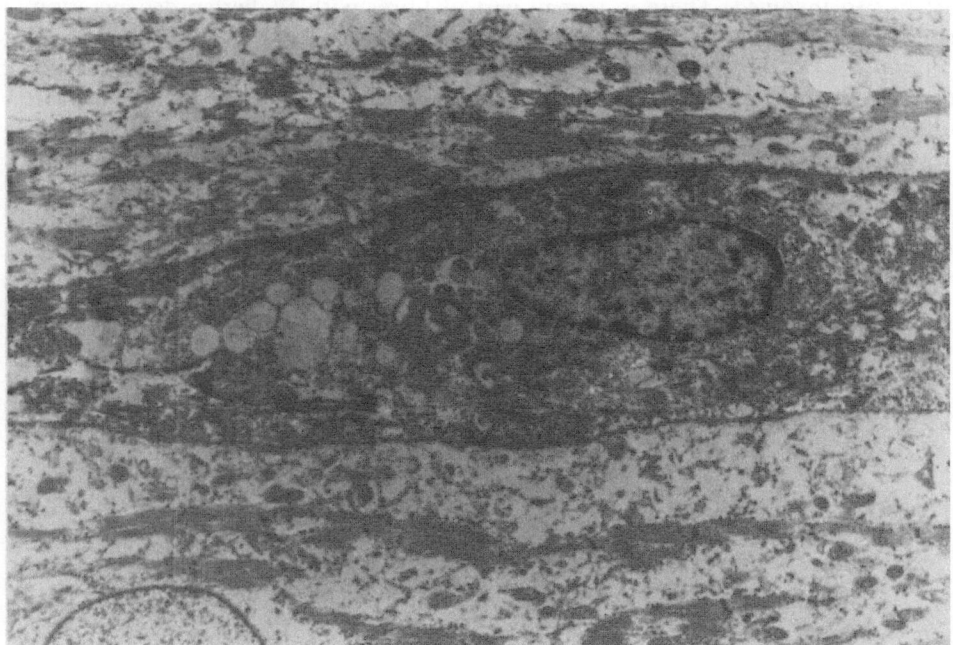

Fig. 10. Another satellite cell at the same period. More richness of myofibrils

## Summary

A study on limb ischemia was performed on 386 rabbits by putting their hind limbs in warm and cold ischemia for 2–4–6–8–12–16 and 20 hours and measuring various parameters of tissues and blood 1–3–5–10–15–30 days after revascularisation.

Light and electron microscope study of these conditions was carried out on muscles, vessels and nerves.

Regeneration of muscles was demonstrated.

The tolerance of muscle to ischemia seems to be 2–3 hours if ischemia is normothermic.

This figure can be multiplied 3 or 4 times for cold ischemia.

In longer ischemia recovery can take place, but with partial regeneration and partial scar substitution proportional to the temperature and elapsed time.

Author's address: Prof. Dr. G. Brunelli, 2ª Ortopedia, Spedali Civili, I-25100 Brescia, Italy.

## Discussion

*Frey:* Your ischemia was produced by a tourniquet. Is there not a possibility of nerve damage by pressure?

*Brunelli:* As you could see in the first slide on nerve alterations, the nerves are not so involved. There is a small part of fibres with Wallerian degeneration and at the 15th day all fibres are well regenerated.

*Holle:* Do you think, that in clinical limb replantations 3 hours of ischemia is the critical time, after which no replantation should be done because of severe muscle damage with all its consequences for the body, for instance toxemia?

*Brunelli:* I can say, that in animals at least 3 hours of ischemia do not show any definitive alterations of the muscle. But 6 hours of ischemia can give some muscular necrosis, some persistance of normal muscles and some regeneration. And if you cool the limb, you can get a good preservation of the limb up to 12 and 16 hours.

# Stimulation of Striated Muscles for Biological Energy Supply

## M. Frey

Department for Plastic and Reconstructive Surgery
of the Second Surgical University Clinic of Vienna, Austria

With 5 Figures

In striving for an energy supply of artificial organs independent from external energy sources, the chronic stimulated, cross-striated muscle is of special interest as an internal generator. Especially in the field of artificial heart replacement (1, 2) it is necessary to have an implantable, external energy source at one's disposal or to make an internal energy source accessible. The whole system "Artificial Heart" consists of the energy source, the transfer of energy, the drive, the control with probes, and the blood pump. Whereas the blood pump is nearly always implanted intracorporeally, there exist only a few solutions to the problem of how to implant the transfer of energy and the drive (3). The additional implantation of both, i. e. the source of energy and the control, was only achieved in some cases. The main problem concerns the source of energy, which up to now was only achieved by a disintegration of radioactive material (4). Because of the high costs and the growing hesitations about the use of atomic power, the search for internal energy production is placed in the foreground. Man is able to produce a mechanical muscle power of about 300 Watts for a short time and of about 50 Watts for a longer period. Compared with the power output of the heart of about 3 Watts, there can be no doubt that this energy can be produced by muscular activity. The muscle should work automatically by means of chronic stimulation using an electric stimulation-generator similar to a pace-maker.

## Material and Methods

To investigate the possibilities of such a biological system of energy production, we used the psoas muscle of the pig. Such a muscle has to satisfy the following conditions:

1. The muscle has to be large enough for adequate output.
2. Physiological adaptation to permanent load is a good condition for chronic electrical stimulation.

3. The use of the muscle should not cause a functional defect.

4. Even if the dimensions of the energy converter and the stimulation unit are reduced as much as is technically possible, enough room is necessary for the implantation in the surrounding tissue.

5. The muscle nerve has to be easily accessible for the fixation of the electrodes and should be free of afferent components, which would probably cause unpleasant sensory effects during electrical stimulation.

6. A defined, circumscript insertion of the muscle is needed for the fixation to the energy converter.

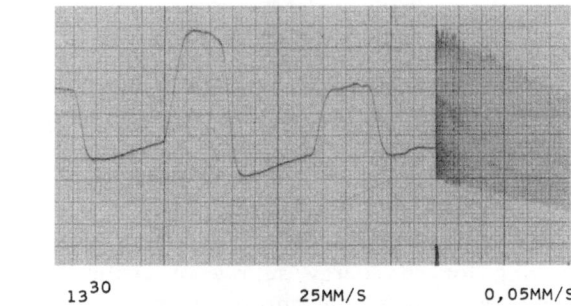

ISOMETRIE-
TENSION

(NON CALIBRATED)

$13^{30}$                        25MM/S               0,05MM/S

Fig. 1. Isometric contractions of the psoas muscle in the pig. Alternating stimulation of the proximal and distal muscle nerve

Similar to Giuzzi and Ugolini (5) in their theoretical considerations, we stated in our practical tests of the different skeletal muscles of the pig that the psoas muscle is the most suitable one for this purpose.

Therefore the chronic stimulation of the psoas muscle was performed in 5 domestic pigs with an average weight of 30 kg. The animals were intubated and anesthetized with a combination of Halothane® and laughing-gas during the whole time of the experiment. By a flank incision the retroperitoneal compartment and the origin of the psoas muscle at the transverse processes and at the bodies of the lumbal vertebrae were exposed. The distal tendinous end of the muscle was cut at its passage under the inguinal ligament. The muscle is supplied by two segmental, plexiform nerves extending from the lumbal plexus. In the first two experiments the tension of isometric contraction was indicated by an elongation measuring strip. In the other three experiments the registration of the distance of isotonic contraction against a constant power of 10 to 15 Newtons enabled us to calculate the energy. This constant tension was applied to the muscle by attaching a weight to the distal, tendinous muscle end. A line sutured to the tendon was turned around a pulley, the excursions of which were registered. Four electrodes were sutured to the proximal muscle nerve and four electrodes to the distal muscle nerve.

To overcome muscle fatigue in stimulation through the nerve, the principles of the "Round About Electrode Stimulation" were applied. An implantable 8-channel stimulator was used, which was supplied with induction current through the skin. A temperature sensor was sutured to the surface of the muscle for registration of the muscle temperature. In the last animal of the series total implantability was simulated by almost complete closure of the wound.

## Results

In the first experiment the psoas muscle was stimulated by pulses of 12 mA, a duration of 1 msec, and a frequency of 1 pulse/sec. Calibration was missing when a creep measuring strip and a Wheatstone bridge were used for the measurement of isometric muscle tension. After simultaneous stimulation of the proximal and distal muscle nerve, an alternating stimulation of both was

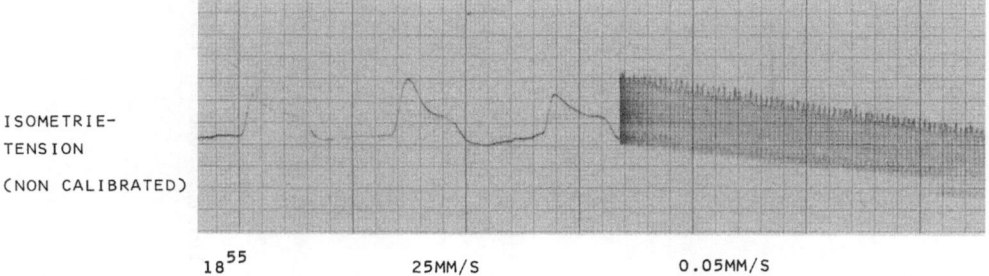

ISOMETRIE-
TENSION

(NON CALIBRATED)

18$^{55}$          25MM/S                    0.05MM/S

Fig. 2. The same experiment as in Fig. 1. Instability of the arrangement of the measurements at the end of the experiments after stimulation for 9 hours

performed then (Fig. 1). Trains of pulses caused a contraction every second, but in this way a working period of half a second and a resting period of 1.5 seconds were achieved for each muscle segment. The instability of the arrangement of the measurements due to a decline of the battery voltage was probably the main reason for the decrease of the amplitude of the distance at the end of the experiment after stimulation for 9 hours (Fig. 2). Similar results were found in the second experiment, in which the technical details were improved.

In experiments 3, 4 and 5 we changed to isotonic conditions. On the average the current was 2 mA at the beginning of stimulation at the proximal and distal muscle nerve. The alternating stimulation of different bundles of muscle fibers by the "Round About Electrode Stimulation" of the muscle nerves led to changing excursions of the muscle, which can be easily seen in the distance diagram (Fig. 3). An interesting observation was made during long term registration under unchanged conditions. For a few minutes the muscle was not able to reach its resting length. This shortening was about 20% of the normal distance of the contraction. After stimulation for 3 hours under identical conditions, there was no important decrease in the distance. Switching off stimulations for 10 minutes caused a short decline in the temperature. Immediately after switching it on again, a short lengthening of the distance was observed. After a few minutes it returned to the earlier value. In evaluating the optimal setting for the current, the cycle was registered during constant increase of the current from 0 to 8 mA. The maximal effect was already gained at 3 mA. One has to consider the extremely long duration of anesthesia for 12 hours

M. Frey:

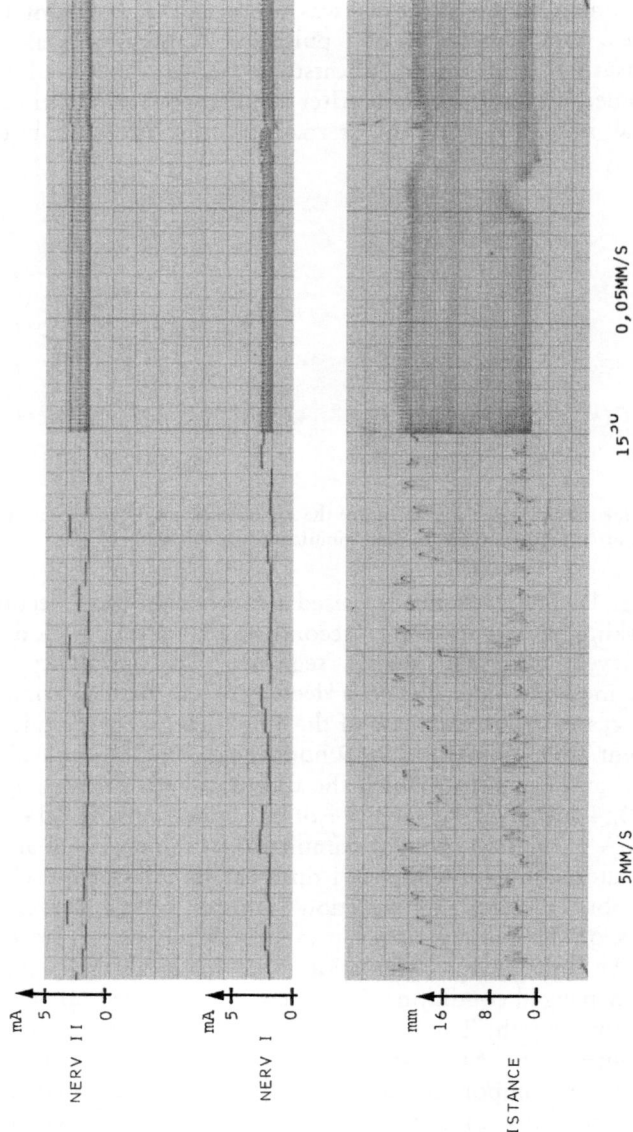

Fig. 3. Experiment No. 5: "Round About Electrode Stimulation" of the muscle nerves. First and second line: Stimulation current. Third line: Excursions of the psoas muscle

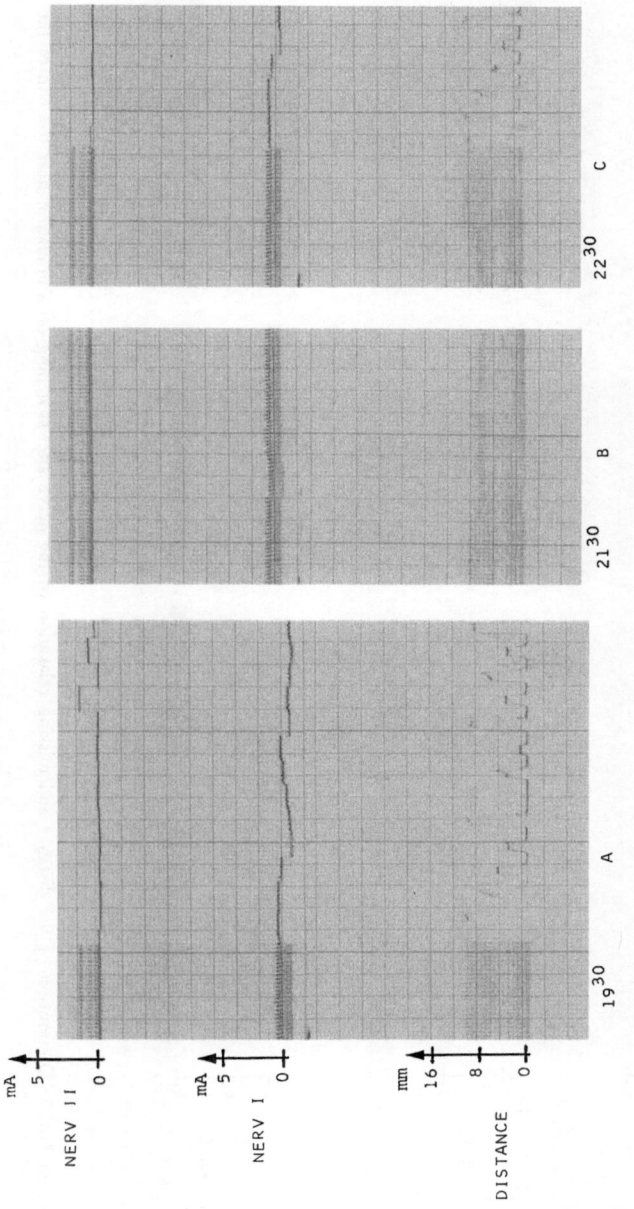

Fig. 4. Experiment No. 5: Long term registration under unchanged conditions

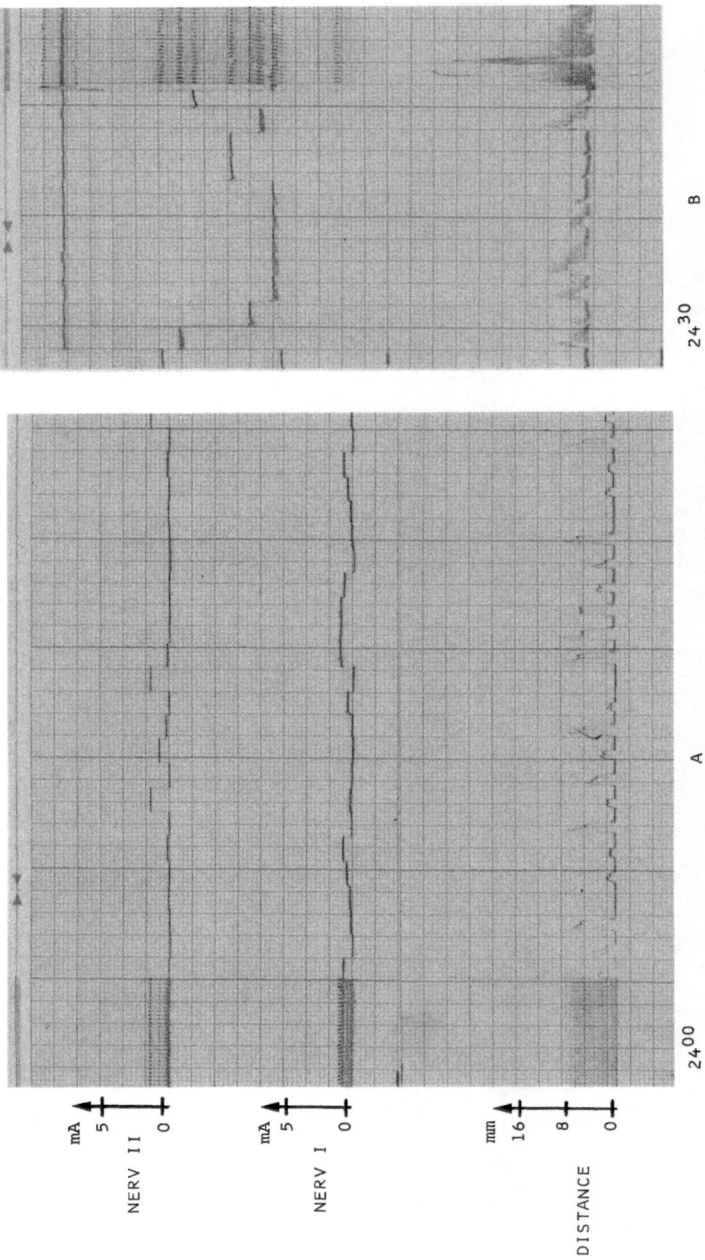

Fig. 5. Experiment No. 5: Diminution of the distance and missing relaxation of the nerve after switching off stimulation near the end of the experiment

when assessing the diminuation of the distance and the missing relaxatior. of the nerve after switching off stimulation near the end of the experiment (Fig. 4, 5). Only a few combinations had a sufficient excursion.

## Discussion

This experimental series intends to show whether such an internal energy supply by muscle stimulation is possible from the surgical point of view, and whether such a system is able to produce enough energy. The results ir.dicated that a power of about 0.2 Watts was gained by stimulation of the psoas muscle in the pig. Considering the body weight of this animal (about 30 kilograms) and the non-optimal arrangement, it should be possible to achieve the desired capacity by continuous improvement of the efficiency as well as by training of the muscle. The fatigue of the psoas muscle at the end of the experiment can be attributed mainly to the long term anesthesia. Prior experimental and clinical experience with functional electric stimulation (6) demonstrated that there is no fatigue of the muscle by loss of transmitted substances at the nerve–muscle junctions. This so called "Round About Electrode Stimulation" consists in a stimulation of single nerve fibres variable in time and location. In our experiments the nonphysiologically high frequency of contractions of 1 Hz may have played a role. The clinical application of this "Round About Electrode Stimulation" for stimulation of the diaphragm by both phrenic nerves was performed up to 160 days and a training effect was seen (7). A similar training effect can be expected for the chronic stimulation of the psoas musc.e.

This pilot study was not performed under ideal muscle-physiological conditions. Therefore we hope that in further experiments in the standing animal and with implantable devices an energy production by chronic stimulation of cross striated muscles will be possible in an order of magnitude sufficient for the supply of an artificial blood pump.

## References

1. Thoma, H.: Assisted Circulation, p. 429. Berlin-Heidelberg-New York: Springer. 1979.
2. Wolner, E., Thoma, H., Deutsch, M., Eckersberger, F., Fasching, W., Horcher, E., Losert, U., Stellwag, F., Stöhr, H., Unger, F., Weisskirchner, R., Polzer, K.: Das Forsch·ungsprojekt „künstliches Herz" an der II. Chirurgischen Universitätsklinik Wien. Wien. klin. Wschr. *91*, 74–81 (1979).
3. Stöhr, H., Horcher, E., Losert, U., Thoma, H., Wolner, E.: Implantierbare automatische Steuerung für künstliche Kreislaufpumpen. Kongr. Ber. Öst. Ges. Biomed. Techn. S. 65–68 (1980).
4. Whalen, R. L., Molokhia, F. A., Jeffery, D. L. Huffmann, F. M., Norman, J. C.: Current studies with simulated nuclear powered left ventricular assist devices. Trans. ASAIO. *18*, 146 (1972).
5. Guizzi, G. L., Ugolini, F.: Proposal for a total, orthotopic, muscle–powered artificial heart system for live application. Digest of the combined meeting: XII. Internat. Conf. on Med. and Biolog. Engineering, V. Internat. Conf. on Med. Physics. *1*, 8.1 (1978).
6. Thoma, H., Benzer, H., Holle, J., Moritz, E., Pauser, G.: Methodik und klinische Anwendung der funktionellen Elektrostimulation. Biomed. Techn. *24*, 4–10 (1979).
7. Thoma, H., Holle, J., Moritz, E., Navratil, J.: Prinzip und Anwendung der Karusselstimulation. Biomed. Techn. *21*, 109–110 (1976).

Author's address: Dr. M. Frey, Abteilung für Plastische und Wiederherstellungschirurgie, II. Chirurgische Universitätsklinik, Spitalgasse 23, A-1090 Wien, Austria.

# Methods of Muscular Electrostimulation

## H. Thoma

Bioengineering Laboratory of the Second Surgical University Clinic of Vienna, Austria

With 6 Figures

## 1. Introduction

Since Galvani 1791 published his experiments on the frog thigh, we have known the principle of functional electric stimulation [1]. There is a hyperbolic connection between the stimulation current and stimulation time. Therefore we need a high current for stimulation with a short impulse. A pulse length of 1 up to 5 ms normally depolarises the fibre. Stimulation is applicable in either muscle or nerve fibre. If we fix the electrodes close to the nerve, stimulation has some advantages:

The inhomogeneous electric field allows a smooth movement.

Less energy for depolarisation of even larger muscle areas (1–5 mA) is necessary.

Knowledge of what kind of fibres we are going to stimulate (afferent and efferent).

Less movement of the electrode area during stimulation.

Less sensivity in most of the cases.

Direct stimulation of the muscle fibre is necessary if we are not allowed to implant electrodes or if there is no nerve fibre existing for the function that we desire. For long-term application we prefer nerve stimulation.

## 2. Electric Parameters

Using functional electric stimulation, we control a biologic function. In cases of heart pacing we need only one impulse to start the whole heart action. But this is the only exception we know. Controlling a biologic function means simulating the process with current impulses.

When stimulating the diaphragm for breathing support, we have to distinguish between (Fig. 1):

the amplitude of current (2 mA)
the duration of the impulse (1 ms)
the frequency of the impulses (25 ms/40 Hz)
the inspiration time (1 s) and
the breathing cycle time (4 s).

The voltage we have to supply depends on the resistance between 2 electrodes. This resistance is from about 200 up to 2000 Ohms.

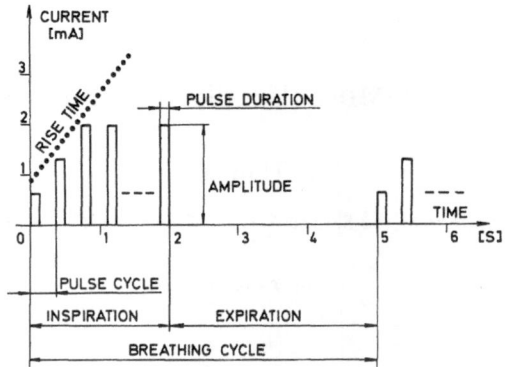

Fig. 1. Stimulation the diaphragm for breathing support

Some philosophies exist for the optimal adjustment of electric parameters. We have had good experience with the following statements:

Optimize the relationship between a minimum of energy and a maximum of information.

Make the duration of the impulse rather longer than amplitude higher (electrode stability depends on the voltage range).

The last remark: We must always minimize the electrolyte component. DC (direct current) is not allowed in case of functional electric stimulation. The effect depends not on the waveform of the current impulse. There is no difference between a triangle, a rectangle or an exponential tail of the impulse.

## 3. Biologic Functions

Methods of electric stimulation are now standard in the field of physiotherapy [2]. However, the *control* of biologic function has not gained a foothold in the clinic up to now except for the method of cardiac pacing. The main reason for that is the problem of fatigue at the neuromuscular junction in the case of long-term stimulation [3]. To overcome the fatigue we developed, in cooperation with Holle, Moritz and Baum (1973), the so-called "round about electrode" (German: Karussellstimulation) [4]. With this new method we simulate the natural rotation of activity by the aid of an electric field around the nerve (Fig. 2). To obtain the desired effect, the stimulation current has to be low enough to prevent stimulation of the whole nerve, and high enough to stimulate a sufficient number of fibres; the electric field must be inhomogeneous. If the

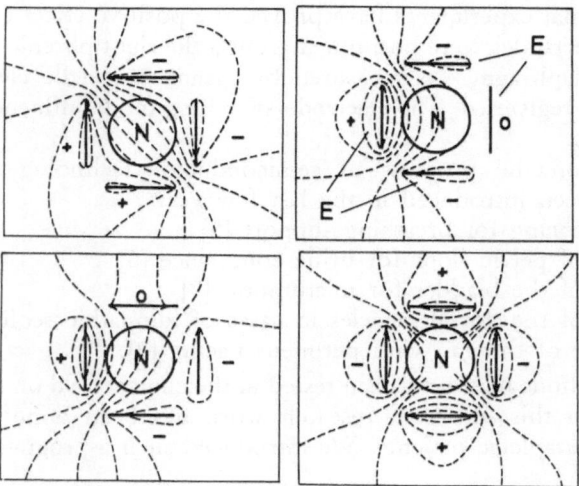

Fig. 2. Flux line distribution in the electrolyte. Selection of electrode combination determines the local potential differences in the nerve cross-section. *N* nerve, *E* electrodes

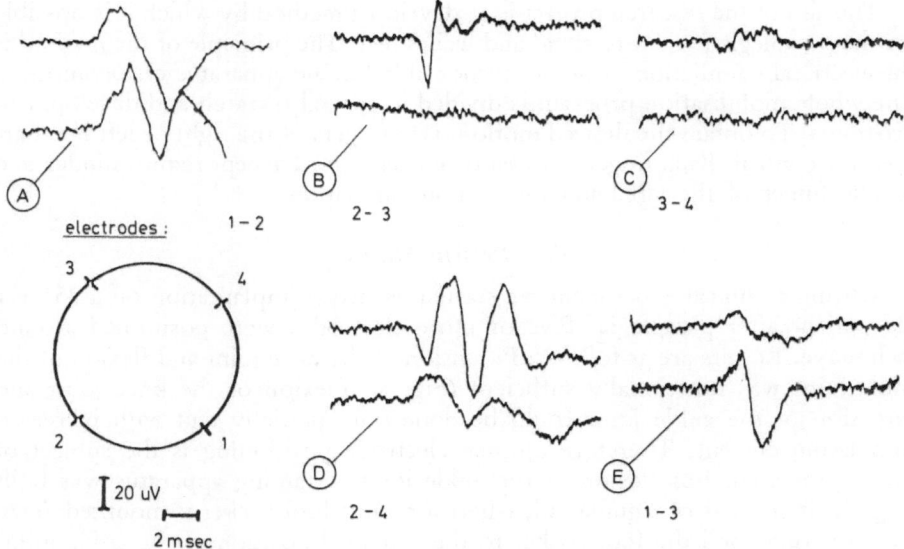

Fig. 3. Muscle reaction due to round about electrode. Selection of electrode combination causes stimulation of various muscles

stimulating electrodes are positioned closer to the nerve, the electric field becomes more inhomogeneous. If, for example, four electrodes are placed around the nerve, one can achieve an intensity variation of the local electric field by different electrode polarization. An automatic switching logic causes a rotating electric field in the cross-section of the nerve; hence "round about electrode". Animal experiments have proved the positive effect of this method (Fig. 3): four electrodes were positioned around the right phrenic nerve. Muscle action of the diaphragm was measured by means of needle electrodes. Two myograms were registered. The electrode-switching mode influences diaphragm muscle reactions.

Depending on the progress of semiconductor technology, some other methods have been introduced in the last few years:

Diaphragm pacing for breathing support [5]

Stimulation of pelvic floor for urine continence [6]

Stimulation of the bladder for micturation [7]

Stimulation of the dorsal muscles in cases of idiopathic scoliosis [8]

Improvement of the gait with peroneus pacing [9].

All these methods have now been tested in the clinical field on some hundred patients. Beyond this, different research work has been done in control of extremities on paraplegic patients. We introduced such a programm 1977 [10].

## 4. Walking After Paraplegia

### 4.1. The Concept

The aim of the research project is to develop a method by which it is possible for the paraplegic patient to stand and walk erect. The principle of the method is the electrical stimulation of nerves responsible for the apparatus of locomotion. The whole mobilisation program is divided in several research and development programs. To obtain the desired motion, two fingers of the right or left hand are used for control. Each finger represents one leg. Our concept requires index and middle finger of the left hand for motion simulation.

### 4.2. Present Status

During a clinical experiment we started electrode implantation on a 25-year old patient after paraplegia. Five or more electrodes were positioned around each nerve. Results are as follows: Extension of the knee joint and flexion of the ankle joint was functionally sufficient (Fig. 4). Flexion of the knee joint and extension of the ankle joint could be done only partially and with increased stimulation current. Therefore optimal electrode positioning is the subject of current research. For flexion of the ankle joint a training apparatus was built (Fig. 5). It consists of a guide rail, where a rotable foot rocker is mounted. Two strong springs pull the foot rocker to the extended position of the ankle joint. Exercise was done under supervision of a medical-physical assistant. Due to this muscle training the circumference of the calf muscles increased by 2.5 cm. This experiment was carried out for four months and proved the efficiency of the round about electrode.

The positive effect of this exercise is the conservation of muscle substance, but it is not deniable that this was a clinical experiment requiring permission of the patient. Motivation of patients is surely one of the important factors. In this case the physiological effect was easily recognizable. The patient was able to move her foot by means of the joystick. Therefore the "eternal paralysis syndrome" disappears in a most important and critical patient's situation, the first month after the accident.

Regarding the technological part, we have just finished a new multichannel stimulation unit (Fig. 6). Presently it is capable of driving eight electrodes, but

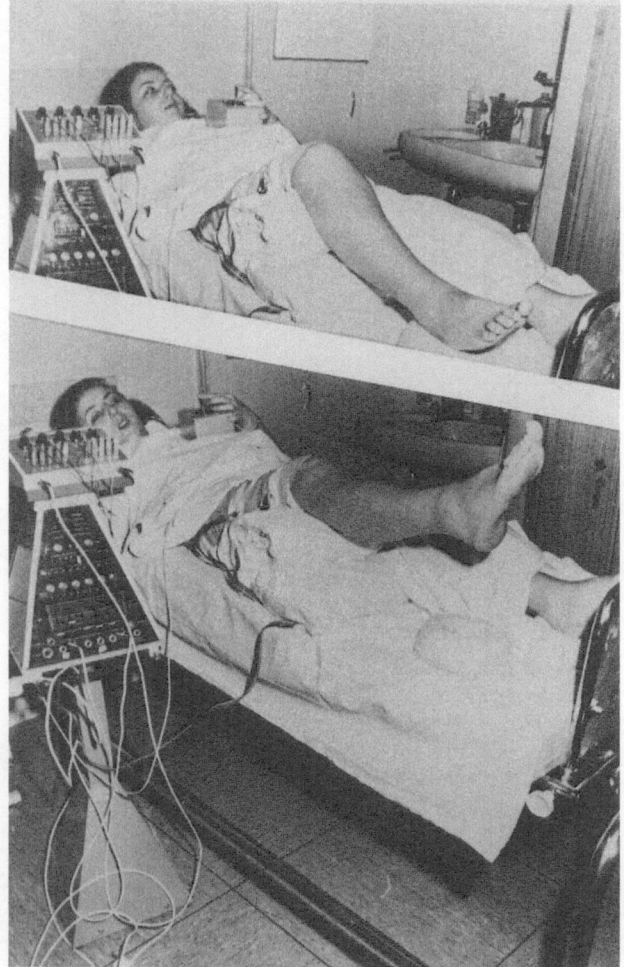

Fig. 4. Functional electro-stimulation of the femoralis nerve

this can be easily expanded. Via a microprocessor program we can determine the electrode combination from one impulse to the next, stimulation current, stimulation duration, frequency and polarity.

Features are:
microprocessor-controlled, freely programmable stimulation;
radio frequency-controlled transcutor;

9    Muscle Transplantation

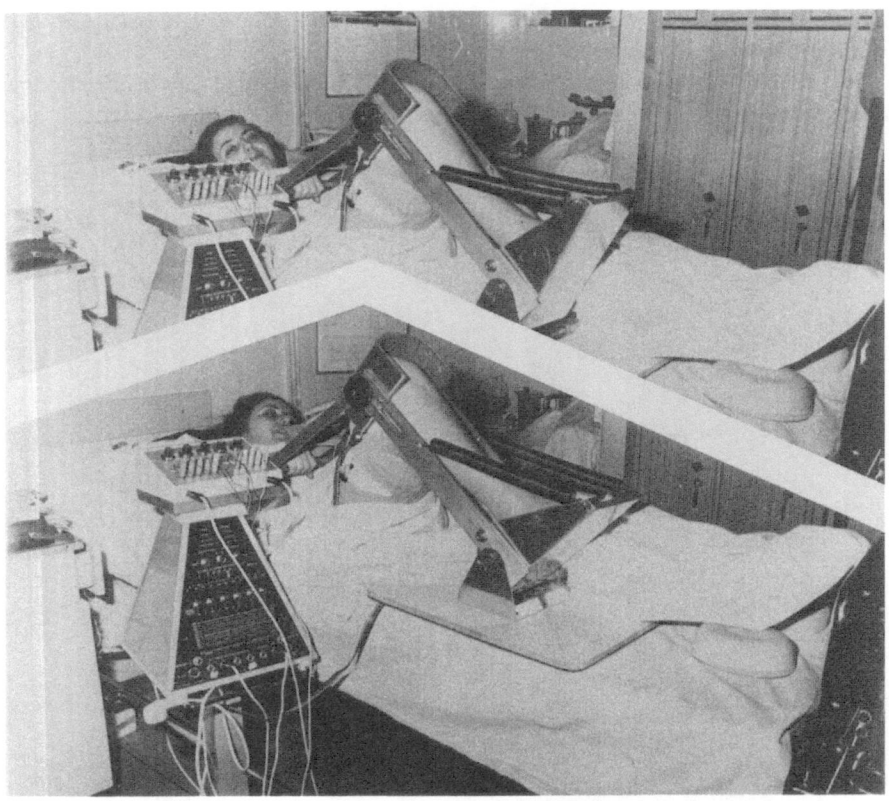

Fig. 5. Functional electro-stimulation of the tibialis nerve

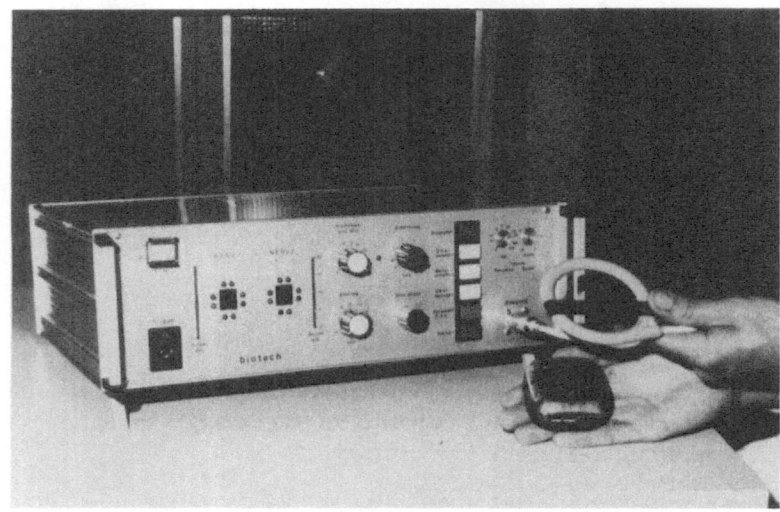

Fig. 6. Multichannel electro-stimulation device

possibility of stimulating 2 nerves simultaneously in the round about electrode-mode (right and left lung); otherwise stimulation of up to 4 nerves; avoidance of inefficient electrode combination;
power failure alarm;
battery-powered for portable applications;
triggerable by external respirator.

### 4.3. Final Remarks

Today we are just at the beginning of functional electrostimulation. By means of our method we can overcome the fatigue of the nerve-muscle complex, and new problems need to be solved. A practical realization will surely take a couple of years, but with the aid of suitable stimulation systems it should be possible to mobilize the paraplegic and support the tetraplegic patient in respect to his quality of life.

### References

1. Galvani, A.: De viribus electricitatis in motu musculari. Commentarius de bononiensi scientiarum et artium instituto atque academia commentarii 7, 363 (1791).
2. Stuart, H. A., Klages, G.: Kurzes Lehrbuch der Physik. Berlin-Heidelberg-New Ycrk: Springer. 1979.
3. Glenn, W., Holcomb, W., Gee, J., Rath, R.: Bulletin de la société internationale de chirurgie 32, 521 (1973).
4. Thoma, H.: Vorrichtung zur örtlich und zeitlich variablen elektrischen Reizstrom-Langzeitstimulation eines Reizobjektes, wie Nerven und Muskeln. OE Patentschrift 330342.
5. Holle, J., Moritz, E., Thoma, H., Lischka, A.: Die Karussellstimulation, eine neue Methode zur elektrophrenischen Langzeitbeatmung; Wien. klin. Wschr. 86, 23 (1974).
6. Caldwell, K. P. S., Cook, P. J., Flack, F. C., James, E. D.: Stress incontinence in females: Report on 31 cases treated by electrical implant. J. Obstet. Gynaec. Brit. Cwlth. 55, 777–780 (1968).
7. Grimes, J., Nashold, B., Anderson, E.: Clinical application of electronic bladder stimulation in paraplegics. J. Urology 113 (1975).
8. Bobechko, W. P., Herbert, M. A., Friedmann, H. G.: "Electro-Spinal Instrumentation". J. Bone Surg. 58 A, 156 (1976).
9. Ship, G., Mayer, N.: Peroneal Nerve Functional Electrical Stimulation For Whom? Proc. 6th Int. Symp. External Control of Human Extremities, pp. 243–256.
10. Thoma, H., Altrichter, C., Hammerschmid, W., Hochmair, I., Holle, J., Schmallegger, H., Stöhr, H.: Anwendung der funktionellen Elektrostimulation bei Querschnittsgelähmten. Österr. Ges. f. Biomed. Technik, 4. Jahrestagung, Juni 1979.

Author's address: Prof. Dipl.-Ing. Dr. H. Thoma, Biotechnisches Laboratorium, II. Chirurgische Universitätsklinik, Van-Swieten-Gasse 1, A-1090 Wien, Austria

## Discussion

Question: Have you used that simulating system in patients with facial paralysis?

*Thoma:* No, we did not use it—it is not an indication for us.

*Carlson:* For chronic implantation in your stimulation experiments, how could you avoid the deposition of connective tissue around your electrodes? I have seen that this often happens.

*Thoma:* This is a problem which has not yet been solved.

*Belgier:* Which sort of electrodes did you use, were these silver-chloride-electrodes? And second question: Can you not only stimulate the nerves in the muscle, but can you also detect action-potentials from muscles by this way?

*Thoma:* We use up to now stainless steel-electrodes, and we can get action potentials of nerves and muscles by these electrodes.

# Myoplastic Operations in Facial Palsy

# Dynamic Reanimation for Facial Paralysis–A Survey

## G. Freilinger

Department of Plastic and Reconstructive Surgery
of the Second Surgical University Clinic of Vienna, Austria

With 6 Figures

An amazing activity regarding neurotisation of denervated muscle tissue, neural neurotisation (Heineke, Steindler, Haberland) as well as muscular neurotisation (Erlacher, Katzenstein, Gersuni) existed already at the beginning of this century. It was, however, reserved to Noel Thompson, independently of Studitsky's work, to report on his experimental and clinical success in transplanting denervated autogenous skeletal muscles in 1971.

Stimulated by these reports, we have started with free muscle transplantation in 1972 and operated a series of patients with unilateral irreversible facial paralysis following Thompson's concept. We have reported our results in several publications 1974, 1975 and 1976. The original Thompson's procedure is based upon muscular neurotisation. A muscle graft is used to re-animate the paralysed half of the face from the healthy side.

Considering modern muscle physiology, we can basically distinguish and logically understand the following myoplastic operations:

1. Free muscle transplantation with muscular neurotisation
2. Free muscle transplantation with neural neurotisation
3. Muscle transposition with muscular neurotisation
4. Muscle transposition with neural neurotisation (Fig. 1).

May I comment, for a moment, on neurotisation. There are two kinds of neurotisation, as we all know, neural neurotisation (n.n.) and muscular neurotisation (m.n.). N.n. can be accomplished by implanting the nerve into the muscle or by nerve-to-nerve suture or by use of a nerve graft as in cross-face nerve transplantation. Nerve-to-nerve suture can be performed either by muscle graft together with a long nerve branch (Thompson) or with only a short stump. M.n. can be accomplished by a muscle graft, as Thompson has used it, or by a muscle flap, which means a transposed and vascularised muscle. Here we have again two possibilities: the denervated muscle flap can be re-innervated from the healthy muscle host to which it is brought in good and direct contact. Or the

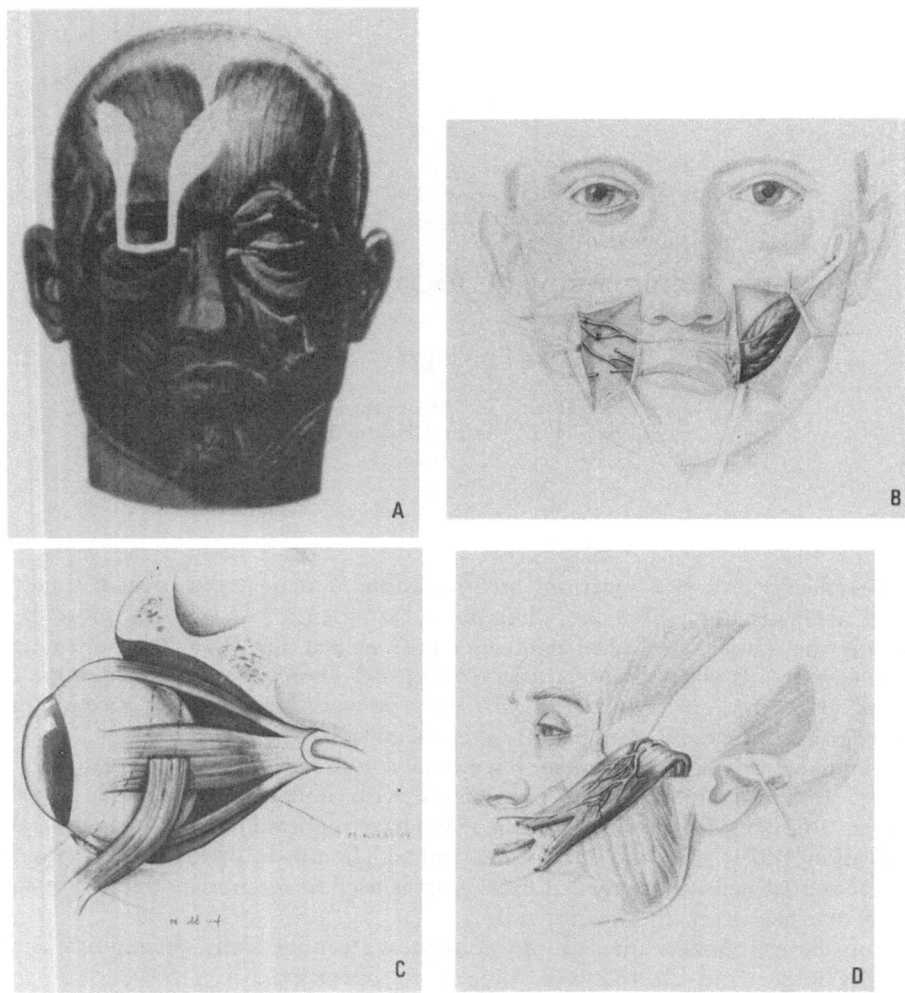

Fig. 1. Four different methods of myoplastic operations. *A* Free muscle transplantation with muscular neurotisation to correct ptosis of the right upper eyelid after traumatological paralysis of right N. oculomotorius and N. frontalis. *B* Free muscle transplantation with neural neurotisation to correct left facial paralysis. *C* Muscle transposition with muscular neurotisation to correct abducens paralysis. *D* Muscle transposition with neural neurotisation to correct left facial paralysis

innervated muscle flap is used to "transport" neural capacity to the paralysed muscle when placed in intimate contact (Fig. 2).

A few cases will demonstrate what was said.

Free muscle transplantation with muscular neurotisation.

This 14-year old girl has the following lesions resulting after a car-accident: skull fracture with lesion of the right nervus oculomotorius and the temporal branches of the right nervus facialis. After a long recovery and intensive care, she was admitted with a complete ptosis of the right upper eyelid. A direct nerve suture was out of question and a commonly used fixation of the upper eyelid to the frontal muscle could not work because of partial paralysis. Therefore, a muscle transplantation seemed to be the only hope for amelioration. The short extensor muscles of the foot were transplanted four weeks after denervation and placed on the frontal muscles. A good contact was accomplished with the left uninjured muscle area and with the lateral part of the right frontal muscles. Electromyography has proved that this lateral muscle tissue was innervated. The tendon was then brought by tunnelling to the tarsus of the upper eyelid and fixed under slight tension. Six months after this operation, re-innervation had occurred so that this girl could freely open and close her eyelid again. This is a classical example of muscular neurotisation.

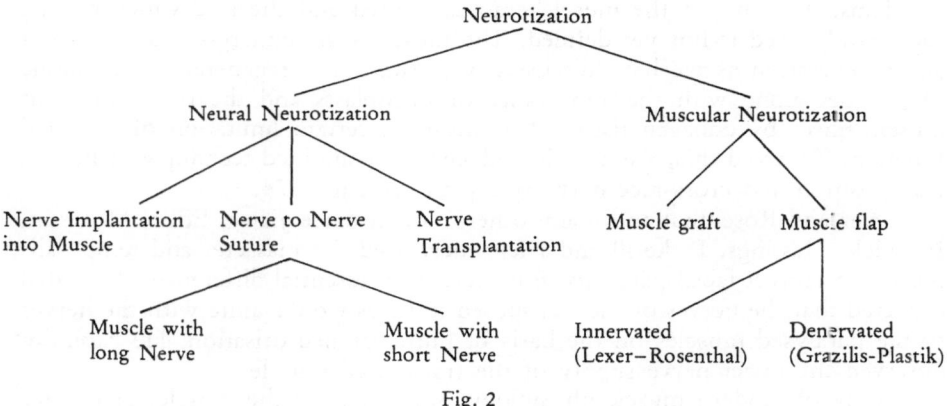

Fig. 2

Free muscle transplantation with neural neurotisation.

This interesting combination is valid for all cases where an irreversible lesion of facial palsy has been diagnosed. Cross-face nerve transplantation, as Smith in New York has introduced in 1971, would not improve the situation since no muscle tissue is left. After axonal growth of the nerve transplant across the upper lip, an additional muscle is used and connected with the nerve. We perform this operation in two steps.

This 20-year old nurse also suffered from a car accident. A decompression of the facial nerve in the Fallopian canal did not improve the situation of a right facial palsy. This patient complained mainly of the lack of mobility of the right corner of her mouth. During a first operation, a sural nerve was transplanted across the upper lip. This transplant was anastomosed to three peripheral branches of the healthy left facial nerve. Six months later, the EMG showed axonal growth through the transplant so that the denervated short extensor muscles of the foot could be transplanted fanlike into the right cheek. By tunnelisation, the graft was placed on top of the atrophic muscles there and fixed close to the corner of the mouth. Under slight tension, their tendons were brought around the zygomatic arch and sutured to themselves. At this stage, a small neuroma from the end of the sural nerve transplant was excised and three small fascicles individualised. They were then separately implanted into each muscle body by 10/O monfilament nylon. Already four months later evoked potentials by use of a concentric needle electrode on the free muscle grafts could be registered after supramaximal stimulation of the facial nerve near the foramen stylomastoideum on the unparalysed side of the face.

Seven months later the girl went back to work with a nearly perfect symmetry of her mouth when in a relaxed state and with good elevations of the right corner of her mouth and normal pursing.

Muscle transplantation with muscular neurotisation:

This method is used in sphincter reconstruction and will be covered by Dr. Holle this afternoon. It is also in use by ophthalmologists as a new technique to correct abducens paresis.

Free muscle transplantation without neurovascular anastomosis has some problems. The size of the muscle graft is limited and the size which can be successfully used is not yet defined. The muscle graft undergoes degeneration and regeneration as we have discussed yesterday. The regeneration of muscle fibres goes along with the appearance of fibroblasts and the replacement of muscle fibres by collagen tissue. This means a certain limitation of the final function. To avoid this, we have introduced the combined technique of muscle transposition and cross-face nerve transplantation in 1974.

Lexer and Rosenthal and many others, for instance Jiany, Eden, Morestin, Fenwick, Hastings, Pickerill and Alexander, used the masseter and temporalis muscle to correct facial paralysis. But there is an essential difference. Rosenthal expected that the nerves of the transposed muscles would unite with the nerves of the paralysed muscles on the basis of muscular neurotisation. He carefully observed the intact nerve supply of the transposed muscle.

Aware of modern muscle physiology, we denervate the muscle, before we transfer it. It is then ready to be re-innervated by the cross-face nerve transplant, which is an extended facial nerve. In doing this, the temporalis muscle changes its characteristic qualities and no longer remains a masticating muscle supplied by the trigeminus nerve, but becomes a mimic muscle supplied by the extended facial nerve.

We fully agree with Niklison, who in 1956 claims that the sound side in facial paralysis is not normal. We all know that there is a pathological tonus and contraction producing a marked over-action of the muscles in that side. This state of functional asymmetry due to marked muscular unbalance needs a correction of both sides. To moderate the sound side and to support and reanimate the paralysed side. Therefore, we denervate the over-active sound side, but do not waste this nerve capacity rather than direct it to the paralysed side.

Muscle transposition with neural neurotisation.

A labourer, aged 29, was seriously injured by a car-accident. As an emergency operation, a bilateral osteoplastic trepanation was performed. An epidural hematoma on the left side and a subdural hematoma on the right side could be treated successfully. Besides a central bilateral complate deafness, a facial paralysis on the left side remained unchanged eight months after injury. After electromyographical proof, the decision of dynamic reanimation of the completely paralysed angle of the mouth was decided. A sural nerve transplant was placed across the upper lip by tunnelisation from one nasolabial to the other. By microsurgical technique, three peripheral branches of the N. facialis on the unparalysed side representing R. buccales were identified and anastomosed with the N. suralis transplant. The exploration of the muscles on the paralysed side, responsible for elevation of the angle of the mouth showed a high grade atrophy. Therefore the M. temporalis was exposed and a central strong part of it freed towards the zygomatic arch. By electric stimulation, the nerve supply to this muscle part was identified and the denervation performed. The central muscle part was then swung down toward the corner of the mouth by several atraumatic sutures. The end of the nervus suralis transplant was then implanted into this transposed temporalis muscle part. Six months later, a clinically nearly normal function of the formerly paralysed muscles was found, no noticeable asymmetry and a strong elevation of the left angle of the mouth.

The use of masseter muscle for transposition is technically easier but maybe not as satisfying for the elevation.

In this 15-year old girl, the irreversible partial facial paralysis on the right side was corrected by masseter transposition and cross-face re-innervation. For years we have used an incision at the nasolabial fold as is generally recommended. Please notice the ugly, symmetrical scars on this young patient. Especially in young persons, the scars are quite obvious. We have now changed our approach. In addition to the face lift incision, the exposure is completed by an incision at the vermilion border around the edge of the mouth. This exposure is perfect, because the skin there is very mobile and allows a good approach towards the buccal region. The final scar is absolutely invisible. We can highly recommend this exposure. It is important not to take end branches of the facial nerve for denervation and connection to the nerve transplant rather than thicker ones. We do distinguish them by minimal faradic stimulation and identify them prior to their course through the parotic gland.

Muscle transplantation by micro-neurovascular anastomosis as introduced by Tamai 1970 and clinically applied by Harii, Ohmori and Torii for facial paralysis can be used on all sizes of muscles. The question and an important point is no more the size rather than the neurovascular supply of the muscle in use. The gracilis muscle is very convenient as a donor for several reasons. It can be removed easily and without functional disability, it is well-shaped and the remaining scar is not too obvious. Many skeletal muscles have multiple innervations, the gracilis has one main neurovascular supply in the upper third of the body, qualified for micro-vascular anastomosis. In our last few cases of irreversible facial paralysis, we have used free muscle grafts with micro-neurovascular anastomosis.

Case report: This 56-year old lady had a facial paralysis on her right side since her first year of life (Fig. 3). In December 1978, a cross-face nerve transplantation, using the sural nerve, was performed. A thick buccal branch of the intact left facial nerve was sutured to the transplant. By a face lift and vermilion border incision, a 15 cm long segment of the right gracilis muscle including the neurovascular supply was used and implanted into the right cheek and fixed under slight tension with the temporalis fascia and rein-like into the upper and lower lip ten months later (Fig. 4 and 5). The artery and vein of the muscle were anastomosed to the temporal artery and vein. Fourteen days later, when the muscle was proved to be intact and bleeding, the nerve to nerve suture between the sural and the gracilis nerve branch was performed in November 1979. This picture and the following film show this lady seven months later with a strong contraction (Fig. 6). For the lagophthalmus, a simple temporalis transfer was used in this case. Please notice the almost invisible scar at the vermilion border. As you have seen in this case, we do not need to take the whole muscle, but only the necessary segment in length, which was about 15 cm.

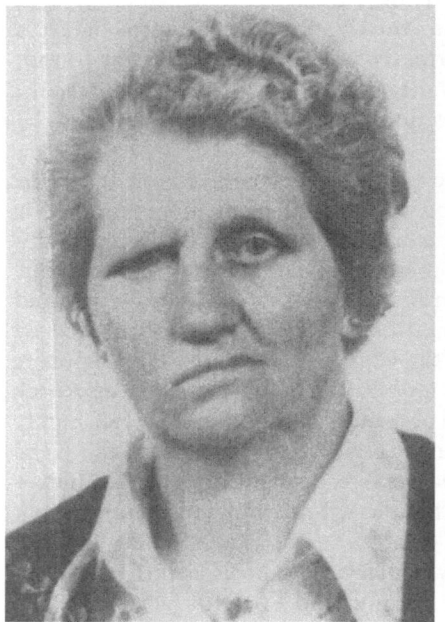

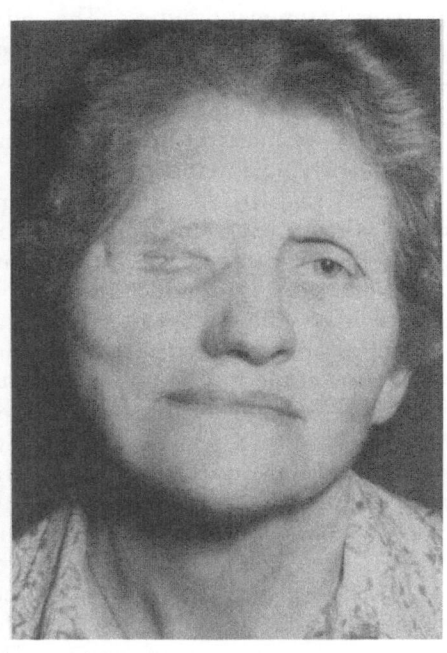

Fig. 3. Right facial paralysis over 50 years duration

Fig. 6. Strong elevation of right corner of mouth 6 months after operation

The next case may show you that we can go even further in dismembering the muscle graft without disturbing its final function or doing dangerous harm to the blood supply.

Case report: This 19-years old boy fell from a scaffold and suffered a fracture of the right temporal bone with a sub-total facial paralysis on his right side. His ocular and oral system of muscles were irreversibly damaged. Two years after injury he came for surgery. We decided to use the Gillies-procedure for his lagophthalmus and a free muscle segment with microvascular anastomosis of the mouth. The re-innervation was expected to take place by muscular neurotisation, since the palsy was incomplete.

This gracilis muscle was sliced twice, once horizontally, since we do not need more than about 10 cm length, and once vertically, since we do not need

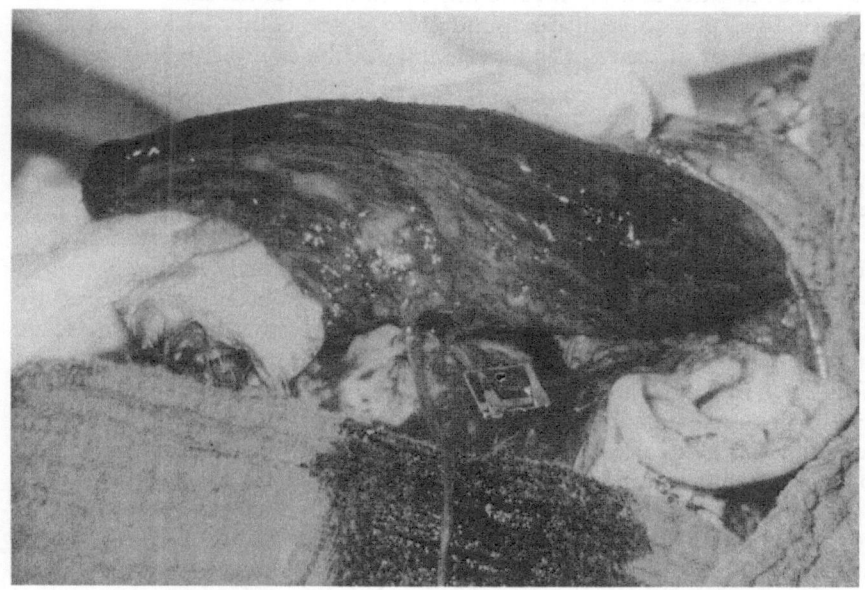

Fig. 5. Free muscle graft microvascular anastomosis

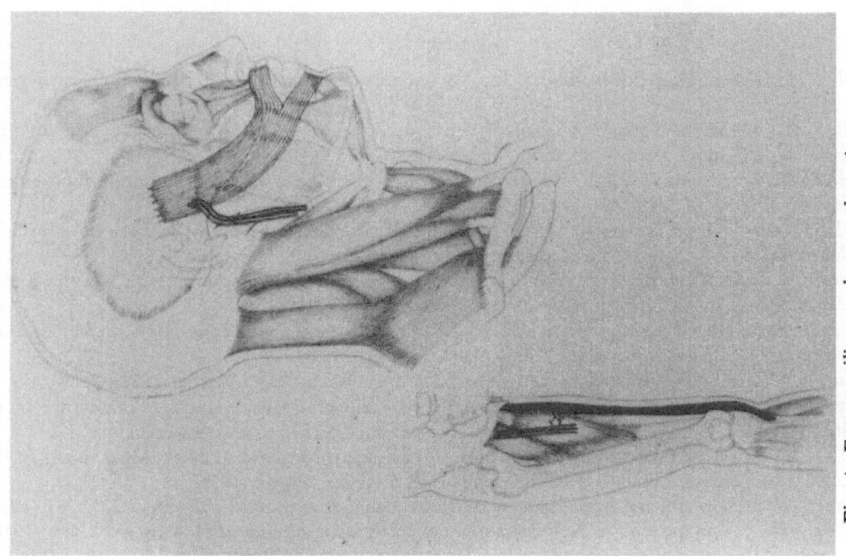

Fig. 4. Free gracilis muscle transplantation with microneurovascular supply–Scheme

the whole thickness of the muscle body. The usual vermilion border incision was used on both sides and the muscle implanted after tunnelisation. The facial artery was located but no vein was found close to the corner of the mouth. A direct anastomosis of the arteries and a vein graft to the external jugular vein was performed.

The mimic muscles consisting of 24 single muscles are a functional unit with three systems, the ocular, the nasal, and the buccal or oral system. The substitution of one muscle, and this is what we actually do to satisfactorily carry out the work of 24 others, is too much too expect. There is indeed very little chance to establish a co-ordinated mimic motion and emotional expression of the face. The controlled balance of these 24 muscles with their infinite shades of expression cannot be expected. Second, and this has been pointed out by Collier, "these thin, delicate muscles lie directly under the flexible and elastic skin" and are inserted either into the skin itself or are attached to the eyelids and lips. This lack of fascia permits the multiplicity of shades of expression by enabling small parts of individual muscles to contract independently.

Therefore, our general concept in handling this real problem of irreversible facial palsy is a combination of many steps and an individual approach. We need the whole armament of procedures to apply individually. We have no priority to any procedures but try to combine denervation on the healthy but over-active side with reanimation of the paralysed side. At present I think we can do a good deal to improve the situation in partial facial palsy and even in complete irreversible cases with our neuromuscular technique. In not leaving any visible scar, we do little harm to the patient.

### References

Heineke, H.: Die direkte Einpflanzung des Nerven in den Muskel. Zentralblatt für Chirurgie *41* (1914).

Steindler, A.: Direct neurotisation of paralyzed muscles, further study of the question of direct nerve implantation. Am. J. Orthop. Surg. *14*, 707–719 (1916).

Harrefeld, A. van: Reinnervation of denervated muscle fibers by adjacent functioning motor units. Am. J. of Physiol. *144*, 477–493 (1945).

Haberland, G.: Diss. Dezember 1913, ref. by P. Erlacher: Hyperneurotisation, musculäre Neurotisation, freie Muskeltransplantation. Zentralblatt f. Chirurgie *1914*, 15.

Erlacher, P.: Experimentelle Untersuchungen über Plastik und Transplantation von Nerv und Muskel. Archiv f. Kl. Chirurgie *106*, 389–406.

Katzenstein, M.: Über Heilung von Schultermuskellähmungen (M. trapezius, bzw. Serratus) durch kombinierte Muskelplastik. Berl. klin. Wschr. *1909*, 2184–2189.

Gersuni, R.: Eine Operation bei motorischer Lähmung. Wien. klin. Wschr. *1906*.

Thompson, N.: Treatment of Facial Paralysis by Free Skeletal Muscle grafts. Transaction of the Fifth Internat. Congress of Plastic and Reconstructive Surgery. Butterworths. 1971.

Studitsky, A. N.: Experimental Surgery of Muscles (Russian). Moscow: Izdatel. Akad. Nauk. 1959.

Lexer, E.: Die gesamte Wiederherstellungschirurgie. Leipzig: Barth. 1931.

Rosenthal, W.: Die bleibende Facialisparese und ihre Behandlung. Dtsch. Z. Chir. *223*, 261 (1930).

Rosenthal, W.: Über musculäre Neurotisation bei Facialislähmungen. Zbl. Chir. *43*, 489 (1916).

Jianu, Amza: The surgical treatment of facial paralysis. Dtsch. Ztschr. Chir. *102*, 377 (1909).

Eden, R.: Über die chirurg. Behandlung der peripheren Facialislähmung. Beitrag zur Kl. Chirurgie *73*, 116 (1911).

Morestin, H.: Section of the facial, lingual and superior maxillary nerves by the same projectile. Tentative improvement of the facial paralysis by muscular anastomosis. Bull. et Mémoires Soc. de Chirurg. de Paris *41*, 1370 (1915).

Fenwick, G.: Surgical treatment of facial paralysis. Brit. Med. J. *2*, 700 (1919).

Hastings, S.: Transplantation of anterior half of masseter muscle for facial paralysis. Proc. Roy. Soc. Med. *13*, 64 (1911–1920).

Pickerill, P.: Facial paralysis, palatal repair and some other plastic operations. Med. J. Australia *1*, 543 (1928).

Alexander, R.: Correction of facial paralysis by muscle transplant. Rocky Mt. Med. J. *38*, 713–716 (1941).

Niklison, J.: Contribution to the subject of facial paralysis. Plast. Reconstr. Surg. *17*, 276–293 (1956).

Tamai, S., Komatsu, S., et al.: Free muscle transplant in dogs, with microsurgical neurovascular anastomosis. Plast. Reconstr. Surg. *46*, 219–225 (1970).

Harii, K., Ohmori, K., Tori, S.: Free gracilis muscle transplantation with microneurovascular anastomosis. Plast. Reconstr. Surg. *57*, 133–143 (1976).

Freilinger, G.: A new technique to correct facial paralysis. Plast. Reconstr. Surg. *56*, 44–48 (1975).

Freilinger, G., Holle, J., Mamoli, B.: Klinische Erfahrungen mit der dynamischen Rekonstruktion nach Facialisparaesen. Österr. Chirurgen-Kongreß, Linz, 1974.

Author's address: Prof. Dr. G. Freilinger, Abteilung für Plastische und Wiederherstellungschirurgie, II. Chirurgische Universitätsklinik, Spitalgasse 23, A-1090 Wien, Austria.

## Discussion

*Holländer:* Is there any scientific proof, that implantation of a nerve into a muscle, as you have shown us in your cases, brings reinnervation of the muscle? Do you have to denervate the muscle which is to be reinnervated completely. Is this opinion still relevant or has it changed?

*Freilinger:* It is difficult to decide, which way of reinnervation of a muscle is better, the implantation of a nerve into the muscle or a simple nerve-anastomosis. We cannot answer this question yet. But there is no doubt that implantation of a nerve into a muscle gives a considerable result.

*Vedun:* In my experiments on cats I put the muscle into the abdomen and into the muscle I implant a nerve, which gives good reinnervation of the muscle. This is in cats, but not in humans.

*Freilinger:* The answer to the second question concerning with the total denervation of the muscle to be reinnervated is that only in denervated muscles can reinnervation take place. Superneurotisation does usually not occur.

*Faulkner:* We have done experiments on monkeys with good evidence that reinnervation takes place by implantation of a nerve into a muscle.

*Tolhurst:* I have used three cases of transposing denervated masseter muscle and putting in a cross-face nerve into the muscle without nerve anastomosis and all three cases were failure cases. So in our experients it does not work.

*Thompson:* I have no doubt, that reinnervation of a transplanted muscle can occur by an implanted nerve.

*Carlson:* If you took a muscle and implanted a nerve into it, would functional connections form earlier or later than after muscular neurotisation, and how much later?

*Freilinger:* I cannot answer this question exactly, but we tend more and more to use muscular neurotisation, if this is possible.

# Free Skeletal Muscle Transfer With Microneurovascular Anastomoses

K. Harii

Department of Plastic Surgery,
University of Tokyo, Japan

With 4 Figures

Tamai *et al.* [1] in 1970 first reported successful free transplantation of a large skeletal muscle in dogs using microneurovascular anastomoses. The rectus femoris muscle was transferred to isotopical and heterotopical recipient sites where the nutrient artery and vein and the motor nerve of the muscle were simultaneously coapted with the recipient vessels and motor nerve. A high rate of functional contraction could be obtained by the transferred muscle, and histological findings showed it to have an almost normal structure at five months postoperatively. The method suggested by this excellent laboratory work would seem to present the greatest potential for free transplantation of skeletal muscles which, since Volkmann's documentation [2], had been believed impossible.

Since 1973, I have carried out various clinical free skeletal muscle transfers, with microneurovascular anastomoses, to reconstruct a paralyzed face or extremity [3]. I would like herein to introduce potential donor muscles, present the provisions for successful transplantation, and describe the clinical materials experienced.

## Donor Muscles

The optimal donor muscle should have one vessel pedicle and a motor nerve. These nourish the entire muscle belly. A muscle which has multiple sources of vascularization and innervation, such as the sartorius muscle, is usually inadequate as a donor muscle. The required muscle also should be easy to isolate and leave no functional disability after removal. Its shape and size should correspond with those of the recipient defect (Fig. 1).

Several skeletal muscles have been transferred to date [4, 5], but I have come to prefer use of either the gracilis muscle or the latissimus dorsi muscle. The former usually well fits defects of the forearm, while the latter has a great advantage in the large caliber of its nutrient vessels and the long stalk they can provide. Such factors contribute to operational ease. Both muscles also are simple to isolate and leave no troublesome functional disability. If such is required, the skin overlying the muscle can be carried together with the muscle to form a musculocutaneous (or myocutaneous) flap.

The extensor digitorum brevis muscle, which has a short original excursion, often cannot display sufficient contraction as each muscle loses one-fourth or one-fifth of its original excursion. Other muscles, such as the tensor fascia lata and gluteus maximus muscles, are mainly used as musculocutaneous flaps to cover skin defects.

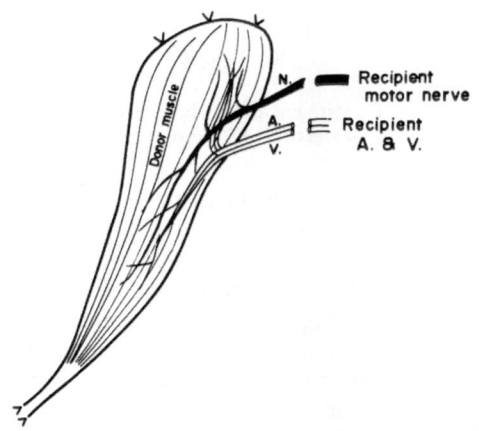

Fig. 1. Optimal type of donor muscles for microneurovascular free transfer

## Criteria for Successful Transfer

### 1. Selection of Recipient Vessels and Nerves

Selection of the recipient vessels is relatively easy. The artery should have sufficient perfusion pressure to nourish the entire muscle belly, and a healthy vascular wall to minimize the possibility of thrombogenesis at the suture site.

The important point on which successful transfer is dependent is selection of a suitable motor nerve in the recipient bed. In an extremity, the stump of the motor nerve which had originally supplied the abrased muscle(s) is selected. In reconstructing a paralyzed face, the facial nerve stump is not available in a majority of cases.

My first clinical case in 1973 was a free gracilis muscle transfer for correction of long-standing Bell's palsy. In this case, as a facial nerve stump was not available in the recipient bed, I used the deep temporal nerve supplying the temporal muscle, and sutured the gracilis motor nerve to it under microscope. The muscle belly was simultaneously vascularized with anastomoses to the superficial temporal artery and vein.

The vascularized muscle was then passed through a subcutaneous tunnel in the cheek and its distal end was split longitudinally in the nasolabial region. The upper division was anchored to the upper paralyzed lip and the lower division to the lower lip. The proximal end of the gracilis was fixed to the temporal fascia, and the wounds were closed. During the operation, the muscle remained moist and muscle ischemic time was less than 90 minutes.

About 6 months after the transfer, the patient felt slight contraction following strong bite action, and contraction reached a maximum 8 to 10

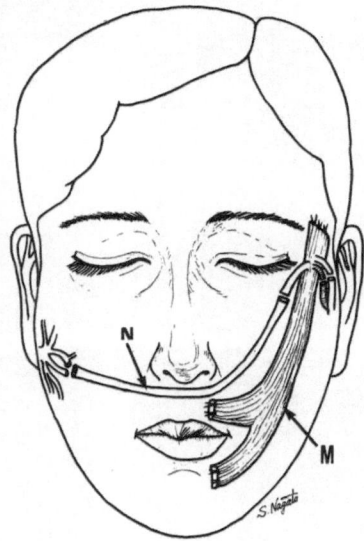

Fig. 2. Our alternative combined with cross-face nerve graft for the treatment of long-standing facial paralysis. Arrow N: sural nerve graft in stage 1. Arrow M: free muscle transfer in stage 2

months after surgery. During this period, the muscle volume was reduced to about one-half it original volume. The patient finally could obtain good contraction of the muscle to make voluntary animation, but the problem obviously was difficulty in achieving a natural facial expression at the involuntary movement. When the patient bit strongly, the muscle showed unnatural contraction.

I therefore have modified the technique to use the stump of a cross-face nerve graft [6] cabled from the healthy facial nerve funiculi in those cases where a facial nerve stump is not available in the recipient bed. A two-stage procedure is necessary for combining cross-face nerve grafting with free muscle transfer (Fig. 2). In the first stage, a long sural nerve graft is cabled from the selected buccal branches of the healthy (opposite) facial nerve to the affected cheek. The terminal stump of the sural graft is placed in the subcutaneous tissue close to the recipient vessels which are planned for selection in the subsequent operation. In the second stage, after Tinel-like signs have advanced to the distal end of the graft (it usually takes 8 to 10 months), the cheek flap is elevated and the sural nerve stump and recipient vessels are exposed. The subcutaneous layer of the cheek is widely undermined to create the tunnel through which the revascularized muscle is passed to the nasolabial region. The suitable donor

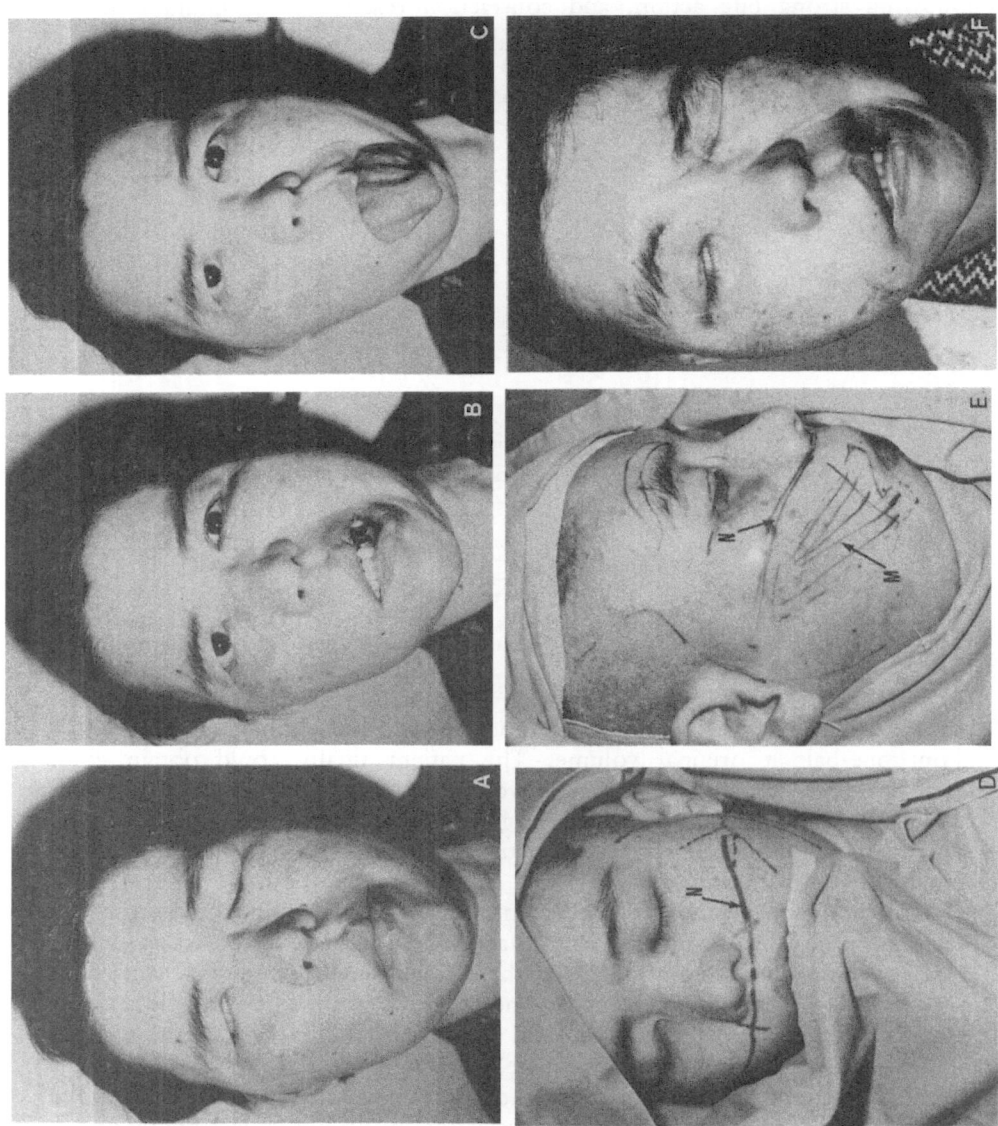

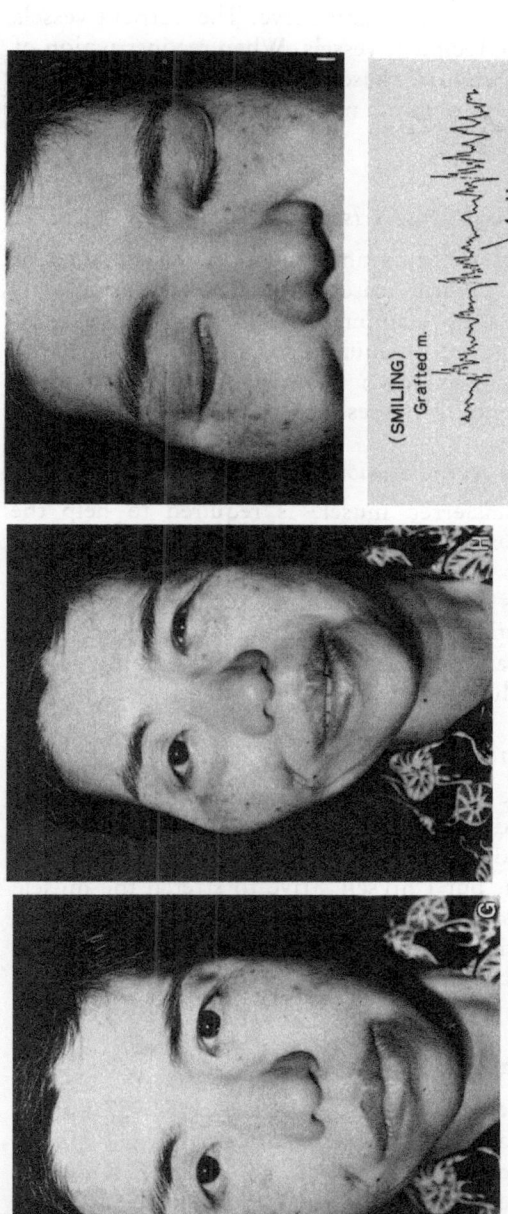

Fig. 3. Clinical case. A 52-year-old female's right complete paralysis after acoustic tumor resection three years prior to reconstruction. Hypoglossal nerve cross-over had been applied without beneficial effects. *A* to *C* Preoperative view, *D* Initial cross-face nerve grafting. Arrow *N* shows the course of the sural nerve graft passed through the upper lip, *E* Design of the second operation, Arrow *M* shows the position of the muscle graft. *F* One month after the muscle transfer. No contraction of the muscle is shown. *G* One year after surgery. Static. *H* On smiling. Note active contraction of the muscle. *I* Eye closure achieved by temporal muscle transposition. *J* EMG led from the muscle

muscle isolated by a second team is then placed in position and its motor nerve is sutured to the refreshed stump of the grafted sural nerve. The nutrient vessels are simultaneously anastomosed to the recipient vessels. When reconstruction of eyelids is required, the conventional temporal muscle transfer is adopted. Using this new alternative, I have been able to obtain a more natural facial expression in cases of long-standing paralysis (Fig. 3).

## 2. Revascularization and Muscle Ischemic Time

It is considered that the shorter the ischemia time, the more degeneration of muscle tissues is minimized. In clinical cases, the muscle usually is revascularized within 90 minutes after clamping of its nutrient vessels. Well-experienced microvascular technique is required for this purpose. If the anastomotic site is patent for as long as seven postoperative days, random capillary connection from the surrounding tissues will occur.

## 3. Neural Neurotization

Smooth neurotization of the transferred muscle is required to help the muscle survive and recover its function. Funicular suture under magnification is applied to coapt the motor nerve of the transferred muscle with the recipient motor nerve. As many funiculi as possible should be coapted to restore sufficient muscle volume and cotractile power. To minimize the distance for regeneration of nerve fibers and obtain smooth innervation, the motor nerves are sutured as close as possible to the point of entry into the muscle.

## 4. Correct Tension

The transferred muscle should be fixed to the recipient bed under proper tension. Too much tension may produce an ischemic necrosis, while too little tension prevents beneficial muscle contracture. In clinical cases, it is actually difficult to decide the proper tension, but I myself strive to stretch the muscle belly to its original length. In cases of facial paralysis, however, the transferred muscle usually elongates due to gravitational pull and some part of the muscle should later be excised to obtain a beneficial contracture.

## Clinical Materials

In 35 clinical cases between September, 1973 and March, 1980, 37 muscle and musculocutaneous flaps were transferred to reconstruct paralyzed muscle function. Thirty-one muscles were applied to correct facial paralysis, while the remaining six muscles were used for extremity defects. Two extensor digitorum brevis muscles were transferred to the face, eight latissimus dorsi muscles (five muscles and three musculocutaneous flaps) were transferred to the face (five muscles and two musculocutaneous flaps) and to a lower extremity (one musculocutaneous flap), while the gracilis muscle was applied in all other cases (twenty-two gracilis muscles to the face, five gracilis musculocutaneous flaps to the extremities).

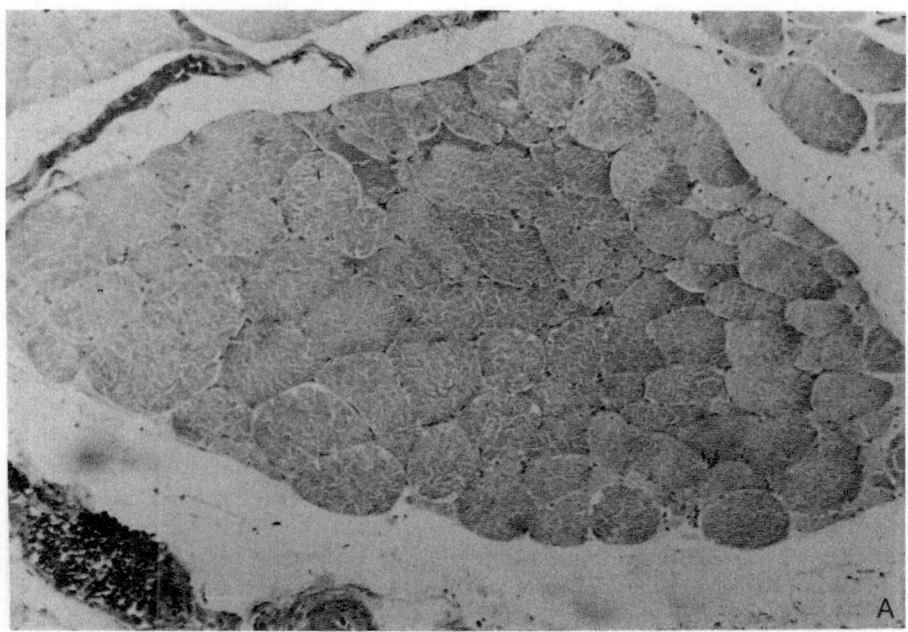

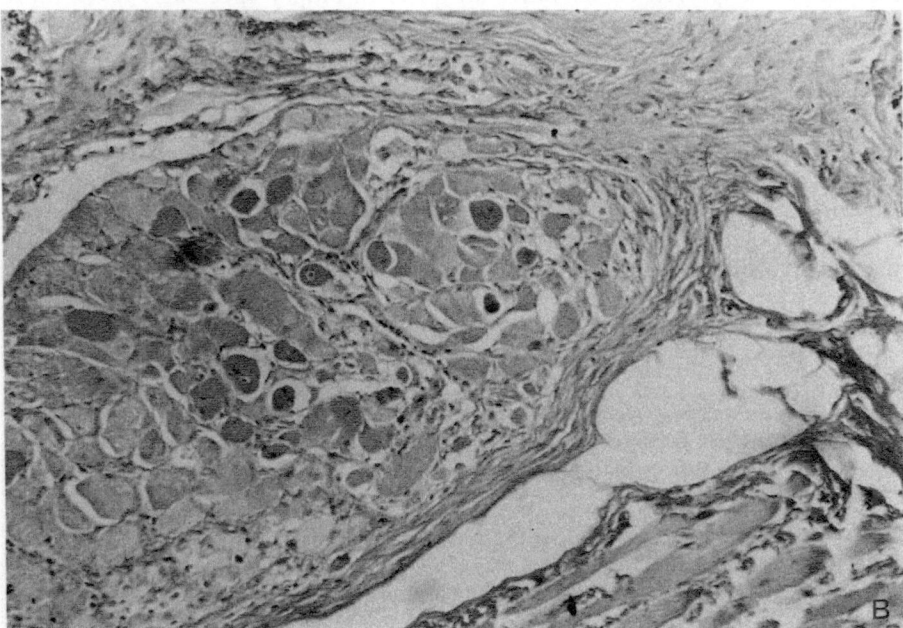

Fig. 4. Muscle biopsied at one year postoperatively. *A* Muscle fibers biopsied from the proximal part show almost normal structure and diameter. *B* Muscle fibers biopsied from the distal part show marked degenerative fibrosis

Of the thirty-one muscles transferred to the face in 29 clinical cases, one flap was lost shortly after the operation due to infection following thrombosis and the remaining thirty obtained initial survival. Three patients with three muscles could not be followed-up, and finally twenty-seven muscles in 25 cases were analyzed. In two of these cases, the initial muscle transferred could not acquire satisfactory contraction (although they had good static suspension), and subsequently additional muscles were transferred. All muscles other than these two showed active contraction.

The initial sign of functional recovery is a slight contraction or twitching of the muscle belly in the fifth or sixth postoperative month on the average. Patients feel some power developing in the cheek. The contractile power then increases up to the eight to tenth postoperative months. Within three to four postoperative months, atrophy of the muscle advances and no positive volitional spikes are displayed by the muscle. In the fifth to sixth postoperative months, an EMG recording of the proximal part of the muscle belly (close to the site of innervation) shows positive volitional spikes but low amplitude (less than 200 micronV) and fewer waves. Following the increase in acquired contraction during the subsequent 6 to 8 postoperative months, the EMG patterns come to display spikes of higher amplitude and evoked potentials are recorded.

Muscle fibers in specimens taken from the proximal part of the muscle in postoperative months 5 to 6 usually showed almost normal structures and diameters with only scattered areas of atrophy, while a large number of fibers in the distal part displayed degenerative atrophy. In biopsy specimens taken more than eight months postoperatively, proximal muscle fibers showed normal structure under light- and electron-microscopes, but a large number of distal muscle fibers had undergone degenerative atrophy and fibrosis. This distal part of the muscle functions like a tendon (Fig. 4).

In my clinical experiences, all transferred muscles lost their original contractile power and underwent a reduction in muscle belly volume during the period of reinnervation. I therefore recommend the transfer of a larger muscle in the case of a muscle defect which is expected to be reconstructed by neurovascular free muscle transfer.

### References

1. Tamai, S., et al.: Free muscle transplants in dogs, with microsurgical neurovascular anastomoses. Plast. Reconstr. Surg. 46, 219 (1970).
2. Volkmann, R.: Über die Regeneration des quergestreiften Muskelgewebes beim Menschen und Säughthier. Beitr. Path. Anat. 12, 233 (1893).
3. Harii, K., Ohmori, K., Torii, S.: Free gracilis muscle transplantation with microneurovascular anastomoses for the treatment of facial paralysis. Plast. Reconstr. Surg. 57, 133 (1976).
4. Ikuta, Y., et al.: Free muscle transplantation by microsurgical technique to treat severe Volkmann's contracture. Plast. Reconstr. Surg. 58, 407 (1976).
5. Manktelow, R. T., McKee, N.: Free muscle transplantation to provide active finger flexion. J. Hand Surg. 3, 416 (1978).
6. Anderl, H.: Reconstruction of the face through cross-face nerve transplantation in facial paralysis. Chir. Plastica 2, 46 (1973).

Author's address: K. Harii, M.D., Assoc. Professor, Department of Plastic Surgery, University of Tokyo, 7-3-1, Hongo, Bunkyo-ku, Tokyo.

## Discussion

*Tolhurst:* How long after the division of a facial nerve does the central stump of the facial nerve retain the ability to sprout axous?

*Harii:* The facial nerves continuously have the ability to sprout axons? I believe from my clinical experiments that 7 years after the lesion has occurred, regeneration can be expected.

*Freilinger:* How many negative results did you have in your cross-face nerve cases?

*Harii:* No negative case.

Question: The question is, how far are the facial nerve nuclei in the brain able to grow their axons? Much futher than the midline? Where is the limit? How far can these axons grow?

*Harii:* I don't know.

*Carlson:* Several years ago I did experiments on limb regeneration, in which I took the hands of salamanders and cut them off and sewed the wrists together. Then I allowed the nerves from one side to grow into the other limb, from which I had excised the nerves at the shoulder level. I found that the nerves could grow much further than their original length, but I don't know the limit.

*Millesi:* I think the Tinell sign is a quite good method for following clinically the regeneration in cross-face transplants. But it does not tell how many fibres are crossing the nerve graft. I must say that I have some good cases with the cross-face nerve grafts and some with poor results. So at this time I cannot answer the question about the value of the method.

# Our Experience With Free Muscle Nerve Graft in Facial Palsy

## Y. Botta-Kauer and D. Montandon

Unit of Plastic and Reconstructive Surgery,
Hôpital Cantonal de Genève, Switzerland

With 7 Figures

Indications for free muscle-nerve grafts in facial paralysis are limited to the long-standing palsy when the local muscles are atrophic and reinnervation is no longer possible. This includes paralysis of traumatic, tumoral and congenital origins. Considering the length of the operation, the importance of the surgical trauma and the long delay between the operation and the first sign of muscular action, we have never practiced this type of surgery on elderly patients or on patients with short life expectancy.

Since 1976 we have performed 6 free neuromuscular grafts with microsurgical anastomosis. Among these cases, 3 concerned patients with a longstanding facial palsy.

All free muscle-nerve grafts have been performed with two surgical teams and all the grafts survived.

## Case Reports

*1st case:* T. A., 10 years old

This child presented a right lower facial paralysis of congenital origin. There was marked asymmetry at rest and a complete absence of muscular contraction below the eyelid region (confirmed by electromyography) (Fig. 1).

A muscle-nerve graft was performed according to Thompson (1976) (Fig. 2). During the first operation a denervation of the extensors brevis pedis was carried out by sectioning the anterior tibial nerve about 10 cm above the ankle. A delay of the skin incision on the dorsum of the foot was also performed in order to obtain a better vascularisation of the flap for the second operation.

Two weeks later, the muscles and nerve were removed as a unit and transferred to the face.

The muscles bellies were attached to the orbicularis oris and their tendons to the zygomatic arch.

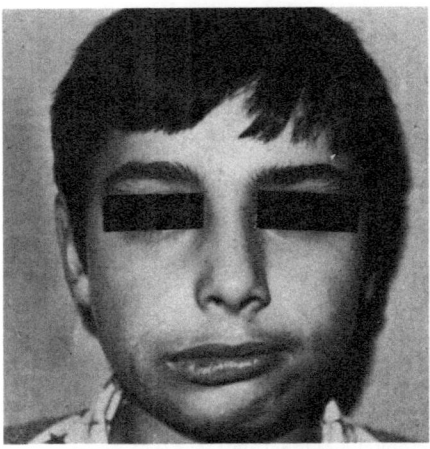

Fig. 1. Child T. A., 10 years old: 10 months after free muscle nerve graft according to Thompson for correction of complete right lower facial paralysis of congenital origin. At rest

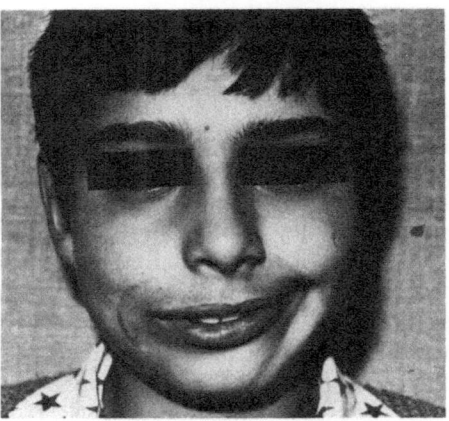

Fig. 2. Ten months after facial reanimation by Thompson free muscle-nerve graft, a voluntary contraction of the transferred muscle can be observed when the patient elevates the normal side of the mouth

    The nerve was brought through an upper labial tunnel to the sound side of the face and anastomosed at the level of the nasolabial fold to previously isolated facial nerve branches.

    At the same time some facial branches were divided in order to diminish the activity of the sound side.

    The postoperative course was uneventful. The young patient, living in a foreign country, was only seen for follow up after 10 months. At this moment the symmetry of the face is still not satisfactory, a voluntary contraction of the transferred muscle can be observed when the patient elevates the normal side of the mouth (Fig. 3).

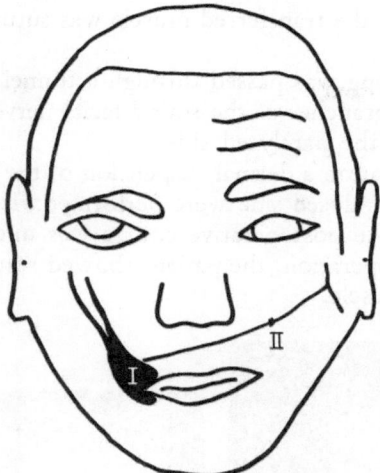

Fig. 3. Schema of the Thompson free muscle transfer technique (1976). The muscles bellies *(I)* were sutured to the angle of the mouth and the tendons to the zygomatic arch. The tibial nerve *(II)* is passed through a tunnel in the upper lip and sutured to some facial nerve branches of the sound side

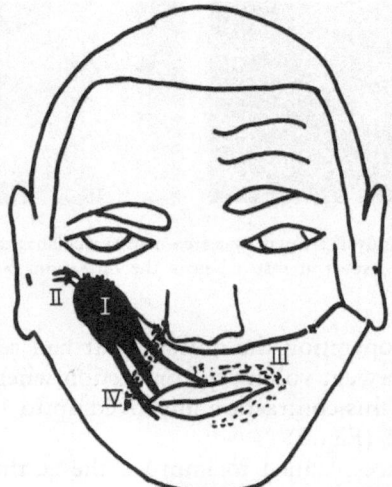

Fig. 4. Operative schema of the 2nd case. *I* muscles bellies; *II* micro vascular anastomosis; *III* nerve graft; *IV* dermal suspension at the nasolabial fold

*2nd case:* Mrs. A. R., 43 years old

This patient presented a complete upper and lower facial palsy, for more than 10 years diagnosed as a Bell's palsy.

In this patient we performed at the lower level in one operative session a cross-facial nerve graft and a free neuro-vascular transfer of the extensor brevis pedis (Fig. 4).

The muscle bellies were sutured to the zygomatic arch, and the tendons to the orbicularis of the lips.

The vascular pedicle of the transferred muscle was sutured to the temporalis superficialis vessels.

A nerve graft 18 cm long was passed through a tunnel in the upper lip and sutured to some isolated branches of the sound facial nerve and to the nerve of the transferred muscle at the paralysed side.

At the end of the operation a dermal suspension of the nasolabial fold and a hemifacial lifting of the paralysed side were performed. The total length of the operation was 7 hours. The postoperative course was uneventful.

Ten months after the operation, the patient showed some movements on the side of the transferred muscle.

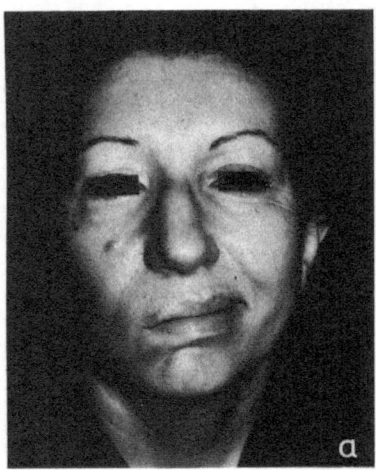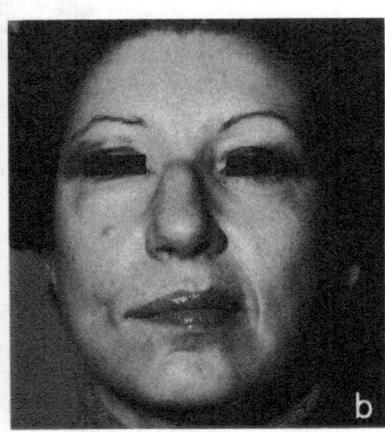

Fig. 5. Mrs. A. R.: Facial paralysis treated by a free neurovascular extensor brevis pedis transfer as shown in Fig. 4. Aspect at rest *a* before the operation, *b* 18 months after

One year after the operation the muscle graft had recuperated clinically its initial volume and underwent voluntary contraction when the patient attempted to smile. The power of this contraction improved up to 18 months after surgery and then became stable (Fig. 5).

Minor corrections are planned to improve the aesthetic result.

*3rd case:* Mrs. B. R., 33 years old

This patient presented a total right facial palsy of unknown origin since the age of 6.

In this case we performed in one operative session a free muscle transfer with a cross-facial innervation similar to the one described for the former patient.

The muscles bellies of the extensor digitorum brevis were sutured to the zygomatic arch and the tendons were inserted into the orbicularis of the sound side of the upper lip and angle of the mouth.

The microvascular anastomoses were performed with the temporal vessels. Twelve cm of the anterior tibial nerve had been removed with the muscle and passed through a tunnel in the upper lip. This nerve being too short for a direct

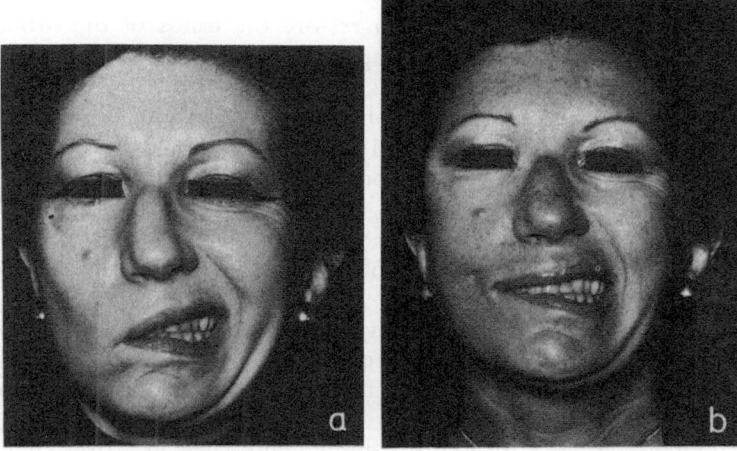

Fig. 6. On smiling *a* before the operation, *b* 18 months after

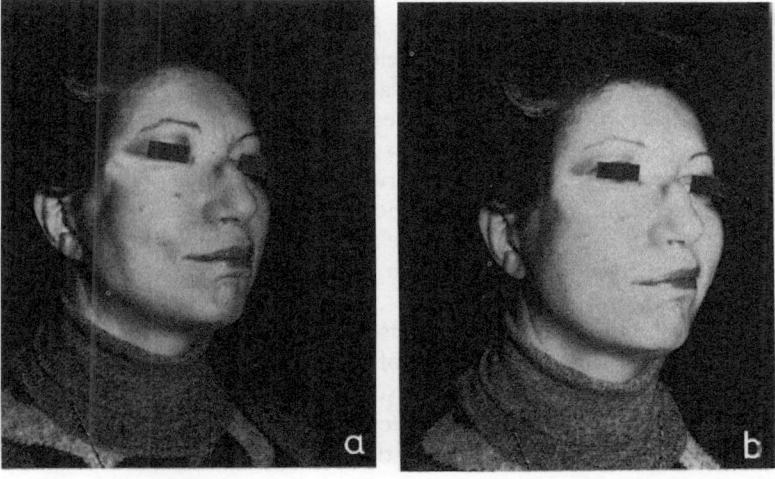

Fig. 7. Muscle volum and contraction power 18 months after a free neurovascular extensor brevis pedis transfer, *a* in contraction, *b* at rest

suture with the facial branches isolated at the sound side, it became necessary to interpose a nerve graft of 6 cm.

In the postoperative period, swelling of the right cheek and upper lip was followed by a purulent discharge. Despite local cleaning and antibiotic therapy, this infection lasted approximately 6 weeks.

One year after operation the muscle mass is still palpable, but there is no sign of muscular contraction.

## Discussion

The aims of facial reanimation are to restore the tonus of the orbicularis muscles, to obtain a good symmetrical appearance at rest and, if possible, a harmonious smile.

The physiological basis and the simplicity of the procedure described by Thompson and Gustavson (1976) (Fig. 1) is seductive, and in our case the transfer performed in a child shows a good muscular contraction.

Advantages of this method are:

1. reduced operative time and trauma;
2. more freedom in the positioning of the muscles by not having to care about their vascular pedicle.

The development of microvascular surgery has however made it possible the revascularisation of isolated muscles. It seems more logical and safer to attempt these anastomoses, than to expect the revival of the muscle by decreasing temporarily its metabolism.

This technique was used by Harii, Ohmori and Torii in 1976. They have published good results using a gracilis muscle graft vascularised by the temporal vessels and innervated by a cross-facial nerve graft.

Among the muscles which can be taken into consideration for the correction of facial palsy we have chosen the extensors digitalis brevis because their volume seems in better harmony with the slim faces of our patients. Moreover, the possibility of laying out several muscle bellies and tendons seems more appropriate for the replacement of the facial musculature than a single unit.

The contractile force of these muscles is good enough; complemented by partial denervation of the normal side as a result of the surgery, it will hopefully provide a satisfactory balance of the perioral region.

For practical reasons we have performed these operations in one session. We think however that it is more appropriate to do a cross-facial nerve graft during a first operation and a muscle graft with vascular anastomosis 6 months later. This will decrease the delay between the transfer of the muscle and its reinnervation and will diminish the phase of atrophy. It will also reduce the length of the operation and the degree of surgical trauma, which is a factor in the postoperative oedema and possible super-imposed infection.

Classical secondary palliative corrections can be always performed in addition to the muscle nerve graft either during the same operative session or at a later stage.

Although still in the experimental phase, the technique of cross-facial muscle nerve graft has given some good results and seems the most physiological for the reinnervation of long standing palsy.

### References

Harii, K., Ohmori, K., Torii, S.: Free gracilis muscle transplantation with microneurovascular anastomoses for the treatment of facial paralysis. A preliminary report. Plast. Reconstr. Surg. 57, 133–143 (1976).

Thompson, N., Gustavson, E. H.: The use of neuromuscular free autografts with microneural anastomoses to restore elevation to the paralysed angle of the mouth in cases of unilateral facial paralysis. Chir. Plast. (Berl.) 3, 165–174 (1976).

Author's address: Dr. Y. Botta-Kauer, 22, chemin Rieu, CH-1208 Genève, Switzerland.

## Discussion

*Harii:* The short extensor muscles of the toe have only a short excursion when they contract. So my impression is that this muscle is not able to give a balance for the strong force of the healthy contracting muscle in the face.

*Botta-Kauer:* Probably a strong muscle can give a better symmetry in collected cases, but in the cases I have shown, the patients had symmetrical balance of the muscles.

*Freilinger:* I would like to ask the anatomists—what is the best way of using a muscle, a partial muscle graft or a transposed masseter or temporalis muscle to get the best results?

*Grim:* I think, the gracilis muscle is very useful, because the motor-end-plates are spread along the whole muscle, which is very important for reinnervation of the muscle, as it had been demonstrated by Carlson.

# Restoration of Emotional Expression to the Unilaterally Paralysed Face

N. Thompson and C. B. Wynn Parry

Regional Plastic Surgery Centre,
Mount Vernon Hospital, Northwood, Middlesex,
and Royal National Orthopaedic Hospital,
London, England

With 9 Figures

Clinical and electromyographic evidence is submitted to support the thesis that facial reanimation in long-standing cases of unilateral facial paralysis is most effectively achieved by the use of autogenous skeletal muscle grafts, used either as free grafts or with microneural anastomosis only.

The facial nerve, supplying motor innervation to the muscles of facial expression, subserves three functions in the latter. First it preserves physiological muscle tone to maintain normal facial expression at rest; facial paralysis results in the characteristic atrophy and sagging of soft tissues on the affected side. Second, it provides a means of voluntary facial movement under conscious control. Third, it is the peripheral nervous mechanism producing the reflex involuntary movements associated with emotional expression.

In the history of the surgical treatment of unilateral facial paralysis the first function was restored by static supporting slings of fascia lata or tendon. The second function was later attempted by homolateral cross-nerve anastomosis of facial nerve with hypoglossal, accessory or phrenic nerves, or transposition of pedicled flaps of temporal or masseter muscle innervated by the trigeminal nerve and therefore producing movement synchronising with activity in the muscles of mastication. The third function of reflex emotional facial expression has however only been attempted in the past decade, by the use of cross-facial nerve grafts first reported by Scaramella in Chicago (1970) and later developed by Smith (1971) in New York and Anderl (1973) in Innsbruck, and also by the use of transplants of skeletal muscle either as free grafts (Thompson, 1971; 1974) or as one-stage pedicled flaps with microneurovascular anastomoses (Harii et al., 1976). These methods are alone in providing the potential means of producing in the unilaterally paralysed face, the bilateral, synchronous, symmetrical and spontaneous reflex (as well as volitional) movements of normal facial expression. But whereas the cross-facial nerve graft is best reserved for use in young patients and early cases of facial paralysis before irreversible atrophy and replacement fibrosis of the paralysed muscles of facial expression have occurred–preferably within a year of onset of the paralysis–free muscle grafts are applicable to such patients regardless of age or the duration of the paralysis.

The principles to be followed in the successful clinical application of free grafts of skeletal muscle initially promulgated (Thompson, 1971) remain in use. Thus:

1. The muscle graft is transplanted as a complete muscle belly to preserve full fibre length; in raising a muscle from its fleshy origin from bone this is not, of course, possible in absolute terms, but it is now known that damage to the distal extremities of muscle fibres has no ill-effects provided the central zone containing the motor endplates is preserved intact (Thompson *et al.*, 1978).

2. The muscle graft, carefully denuded of all fascia, fat and ligamentous tissue is sutured in direct contact with fully innervated and vascularized host muscle at the recipient site, from which revascularization and reinnervation of the graft proceeds.

3. The muscle graft is denervated 14 days before transfer. Although the effects of denervation are incompletely understood, it is known that it produces a change of muscle fibre metabolism reducing nutritional requirements (Hogan *et al.*, 1965; Romanul and Hogan, 1965); it also increases the effectiveness and speed of axonal regeneration (Gutmann, 1942; Ducker *et al.*, 1969; McQuarrie and Grafstein, 1973), as well as greatly improving the machinery of protein synthesis accompanying that process (Lieberman, 1971).

Free muscle grafts have been used to restore three reflex movements to the unilaterally paralysed face: to afford corneal protection and relieve conjunctivitis and blepharitis by restoring movement to the paralysed eyelids by reconstructing orbicularis oculi muscle activity; to restore sphincteric activity to the paralysed mouth by reconstructing the orbicularis oris muscle, to enable drinking of fluids without dribbling; and to restore spontaneous elevation to the paralysed elevators of the mouth, as in smiling, laughter etc.; where necessary all of these can be carried out simultaneously on the same patient. No need has been found to restore frontalis muscular activity to the forehead, provided the ptotic eyebrow is elevated by excision of a crescent of skin from above the eyebrow and an upper eyelid blepharoplasty is done to remove redundant skin.

## Operative Procedure

The muscles used as free grafts are the palmaris longus of the forearm and the extensor digitorum brevis of the foot. Both are readily accessible, dispensible in that they leave no residual dysfunction at the donor site, and of useful size for transplantation. The extensor digitorum brevis muscle is exceedingly versatile and adaptable in that it consists of four muscle bellies supplying the medial 4 toes, all of varying size so that by selecting one, two or all bellies a graft of appropriate volume can be applied, according to requirements. Denervation is carried out under a pneumatic tourniquet and employing a nerve stimulator,

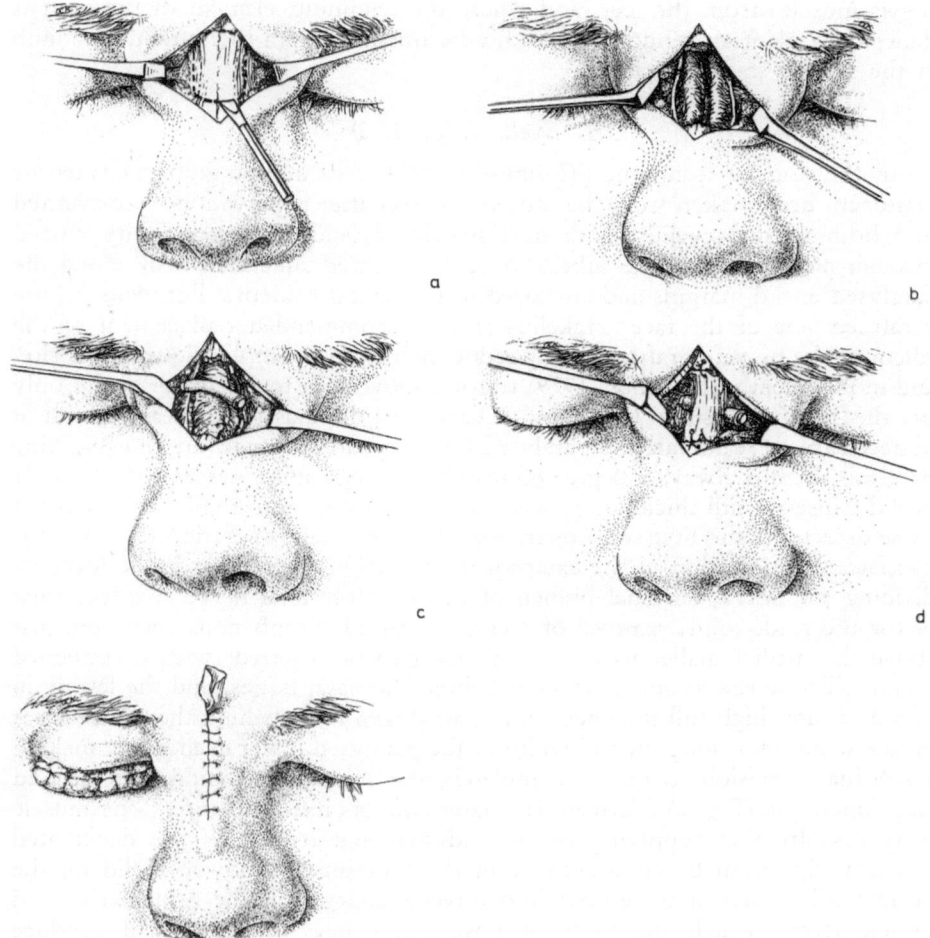

Fig. 1. First Stage Operation to correct unilateral paralysis of the eyelids. *a* An upper mid-line nasal incision is used. The nasal mucosa is widely infiltrated by intranasal injection of local anaesthetic to elevate it off the deep surface of the nasal bones, which can then be easily removed leaving intact nasal mucosa. *b* The intact domes of nasal mucosa displayed. The lateral nasal processes of maxilla will be removed by rongeurs to make a bed for the vein graft; the septal cartilage and vomer have already been removed anteriorly. *c* The nasal mucosal domes are plicated, and the vein graft enclosing a silicone rod space retainer, placed obliquely from lower canthus on the normal side to upper canthal ligament on the paralysed side. *d* The nasal bones after selective removal of bone overlying the vein graft are replaced. If unstable they can be retained accurately in position by suture. *e* The wound closed with drainage. The paralysed lower eyelid, after a transverse incision completely relieving ectropion, has a full thickness post-auricular skin graft inserted into the defect: here shown with dressing in position retained by classical tie-over sutures

care being taken to make the denervation complete and to preserve the blood supply intact, and the graft is transplanted fourteen days later. If the palmaris longus muscle is absent, it may be necessary to use both extensor digitorum brevis muscles from the feet, and where the tendinous element of the graft is deficient, a plantaris tendon can readily be obtained from the same donor limb at the second stage operation.

## 1. Eyelid (Figs. 1, 2)

In the original technique (Thompson, 1974) free muscle grafts of extensor digitorum brevis taken from the foot at 2 weeks after denervation were inserted into both normal eyelids, and their associated tendons in continuity passed through post-nasal silicone tubes, to be transmitted subcutaneously along the paralysed eyelid margins and anchored to the lateral palpebral ligaments on the paralysed side of the face. Hakelius (1974) recommended replacement of the silicone tube by vein grafts, thereby reducing infective complications at this site, and more recently (Hakelius, 1979) restores movement to the upper eyelid only on the paralysed side. Like him I have for the past two years found it unnecessary to reanimate the paralysed lower eyelid, but since in long-standing paralysis there is always a degree of atrophy and ectropion present in the lower eyelid I insert a full thickness post-auricular skin graft into the latter to correct these defects, at the first stage operation. The first stage operation (Fig. 1) thus consists of denervation of the extensor digitorum brevis muscle in the foot, by dividing the lateral terminal branch of the anterior tibial nerve at a level just below the ankle joint, removal of 4 cms, of the long saphenous vein from just above the medial malleolus of the same leg to be inserted (with a contained 3 mm. silicone rod as space retainer) behind the nasal bones, and the letting in of a 3–5 mm. high full thickness skin graft (taken from behind the adjacent ear on the same side) along the full width of the paralysed lower eyelid after making a subciliary incision to relieve completely the existing ectropion. The second stage operation (Fig. 2) fourteen days later consists in transplanting one muscle belly (usually that supplying the second toe) and tendon of the denervated extensor digitorum brevis muscle from the foot into the lower eyelid on the normal side where it is sutured into direct contact with the orbicularis oculi muscle (from which ingrowth of host axons into the graft will produce reinnervation) while the tendon of the graft is passed through the retro-nasal vein graft and across the full width of the paralysed upper eyelid to be sutured to the lateral palpebral ligament on the paralysed side.

## 2. Oral Sphincter (Fig. 3)

The palmaris longus muscle is still preferred (Thompson, 1971), the muscle belly being split along the length of its fibres up to its tendinous attachment. Using small local incisions just lateral to each angle of the mouth the skin of both lips is undermined by blunt scissors dissection across their full width, and half the muscle belly is inserted into each lip so as to completely surround the mouth. The muscle graft is sutured to local soft tissues at each extremity, so that when the tendon in continuity is slung from the zygomatic arch on the paralysed side (exposed through a pre-auricular incision) under positive tension to correct the static droop of the paralysed angle of mouth, the pull exerted is not transmitted to the muscle graft which is preserved under "normal" tension.

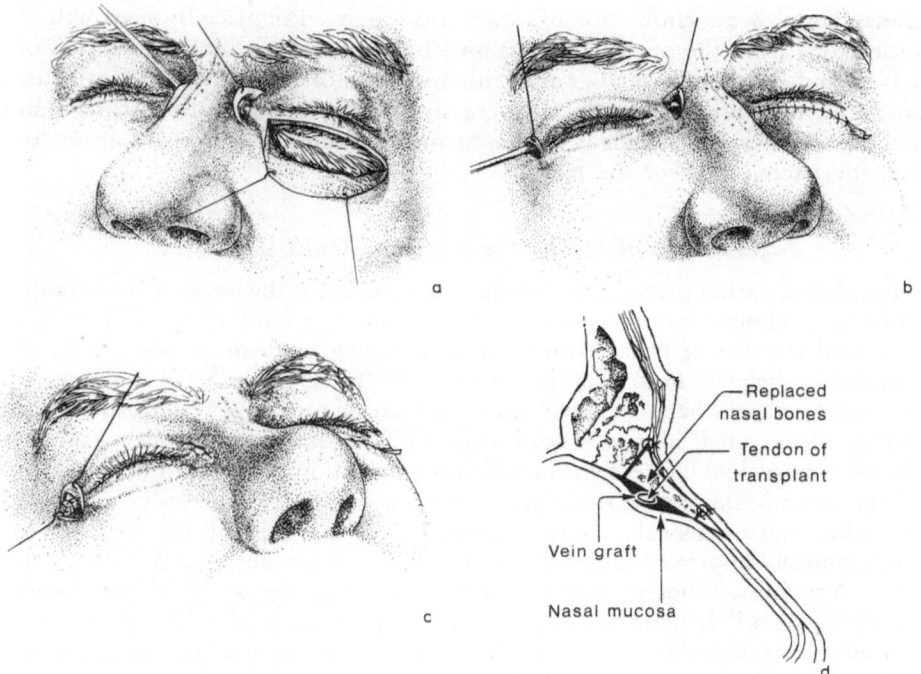

a                                                                                b

c                                                                                d

Fig. 2. Second stage operation to correct unilateral paralysis of the eyelids. *a* The skin graft to the paralysed (right) lower eyelid has completely corrected the ectropion of this eyelid. The normal lower eyelid (left) has been reflected as a musculocutaneous flap, the 2nd belly of the denervated extensor digitorum brevis muscle has been inserted and sutured to the deep surface of the orbicularis oculi muscle; the silicone rod spacer has been removed, and the graft tendon has been passed through the post-nasal vein graft. *b* The tendon of the graft has been passed onwards beneath the skin of the right eyelid at the level of the upper border of the tarsal plate. *c* The tendon of the graft is anchored by suture to the lateral palpebral ligament on the paralysed side. The bed in which the muscle graft is placed is drained for 24–48 hours. *d* A sagittal section shows the siting of the graft tendon, behind the nasal bones, lying on nasal mucosa in the plane of the eyelids

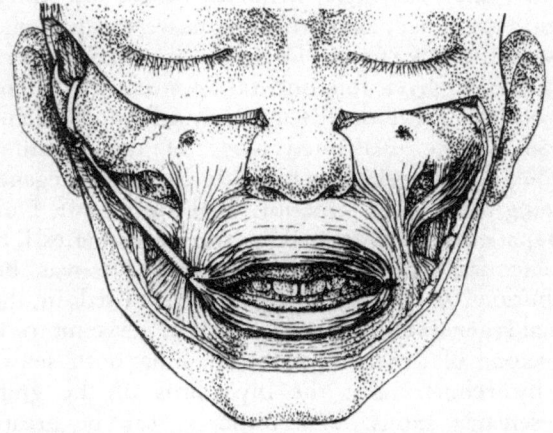

Fig. 3. Diagrammatic representation of palmaris muscle graft to reconstruct the oral sphincter. [By courtesy of Plast. Reconstr. Surg. *48*, 167 (1971)]

Reinnervation of the entire circum-oral muscle graft takes place by ingrowth of motor axons from the orbicularis oris muscle fibres on the unparalysed side of the face, and serial electromyographic investigations of the muscle graft over the next 3 to 9 months demonstrates a progressive wave of reinnervation of the graft on the paralysed side which is maximum near the mid-line but progresses to reach the lateral angle of the mouth.

### 3. Elevation of the Angle of the Mouth (Fig. 5)

In cases of partial paralysis of the elevator muscles of the angle of the mouth, considerable clinical improvement can be obtained by reinforcing the partially denervated muscles of facial expression by applying to them an onlay graft of denervated skeletal muscle (Thompson, 1974). The graft of previously denervated extensor hallucis brevis muscle is sutured into direct contact with the partially denervated levator anguli oris and zygomaticus muscles exposed through a nasolabial incision, from which reinnervation of the graft occurs. The graft gives static support to the slightly drooping angle of the mouth by passing its tendon subcutaneously to be anchored to the temporal fascia. Electromyographically improved muscle activity at the graft site becomes demonstrable after 3–6 months. Where, however, the paralysis is of appreciable degree (more than 80%) then it is better to employ a neuromuscular graft with microneural anastomosis, as described below, to add an element of "neural" neurotization to the "muscular" neurotization of the graft, with correspondingly improved contractile function in the graft resulting from the dual mode of reinnervation. The technique for using such neuromuscular grafts is given below.

In its original form (Thompson and Gustavson, 1976) the use of a composite neuromuscular graft with its motor nerve of supply in continuity with the graft, consisted of one, or at most two bellies of the extensor digitorum brevis muscle taken as a composite transplant together with 10 cms. of its attached anterior tibial nerve, at two weeks after preliminary denervation. The muscular element of the graft was inserted into the paralysed cheek through a nasolabial incision to be sutured to the paralysed angle of mouth below and slung by its tendon from the zygomatic arch above, after which its nerve was passed subcutaneously across the full width of the upper lip as a cross-facial nerve graft for its constituent fasciculi to be given microneural anastomosis to terminal filaments of the contralateral facial nerve on the unparalysed side, which on stimulation produced elevation of the unaffected angle of the mouth on that side. Reinnervation of the muscle graft then followed by axonal regeneration of facial nerve axons replacing those in the anterior tibial nerve graft. During the period 1975 to 1978, 34 patients were treated in this way (Series I below) but the results, though encouraging, were disappointing. It was believed that a significant contribution to the mediocre results existed in the difficulty of ensuring that axonal regeneration by invading facial nerve motor axons replacing the degenerating axons of a nerve graft containing both sensory and motor elements, ended by reinnervating the myofibrils of the graft and not by replacing useless sensory axons. This difficulty can be greatly reduced by locating the distribution and predominance of motor axons in the nerve graft

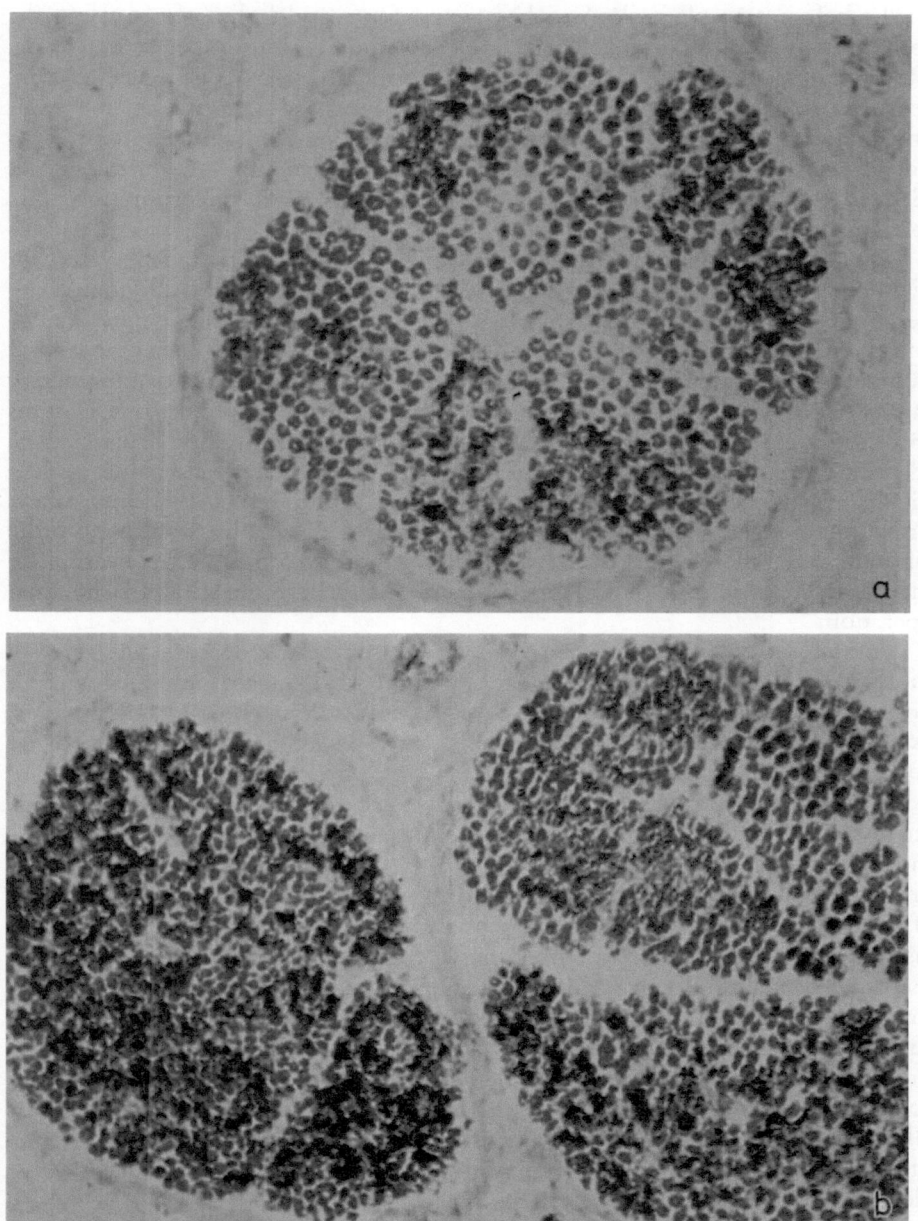

Fig. 4. Cross-sections of fasciculi of anterior tibial nerve stained for acetylcholinesterase. *a* Motor axon content about 30 %. Not used for microneural anastomosis. *b* Two fasciculi, one containing 35 % and the other 50 % of motor axons. These were used for microneural anastomosis

fasciculi by taking an anterior tibial nerve biopsy at the time of denervation (two weeks before transplantation) to be stained for acetylcholinesterase using the technique of Karnovsky and Roots (1964) as modified by Gruber *et al.* (1971). Motor axons take up the brown stain (Fig. 4) and are clearly distinguished from sensory axons which remain unstained. Only those fasciculi in the graft containing the greatest concentration of motor axons are selected for microneural anastomosis to contralateral facial nerve fasciculi. A further series (Series II) was completed in the period 1978–1979, incorporating this refinement, as described below.

The extensor digitorum brevis muscle of the foot is first denervated by dividing the anterior tibial nerve at a level 10 cms. above the ankle joint. The nerve after exposure is lifted from its bed, the epineureum slit longitudinally, and the nerve trunk carefully split into its constituent fasciculi–usually 3 to 5 in number; an optical loupe is helpful but the operating microscope is unnecessary at this stage. Each individual fasciculus is then labelled by applying to it ligatures (5/0 Supramid) one or two or three etc. in number to allow later specific identification of each at the second stage operation. Each fasciculus is then divided proximal to the identifying sutures at two levels 1–2 cms. apart, providing biopsies which are placed in separate frozen containers and sent to the laboratory for acetylcholinesterase staining of motor axons. Weight bearing on the operated foot is avoided for 10 days, and kept minimal until the final operation.

At the second operation 2 weeks later, two teams of surgeons operate simultaneously, one working on the foot and the second team (equipped with an operating microscope) on the face. At the lower limb site, a long incision extends from the previous incision 10 cms. above the ankle joint along the distal course of the anterior tibial nerve and onto the dorsum of the foot to allow exposure of the extensor digitorum brevis muscle bellies; four separate small incisions over the roots of the medial four toes are used to divide the associated short extensor tendons from their points of insertion, which are then mobilised proximally to present in the main wound. The site of earlier section and biopsy of the nerve is dissected free, carefully preserving the identifying sutures on each fascicle, and the distal anterior tibial nerve dissected free from its bed between the extensor hallucis longus and tibialis anterior muscles, then from beneath the former's tendon at the level of the ankle joint, to its termination on the deep surface of the extensor digitorum brevis muscle on the dorsum of the foot. The medial sensory terminal division of the nerve supplying the first interdigital web space is divided 2 cms. from its origin, and the entire tissue block consisting of all 4 bellies of extensor digitorum brevis muscle and their tendons, with 12 cms. of nerve trunk in continuity, removed for transplantation to the face, after cleansing it of all fascia, fat etc. (Fig. 5).

Meanwhile, the team working on the face has through bilateral nasolabial incisions prepared a bed for the muscle graft overlying the zygomaticus muscles on the paralysed side of the face, and dissected out the terminal filaments of the buccal branch of the facial nerve on the contralateral (normal)side. These lie on a deep plane and are located at the lateral border of the zygomaticus muscles entering their deep surface. Usually 2 to 4 nerve filaments are found which on electrical stimulation cause elevation of the adjacent angle of mouth, and all can be safely divided and their central ends used for microanastomosis to fasciculi in the nerve graft, selecting those with a high concentration of motor axons (as disclosed by acetylcholinesterase staining of the earlier nerve biopsy) for this purpose. Microdissection is used to locate the labelling sutures on the constituent fasciculi of the anterior tibial nerve graft, and usually 2 or 3 of these (Fig. 4) have been reported on by the histologist as containing a major content of motor axons. No discoverable weakness of the normal side of the face has resulted from using all available facial nerve filaments as donors for reinnervation: indeed the overactivity of contralateral muscles in cases of

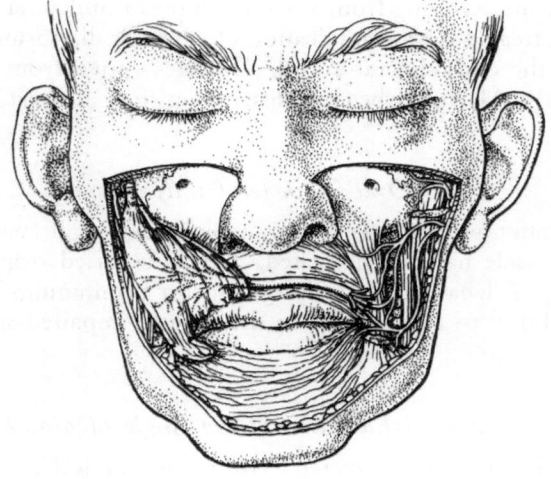

Fig. 5. Diagrammatic illustration of extensor digitorum brevis muscle graft (from right foot) inserted into paralysed right face. All 4 muscle bellies are used, with the tendons slung from the zygomatic region above by suture to fascia and periosteum, and the muscle bellies sutured to the angle of mouth below by their ligamentous origins. The nerve graft of anterior tibial nerve is passed subcutaneously to the left face, where three fasciculi of high motor axon content are given microneural suture to terminal filaments of the contralateral facial nerve: nerve graft fasciculi of low motor axon content are left unused

unilateral facial paralysis is decreased by this selective neurectomy and so improves the final overall clinical result. It is rare for the sensory division fasciculi (in the medial terminal branch) of the anterior tibial nerve graft to be separable from the main nerve trunk due to the large number of intercommunicating nerve filaments existing between the two; usually, therefore, the sensory branch is implanted into the muscle graft to allow any transmitted motor axons to play their part in reinnervation of the graft myofibrils. The microneural anastomosis is by perineural atraumatic 10/0 nylon sutures. The nasolabial incisions are closed with suction drainage to the recipient site of the muscle graft only, and elastoplast pressure to both cheeks and upper lip is maintained for 5 days.

In a final series (Series 3), in an attempt to assess whether the clinical results in the neuromuscular grafts with microneural anastomosis might be improved by the addition of a microvascular anastomosis at the same operation, the procedure described above was repeated in detail but with the anterior tibial artery and vein included as graft constituents at the time of transplantation to be given end-to-end microvascular anastomosis to the facial artery and vein on the paralysed side.

## Clinical Material and Methods
### 1. Eyelid Paralysis

Sixty-two patients suffering from a major degree of unilateral paralysis of the eyelids have been treated by the application of extensor digitorum brevis muscle grafts applied to the contralateral eyelid. The ages varied from 10 to 74 years (average 30 years). All have been followed up for at least 2 years post-operatively.

### 2. Oral Sphincter Paralysis

Forty-nine patients suffering from major unilateral paralysis of the orbicularis oris muscle have been treated. The ages varied from 7 to 70 years (average 28 years). All have been followed up for a minimum of 2 years. All suffered from inability to retain fluids in the mouth, impaired speech, or both.

### 3. Paralysis of Elevation of the Angle of Mouth

*a) Series I.* These were treated over the period 1974–8 with a neuromuscular composite graft of extensor digitorum brevis muscle and anterior tibial nerve, with microneural anastomosis only, and no histochemical localization of motor axons in the graft fasciculi. Of the thirty-four patients in this group, 14 were male and 20 female. The age varied from 9 to 59 years (average 26 years), and the duration of paralysis from 2 to 27 years (average 9.6 years). The causes of paralysis were Bell's palsy (11), congenital (7), fractured base of skull (4), cerebral tumour (5), mastoidectomy (3), an 1 case each of parotidectomy, buccal epithelioma, and cholesteatoma; in 1 case the cause was unknown.

*b) Series II* (Table 1). Ten patients were dealt with as in Series I, by composite neuromuscular grafts of extensor digitorum brevis and anterior tibial nerve, but with the addition of histochemical localization of motor axons in the nerve graft fasciculi. The average age was 23.8 years, and the duration of paralysis 14.7 years.

The laboratory procedure was as follows: the nerve biopsies are transported frozen to the inner walls of glass containers placed in a thermos flask of ice, with each biopsy in an individual receptacle labelled with the number of the fasciculus (1 to 5) in the nerve trunk. The specimen is embedded in gelatine oriented vertically, frozen using $CO_2$ snow, and accurate transverse sections are cut at 8 microns thickness. The sections are fixed in formalin and incubated for

Table 1. (series II) *Muscle-nerve* grafts with microneural anastomoses only (using cholinesterase staining)

| CASE | AGE (YEARS) | CAUSE OF PARALYSIS | DURATION OF PARALYSIS (YEARS) | DEGREE OF PARALYSIS |
|---|---|---|---|---|
| 1.  LS | 9 | Excision lymphangioma cheek | 8 | Complete |
| 2.  JD | 17 | Cholesteatoma | 15 | Partial |
| 3.  RF | 51 | Rad. Mastoidectomy | 42 | Partial |
| 4.  NB | 18 | Bells Palsy | 6 | Partial |
| 5.  OSY | 33 | Congenital | 33 | Partial |
| 6.  MA | 10 | Cholesteatoma | 6 | Partial |
| 7.  KC | 41 | Radical Parotidectomy | 9 | Complete |
| 8.  DH | 35 | Fract. Base Skull. | 4 | Partial |
| 9.  ME | 14 | Congenital | 14 | Partial |
| 10.  SM | 10 | Congenital | 10 | Partial |

Table 2. (series III) *Muscle grafts* with microneuro-vascular anastomoses (using cholinesterase staining)

| CASE | AGE (YEARS) | CAUSE OF PARALYSIS | DURATION OF PARALYSIS | DEGREE OF PARALYSIS |
|---|---|---|---|---|
| 1.  MM | 48 | Acoustic neuroma | 5 | Complete |
| 2.  CG | 34 | Bells Palsy | 4½ | Partial |
| 3.  NS | 24 | Excision haemangioma | 18 | Partial |
| 4.  JC | 26 | Congenital | 26 | Complete |
| 5.  AT | 29 | Mastoidectomy | 13 | Partial |
| 6.  PH | 37 | Bells Palsy | 10 | Partial |
| 7.  GD | 19 | Congenital | 19 | Partial |
| 8.  CL | 22 | Congenital | 22 | Complete |
| 9.  PC | 45 | Congenital | 45 | Complete |
| 10.  MW | 29 | Mastoidectomy | 29 | Partial |

4 hours at 37°C in a phosphate buffered solution of acetylcholinesterase iodide, trisodium citrate, cupric sulphate and potassium ferricyanide (Karnovsky and Roots, 1974). The sections are counterstained with Mayers haemalum; motor axons contain acetylcholinesterase and are stained brown in the centre of the myelin sheath while nuclei are stained blue. An axon count allows expression of motor axon content of each fasciculus as a percentage (Fig. 4).

c) *Series III* (Table 2). Three of my registrars at Mount Vernon Hospital treated 10 patients as in Series II, but added to the microneural anastomosis an immediate restoration of vascular circulation to the muscle graft by micro-surgical anastomosis of the anterior tibial vessels of the graft to facial vessels at the recipient site (Mayou *et al.*, 1981). The grafts had undergone preliminary denervation 2 weeks before transplantation, and microneural anastomosis with the assistance of acetylcholinesterase localization of motor axons in the nerve graft to enhance reinnervation. It was hoped to establish whether the immediate restoration of blood circulation in the graft at the time of transfer (as opposed to the more gradual establishing of circulation in the graft by direct anastomosis of the graft and host vessels during the 72 hours following transfer to be subsequently reinforced by the direct ingrowth of host vessels) assisted its survival with consequent improvement in clinical results.

The patients in Series III were comparable to Series II in average age (31 years as compared with 24 years) and average duration of paralysis (19 years as compared with 15 years).

*Clinical Assessment* is based upon serial photographs at rest and on voluntary movements beginning with preoperative views and continuing at three monthly intervals throughout the period of follow-up, combined with the personal reactions of the patient. The results are classified into 3 groups:

*1. Good.* There is loss of chief complaint, and restoration of function to essentially normal levels. Eyelids lose all signs of irritation and epiphora, and are capable of complete voluntary occlusion of the palpebral fissure. The mouth sphincter is quite competent, there is no dribbling of fluids, and speech is restored to normal. In cases treated by neuromuscular grafts to restore elevation to the angle of mouth on smiling, the range of muscular movement restored is in excess of 50% of normal.

*2. Improved.* Here the improvement in function and loss of complaints is distinct and appreciable, but short of restoration to normal. In the eyelids epiphora is minimal and they lack only 2–3 mms. of full voluntary occlusion; there is complete corneal protection and major relief of irritation. In the mouth dribbling of fluids is eliminated almost if not absolutely completely, but the force of sphincter contraction is distinctly less than normal. In the cases of neuromuscular grafts to restore elevation to the angle of the mouth there is distinct improvement but the improved muscular activity is only 20%–40% of normal.

*3. Unimproved.* There is no improvement in muscular activity or relief of complaints, but the patients state is not worsened. The commonest cause is failure of graft take due to failure to develop an anastomotic vascular circulation by connection of graft with host vessels in the bed on which the graft is placed at the recipient site, or failure of reinnervation.

*Electromyography* has been carried out in selected cases throughout all varieties of paralysis, but those patients with paralysis of the elevators of the angle of mouth, in Series II and III have received particularly intensive study, reported below in detail.

Concentric electrodes were inserted into the muscle grafts at the recipient site. Spontaneous activity was looked for at rest in the form of fibrillation and the patient was then asked to attempt voluntary contraction as in smiling, showing the teeth and grimacing, and photographic records were made of any volitional activity that ensued. Amplitudes and duration and number of units were recorded. In addition the nerve was stimulated electrically both at the microneural anastomosis and the stylo-mastoid foramen on the contra-lateral (unparalysed) side in an attempt to obtain a motor conduction velocity.

## Results

### Eyelid Paralysis (Fig. 6)

Of 62 patients treated, the results were Good in 32 (51.6%), Improved in 23 (37.1%) and Unimproved in 7 (11.3%). Complications followed in 6 patients (9.6%) consisting of graft absorption in 3, tendon necrosis inside the vein graft in 1, and infection in 2. Secondary operations were required in 18 patients

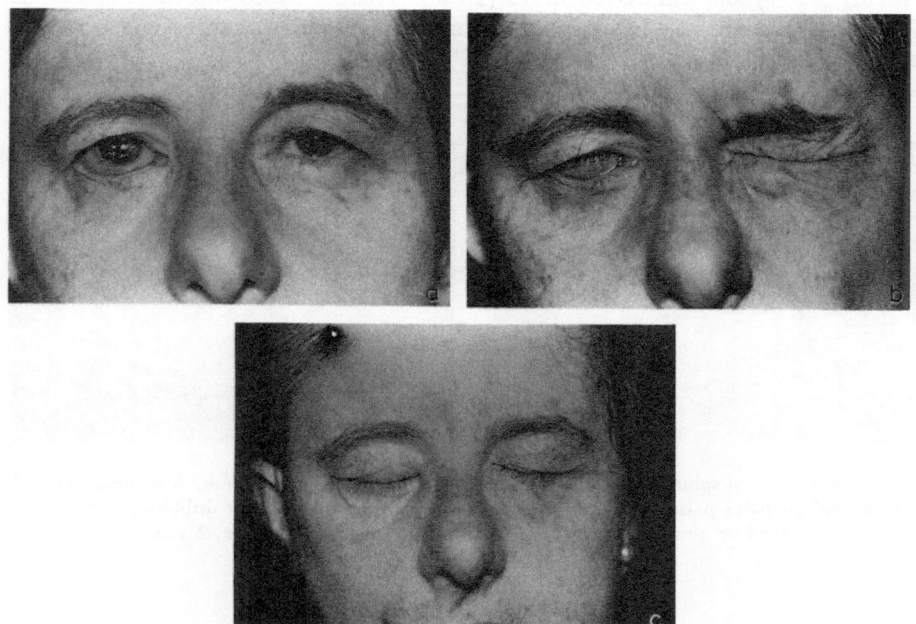

Fig. 6. Paralysed eyelids treated by muscle grafts. A woman, age 50, with unresolved Bell's palsy of 10 years' duration. Severe corneal ulceration so impaired vision that a corneal graft had been applied. *a* Preoperative. At rest. Corneal graft in situ. *b* Pre-operative. On attempted closure of eyelids. *c* Post-operative, 2 years, following insertion of full thickness skin graft to correct ectropion of lower eyelid, and insertion of extensor digitorum brevis muscle graft into the left lower eyelid, its tendon inserted into paralysed right upper eyelid

(29%) and consisted of tenolysis to free tendons at the post-nasal site or tightening of tendons in 12 patients (19%), replacement of the absorbed muscle graft by a new graft in 3 (4.8%); in 3 patients an upper eyelid blepharoplasty and raising of the eyebrow (by excision of a crescent of skin from above the eyebrow) was carried out to improve cosmetic appearance.

The appearance was satisfactory and accepted by the patient in the great majority of cases, although minor asymmetry of the palpebral fissures between the two sides was not infrequent, but in only 3 patients was it of sufficient degree to warrant a secondary operation to attempt correction.

## Oral Sphincter Reconstruction (Fig. 7)

Fifty-seven patients have been treated and followed up. Of these 49 received palmaris longus grafts, but in the remaining 8 patients no palmaris longus muscle was found on clinical examination and the extensor digitorum brevis muscle of the foot was used in association with the plantaris tendon (or in 1 patient where this was not present, an extensor digitorum longus tendon) to sling the graft up to the zygomatic arch. The results were classified as Good in 30 patients (52%) and Improved in 15 (26%). There was no improvement in 12 (22%) and in 2 of these fibrotic contracture of the graft was sufficient to require later division of the constricting bands.

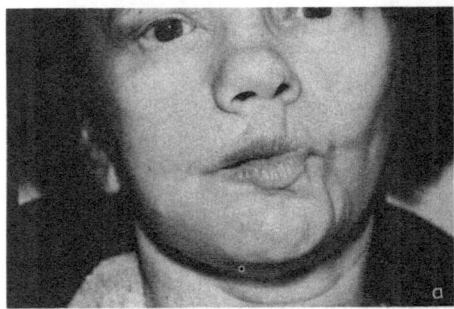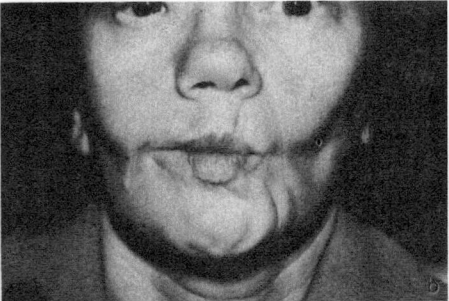

Fig. 7. Paralysed oral sphincter reconstructed by palmaris longus muscle graft. A woman, aged 58, with unresolved Bell's palsy of 12 years' duration, suffering from constant dribbling of fluids and saliva on pursing the lips: *a* Pre-operative. *b* Post-operative, 2 years

## Elevation of Angle of Mouth

*Series I* (Fig. 8 a, b). In the 34 patients in this group observed for periods of 1 to 4 years postoperatively, clinical assessment showed Good results in 9 (26.5%) and Improvement in 9 (26.5%). This left 16 patients (47%) unimproved. It was noteworthy that in this group treated by microsurgery in the early days following the introduction of this technique into the Mount Vernon Hospital plastic surgery centre, the complication rate was high (18%): infection in 5 and haematoma in 1, all the more important since in such cases graft failure was usual. With increasing experience however the complication rate has been reduced to 8% in the last 20 cases treated, a trend improved by reduction of operating time at the second staged operation from 6 hours in the early cases, to 2½ hours (with two teams of surgeons) in the most recent. It is also noteworthy that progressive improvement results from more prolonged follow-up. It is usual in successful cases to find the Tinel sign positive on percussion over the point of microneural suture after 2 or 3 months, and clinical movement at the muscle graft site to be established by 6 months, increasing steadily up to 1 year. It is however by no means rare to find clinically increasing movement progressing for up to 2 years.

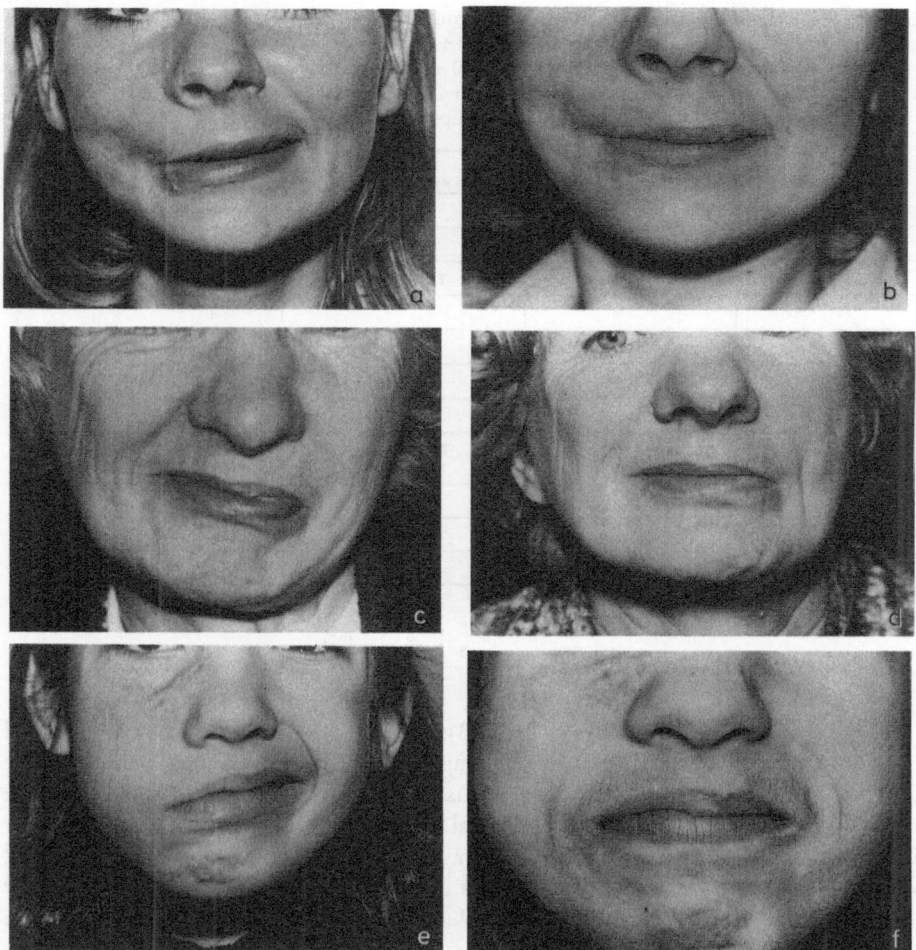

Fig. 8. Patients illustrating use of neuromuscular grafts of extensor digitorum brevis muscle and anterior tibial nerve grafts with microneural anastomosis to correct paralysis of elevators of the angle of the mouth. Activity illustrated in all photographs during the act of smiling. *a* Series I. Woman aged 27, with paralysis of right lower face following receipt of fractured base of skull in a road traffic accident 8 years earlier. Pre-operative. *b* Post-operative, 1 year. Scarring of lower lip relieved by small skin graft. Note that loss of right nasolabial groove is traumatic in origin, was present pre-operatively, and is not due to the muscle graft inserted at this site. *c* Series II. Case 3. Woman aged 51. Paralysis of left face following mastoidectomy at age 9 years. Pre-operative. *d* Post-operative 1¹/₂ years. *e* Series II. Case 1. Girl age 9 years. Complete paralysis of lower right face following excision of lymphangeoma of cheek in infancy at age 6 months. (Confirmed by EMG) *f* Post-operative 2 years

Further improvement in results became evident in Series II and III, probably attributable to the preliminary histochemical identification of motor axons allowing microsuture of fasciculi containing increased concentrations of motor axons, thus improving reinnervation of the graft.

Table 3. (series II) *Muscle-nerve* grafts with microneural anastomoses only (using cholinesterase staining). In column 4, note that: EMG results: + = one or two units firing in muscle graft. ++ = several units firing. Cases 1, 3, 5, 8 and 10 showed activity in muscle graft on stimulation of contra-lateral (normal) facial nerve, but no activity on stimulation of homolateral facial nerve. Clinical results: + = Improved. ++ = Good

| CASE | PERIOD FOLLOW-UP (MONTHS) | COMPLICATIONS | RESULTS EMG | RESULTS CLINICAL |
|---|---|---|---|---|
| 1. LS | 25 | | ++ | ++ |
| 2. JD | 18 | Infection | + | 0 |
| 3. RF | 18 | | + | + |
| 4. NB | 15 | | + | 0 |
| 5. OSY | 14 | | + | + |
| 6. MA | 12 | | + | ++ |
| 7. KC | 9 | Haematoma Infection | 0 | 0 |
| 8. DH | 9 | | ++ | ++ |
| 9. ME | 8 | | 0 | 0 |
| 10. SM | 8 | | + | + |

GOOD RESULT 3 ⎫
IMPROVED 3 ⎬ 6 = 60%

*Series II* (Figs. 8 c, d, e, f and Table 3). In this group of 10 patients followed up for periods of 8 to 25 months (average 13.6 months) all four bellies of the denervated extensor digitorum brevis muscle were utilised in the transplant with microneural anastomosis of contralateral facial nerve filaments to the anterior tibial nerve graft after acetylcholinesterase localisation of motor axons. Blood supply to the transplant was derived as a direct anastomotic circulation from the host tissues in the graft recipient site. Clinical examination showed that 60% were benefitted, equally divided between Good and Improved. Two patients suffered complications from infection (one at the site of a haematoma). The correlation between clinical and electromyographic findings was complete except in 2 patients where EMG volitional activity is not clinically evident at 15 to 18 months follow-up, and may well therefore become so over a further period of time. This conjecture is reinforced by the presence of a positive "Tinel" sign on percussion over the microneural anastomosis in all patients except the 2 failing to demonstrate any EMG activity in the graft (cases 7 and 9). It will be seen that the bilateral nasolabial incisions (Fig. 8) leave essentially inobvious scars, and are, I believe, to be preferred to the muco-cutaneous incisions advocated by Freilinger (see elsewhere in this volume).

## Electromyography

In Table 3 demonstrating the results of electromyography compared with clinical findings, + indicates one or two units firing: ++ indicate several units firing. In all cases the amplitudes and the motor units action potential varied

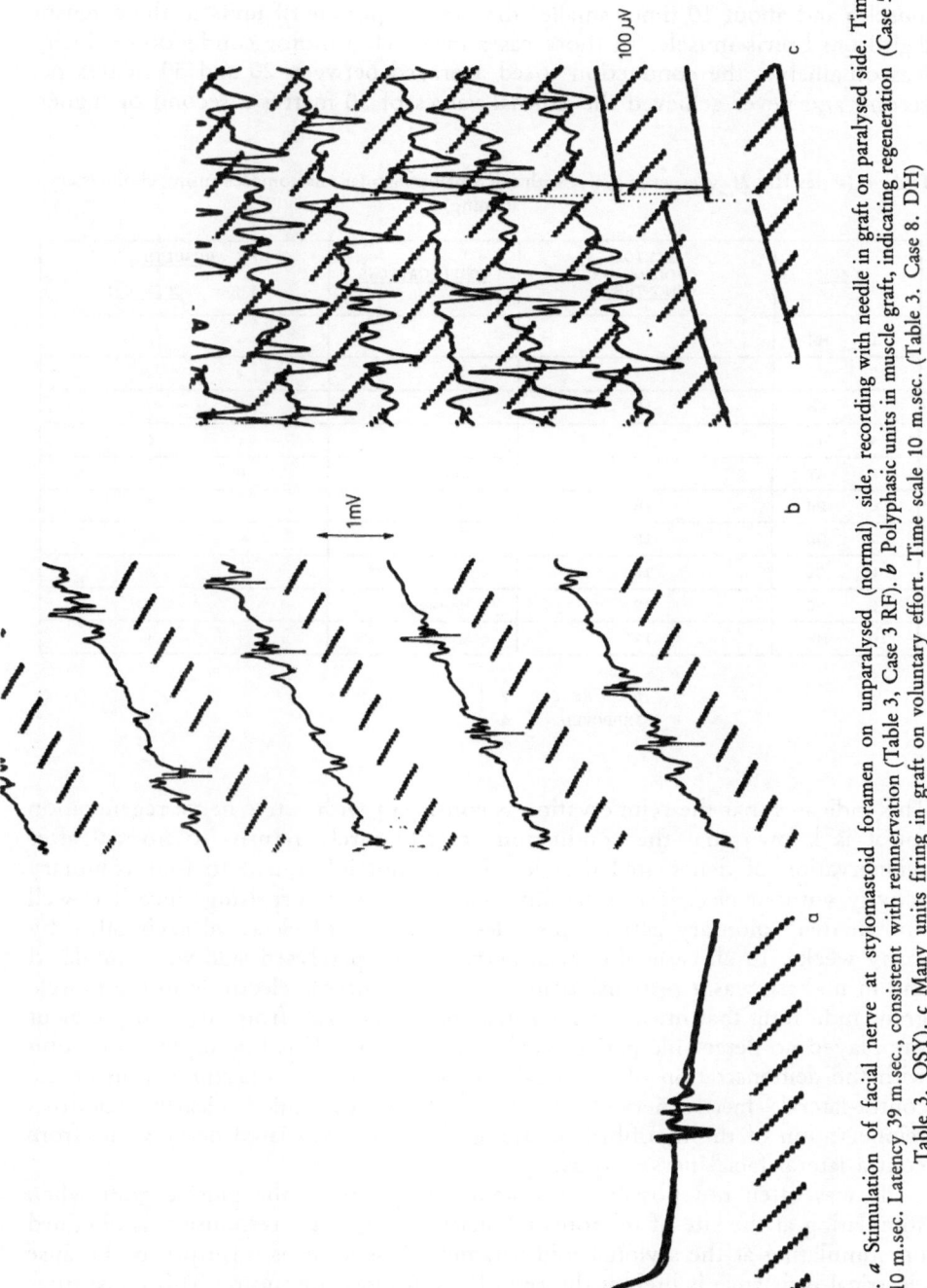

Fig. 9. *a* Stimulation of facial nerve at stylomastoid foramen on unparalysed (normal) side, recording with needle in graft on paralysed side. Time scale 10 m.sec. Latency 39 m.sec., consistent with reinnervation (Table 3, Case 3 RF). *b* Polyphasic units in muscle graft, indicating regeneration (Case 5, Table 3. Case 8. DH)

between 200 and 300 microvolts, which is the average amplitude of normal facial muscles and about 10 times smaller than the amplitude of units in the extensor digitorum brevis muscle. In those cases in which a motor conduction velocity was obtainable, the conduction speed averaged between 20 and 30 metres per second and never achieved the normal values of 50 metres a second or higher.

Table 4. (series III) *Muscle-nerve* grafts with microneurovascular anastomoses (using cholinesterase staining)

| CASE | | PERIOD FOLLOW-UP (MONTHS) | COMPLICATIONS | RESULTS | |
|------|---|---|---|---|---|
| | | | | EMG | CLINICAL |
| 1. | MM | 19 | | + | + |
| 2. | CG | 19 | | + | + |
| 3. | NS | 16 | | | + |
| 4. | JC | 12 | | + | 0 |
| 5. | AT | 12 | Haematoma | 0 | 0 |
| 6. | PH | 18 | | 0 | 0 |
| 7. | GD | 18 | | ++ | ++ |
| 8. | CL | 15 | | + | ++ |
| 9. | PC | 18 | Haematoma | + | 0 |
| 10. | MW | 12 | | + | + |

GOOD RESULT   2 ⎫
                     ⎬ 6 = 60%
IMPROVED      4 ⎭

This indicates that the reinnervation is consistent with active nerve regeneration for it is known that the conduction velocity rarely returns to normal after reinnervation of denervated muscles. It was not infrequent to find voluntary activity without electrical excitability and this is not surprising since it is well known that voluntary activity precedes the return of electrical excitability by many weeks. In all cases the facial nerve on the paralysed side was stimulated and in no case was a response detected with the needle electrode in the muscle graft, indicating that muscular neurotisation of the graft from the host recipient site played no detectable part in graft reinnervation. This finding in association with the demonstration of electrical activity in the graft on stimulation of the contra-lateral facial nerve on the unparalysed side, clearly confirms reinnervation of the myofibrils of the graft via its associated nerve graft, from contra-lateral facial nerve axons.

It was often not possible to obtain a response in the muscle graft when stimulating at the site of microneural anastomosis, yet a response was obtained on stimulating at the stylomastoid foramen. This again is unsurprising because electrical resistance is high at the site of anastomosis or suture. This constitutes further proof that the activity in the graft is due to nerve regeneration and not local spread to partially paralysed muscles.

*Series III* (Table 4). In this group of 10 patients followed up for periods of 12 to 19 months (average 15.9 months) treatment was exactly as in Series II but with the addition of a microvascular anastomosis of anterior tibial to local facial vessels (usually facial artery and vein but occasionally the superficial temporal vessels), on the paralysed side. Clinical examination showed that 60% were benefitted (2 Good and 4 improved) with 2 patients suffering complications from haematoma. The correlation between clinical and electromyographic findings is identical with Series II.

## Discussion

In a recent review of the present status of muscle grafts (Thompson 1979) it is clear that there exists remarkable unanimity in clinical and experimental reports from a significant number of centres in different countries on the successful results obtained following skeletal muscle autotransplantation in animals and man, and that two dissentient views are based upon demonstrably inadequate assimilation of available evidence (Miller, 1978) or defective experimental design (Watson and Muir, 1976).

The relative merits of free muscle grafts (with or without microneural anastomosis) and one-stage free pedicled muscle flaps with microneurovascular anastomoses requires further evaluation. Harii *et al.* (1976) reported first on the second of these, describing 2 patients in which the gracilis muscle was used in the treatment of unilateral facial paralysis. The gracilis vessels were united with the superficial temporal vessels and the motor nerve to the muscle was anastomosed to a deep temporal nerve, producing exaggerated muscle movements in the face due to the massive amount of muscle tissue transplanted, such movements being inevitably synchronous with masticatory jaw movements and unrelated to contralateral facial expression. To overcome these fundamental defects Harii (1979) has more recently used a two staged operation, comprising an initial conventional cross-facial sural nerve graft given microneural anastomosis to contralateral facial nerve elements on the unparalysed side of the face, followed 6–8 months later by the transplantation of a segment only (to reduce muscle bulk and over-activity at the recipient site) of gracilis muscle with microneural anastomosis of the obturator nerve supplying the muscle graft (to the distal stump of the sural nerve graft) and microvascular anastomosis of gracilis vessels with facial vessels to complete the operation. Of 3 patients with Bell's palsy so treated all yielded good results. The technique reduces the grotesque over-activity so often resulting from complete gracilis transfer, but must also militate against complete reinnervation in that a segment of muscle may not necessarily be innervated by those motor axons in the obturator nerve selected for the microneural anastomosis. Further trial is reported elsewhere in this volume. O'Brien (1980) also prefers two-staged cross-facial nerve grafts in association with gracilis transplantation and microneurovascular anastomoses, regarding the substitution for the gracilis of extensor digitorum brevis as unsatisfactory because of the limited volume of muscle tissue in the latter, and its inadequate reinnervation when used as a neuromuscular graft. Although Terzis *et al.* (1978) have demonstrated in rabbits that transplanted muscle grafts lose 75 % of their contractile function, this has yet to be demonstrated in human beings, and the muscles of facial expression are being replaced in extensor digitorum brevis muscle grafts by a muscle mass many times the volume of the muscles of facial expression being replaced. It is of particular interest that the EMG electrical activity in the mature muscle graft equalled that occurring in normal facial muscles, on voluntary movement, and use of all 4 bellies of the extensor digitorum brevis produces a muscle volume comparable to the segmental gracilis transplant. The degree of reinnervation whith acetylcholinesterase localisation of motor axons in the nerve graft produces clinical results of at least comparable contractile activity. The present report suggests that provided the muscle graft is first denervated the limiting factor to success is reinnervation rather than revascularisation, and that preliminary denervation of gracilis muscle transplants might well improve the degree of final clinical activity at the recipient site.

The results reported in cases requiring reconstruction of the sphincter muscles of the eyelids and mouth (with acceptable improvement of function in 88 % of the former and 78 % of the latter) confirm a number of similar earlier reports suggesting that simple two-stage free muscle autografts probably represents the treatment of choice in cases of chronic unilateral facial paralysis affecting these sites.

### References

1. Anderl, H.: Reconstruction of the face through cross-face nerve transplantation in facial paralysis. Chir. Plast. (Berl.) 2, 17 (1973).
2. Ducker, T. B., Kempe, L. G., Hayes, G. J.: The metabolic background for peripheral nerve surgery. J. Neurosurg. 30, 270 (1969).
3. Gruber, H., Zenker, W., Hohberg, E.: Untersuchungen über die Spezifität der Cholinesterasen in peripheren Nervensystem der Ratte. Histochemie 27, 78 (1971).
4. Gutmann, E.: Factors affecting recovery of motor function after nerve lesions. J. Neurol. Psychiat. 5, 81 (1942).
5. Hakelius, L.: Transplantation of free autogenous muscle in the treatment of facial paralysis. A clinical study. Scand. J. Plast. Reconstr. Surg. 8, 220 (1974).
6. Hakelius, L.: Free muscle grafting. Clin. Plast. Surg. 6, 301 (1979).
7. Harii, K., Ohmori, K., Torii, S.: Free gracilis muscle transplantation with microneurovascular anastomoses for the treatment of facial paralysis. Plast. Reconstr. Surg. 57, 133 (1976).
8. Harii, K.: Microneurovascular free muscle transplantation for reanimation of facial paralysis. Clin. Plast. Surg. 6, 361 (1979).
9. Hogan, E. L., Dawson, D. M, Romanul, F. C. A.: Enzymatic changes in denervated muscle. II. Biochemical studies. Arch. Neurol. 13, 274 (1965).
10. Karnovsky, M. J., Roots, L.: A "direct-coloring" thiocholine method for cholinesterases. J. Histochem. Cytochem. 12, 219 (1964).
11. Lieberman, A. R.: The axon reaction. A review of the principal features of perikaryal responses to axon injury. Int. Rev. Neurobiol. 49, 124 (1971).
12. McQuarrie, I. G., Grafstein, B.: Axon outgrowth enhanced by a previous nerve injury. Arch. Neurol. (Chic.) 29, 53 (1973).
13. Mayou, B. J., Watson, J. S., Harrison, D. H.: Brit. J. Plast. Surg. Under publication. 1981.
14. Miller, T. A.: Are free muscle grafts a reliable reconstructive method? Editorial. Plast. Reconstr. Surg. 62, 597 (1978).
15. O'Brien, B. M., Franklin, J. D., Morrison, W. A.: Cross-facial nerve grafts and microneurovascular free muscle transfer for long established facial palsy. Brit. J. Plast. Surg. 33, 202 (1980).
16. Romanul, F. C. A., Hogan, E. L.: Enzymatic changes in denervated muscle. I. Histochemical studies. Arch. Neurol. 13, 263 (1965).

17. Scaramella, L. F., Preliminary report on facial nerve anastomosis. Read before the Second International Symposium on Facial Nerve Surgery, Osaka, Japan. 1970.
18. Smith, J. W.: A new technique of facial animation. Trans. 5th Internat. Congr. Plast. Reconstr. Surg. London: Butterworths. 1971.
19. Terzis, J. K., Sweet, R. C., Dykes, R. W., Williams, H. B.: Recovery of function in free muscle transplants using microneurovascular anastomoses. J. Hand. Surg. 3, 37 (1978).
20. Thompson, N.: Investigation of autogenous skeletal muscle free grafts in the dog. With a report on a successful free graft of skeletal muscle in man. Transplantation 12, 353 (1971).
21. Thompson, N.: Autogenous free grafts of skeletal muscle. A preliminary experimental and clinical study. Plast. Reconstr. Surg. 48, 11 (1971).
22. Thompson, N.: A review of autogenous skeletal muscle grafts and their clinical applications. Clin. Plast. Surg. 1, 349 (1974).
23. Thompson, N.: Free muscle graft pharyngoplasty with palatal retroposition in the treatment of velopharyngeal incompetence. With a note on the present status of free muscle autografts. Chir. Plast. (Berl.) 5, 1 (1979).
24. Thompson, N., Gustavson, E. H.: The use of neuromuscular free autografts with microneural anastomosis to restore elevation to the paralysed angle of the mouth in cases of unilateral facial paralysis. With an analysis of late results of muscle grafts in the treatment of 103 cases of facial paralysis. Chir. Plast. (Berl.) 3, 165 (1976).
25. Watson, A. C. H., Muir, A. R.: Failure of free muscle grafts in dogs. Brit. J. Plast. Surg. 29, 27 (1976).

Author's address: Mr. N. Thompson, 26 St. Andrews Mansions, Dorset Street, London W1H 3FD, England.

## Discussion

*Miller:* What is the value of muscular neurotisation and the direct nerve-muscle neurotisation?

*Thompson:* The indications for a muscle transplantation with muscular neurotisation and a muscle transplantation with neural neurotisation are different. In a partial facial palsy muscular neurotisation can occur and therefore a free graft put onto partially functioning muscles in the paralyzed face can give recognizable results. But if a total facial palsy is evident, the muscle graft has to be reinnervated by nerves. And this can occur very nicely as our myographic investigation have proved.

*Harii:* How are the success rates, Mr. Thompson, at your cases with total facial palsy?

*Thompson:* There is no difference in the results in patients with total or partial facial palsy, because the source of muscular neurotisation in the cases of oral sphincter reconstruction or reconstruction of the orbicularis occuli, the source of reinnervation is the normal functioning muscle on the healthy side; therefore muscular neurotisation takes place in the usual way. But according to the angle of the mouth, there is no doubt that the results in partial facial palsy are better, because of the reinnervation of a muscular neurotisation, which is better than the cross-face neurotisation.

# Experience With Thompson's Free Muscle Grafts*

## I. Miyake

Department of Plastic and Reconstructive Surgery,
Juntendo University Hospital,
Tokyo, Japan

With 6 Figures

Thompson's free muscle grafts were performed on 8 patients with unilateral facial palsy, and their results were assessed regarding the effects on closure of the eyelids and elevation of the drooped corner of the mouth.

Following Thompson's [1] (1971) method, free muscle grafts were performed on 8 patients with unilateral facial palsy—7 during 1975 to 1976 and one in 1979. Most of the cases have now been followed up for more than 3 years.

The advantages and disadvantages of this method have already been reported by Thompson [2] (1974) himself and others (Hakelius [3], 1974; Mazzola [4], 1975), so that there is little left to be added. This paper confirms their observations, with some racial characteristics of Japanese being noted.

## Cases

Details of the 8 patients are listed in Fig. 1, according to Mazzola's [4] (1975) manner of presentation. All patients are cases of long-standing facial palsy, with more than 2 years between the onset of palsy and the operation. These patients were arbitrarily divided into three groups, depending upon the muscles on which the grafts were transplanted.

*Group I.* Two patients are included in this Group. The denervated muscles were grafted on orbicularis oculi muscles of the unaffected side, that is the contralateral side, and their tendons went through a hole made in the nasal root and then into the margins of the upper and lower eyelids up to the lateral canthus of the affected side, i.e. the ipsilateral side. There they were fixed.

*Group II* Five cases are included in this Group. The muscle grafts were on the temporal muscle of the ipsilateral side and their tendons went through the

---

* Some cases presented here were already reported in The Japanese J. Plast. and Reconstr. Surg. 20, 554–562 (1977).

margins of the upper and lower eyelids and were fixed at the ipsilateral median canthal ligament.

In all cases except case 7, free muscles were also grafted around the mouth, having been placed in contact with the orbicularis oris muscles of the contralateral side.

*Group III.* In this case, added to the operation of Group II, one more pair of muscles was grafted on the upper part of the masseter muscles of the ipsilateral side.

| Case | Name | Sex | Age | Etiology | Interval between paralysis and operation | Group |
|------|------|-----|-----|----------|------------------------------------------|-------|
| 1 | S. I. | w. | 36 | Bell | 11 years | I |
| 2 | Y. S. | m. | 24 | congenital | 24 years | I |
| 3 | M. N. | w. | 25 | neurinoma | 4 years | II |
| 4 | K. K. | w. | 50 | Bell | 10 years | II |
| 5 | K. Y. | w. | 18 | congenital | 18 years | II |
| 6 | E. A. | w. | 22 | Bell | 5 years | II |
| 7 | F. T. | w. | 54 | nerve block for spasm | 2 years | II |
| 8 | H. H. | w. | 26 | cholesteatoma | 6 years | III |

Fig. 1. List of the operated cases

## Operation

Extensor digitorum brevis or palmaris longus muscles were denervated 2 weeks before transplantation. The denervation was confirmed by EMG, which was taken before and after the severance of the nerve. After 2 weeks, those muscles were transplanted on the ipsi- or contra-lateral mimetic or masticatory muscles as mentioned already.

After the operation, EMG's of the grafted muscles were taken monthly, but after about 6 months the grafted muscles seem to have atrophied and it became rather difficult to confirm them from the outside. At this time it was also difficult to differentiate the EMG of the grafts from that of the normal muscles underneath. Thus the last results of this operation were only evaluated clinically.

## Results

The results of this operation were assessed from two different aspects; one is to achieve complete eyelid closure and the other is to elevate the drooped corner of the mouth.

Group I, in which the grafts were applied on the contra-lateral orbicularis oculi muscles, includes two patients-cases 1 and 2. Both patients showed only incomplete eyelid closure even with tight squeezing of the contralateral orbicularis oculi muscles (Fig. 2).

This may be the result of a technical failure, but also because we Japanese have rather flat noses, compared with European races, so that it is difficult to get enough space for a tunnel in the nasal root.

Group II, in which the grafts were applied on the ipsi-lateral temporal muscles, includes 6 patients—cases 3 through 8. All patients of this group except one could close the eye completely (and the one incompletely) when they contracted the temporal muscles. Movement of the eyelids during mastication

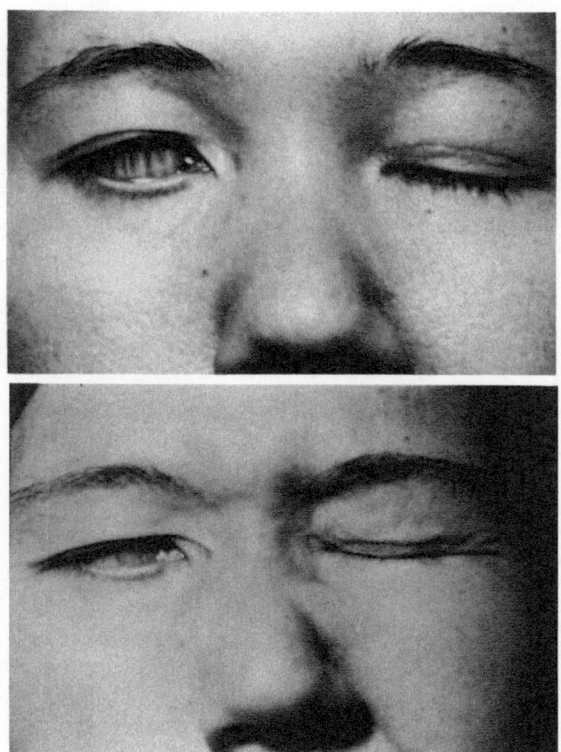

Fig. 2. Case 1 operated as Group I; Above—before the operation. Below—after the operation. The closure of the eyelids is not complete

did not cause much trouble for them, even though some authors have reported that it was quite annoying in some cases (Fig. 3).

The only trouble here was that the movement of the eyelids is rather slow and it takes about one to two seconds to close the eyelids completely. It is impossible to expect them to blink briskly. In order to explain this slowness, the author tried to prove the lag in the time of the contraction of the grafted muscles, compared with that of the normal muscles underneath. But EMG examinations showed simultaneous contraction of the supposedly grafted muscles with the normal muscles underneath. This may be the difference between mimic muscles and skeletal muscles which need tendons to transmit their movements.

As to the effect of elevation of the drooped corner of the mouth, the results were rather unsatisfactory as already reported by the author [5] (Miyake, 1977). When the patients try to purse the mouth, the corner of the paretic mouth is definitely elevated as shown in Fig. 4. But when they laugh (i.e., at the time of

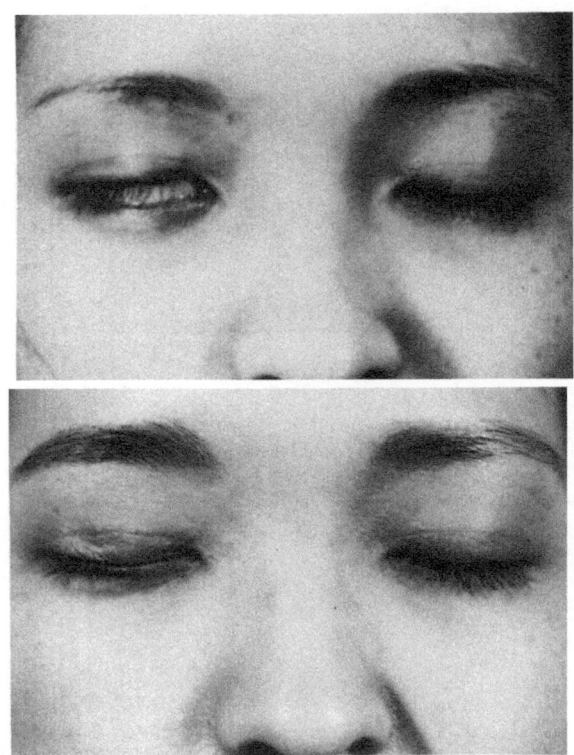

Fig. 3. Case 3 operated as Group II; Above–before the operation. Below–after the operation. The closure of the eyelids is complete

the relaxation of the orbicularis oris muscles), deformity becomes conspicuous (Fig. 5).

In order to compete with this deformity, in case 8 of Group III, added to the operation of Group II, one more pair of extensor digitorum brevis muscles was grafted on the upper part of the ipsilateral masseter muscle. Unfortunately these grafts had no effect on the angle of the mouth, but at the time of clenching they pressed the mucous membrane of the cheek to the teeth, preventing an accumulation of the food in the prealveolar space, which was the complaint of the patient before the operation.

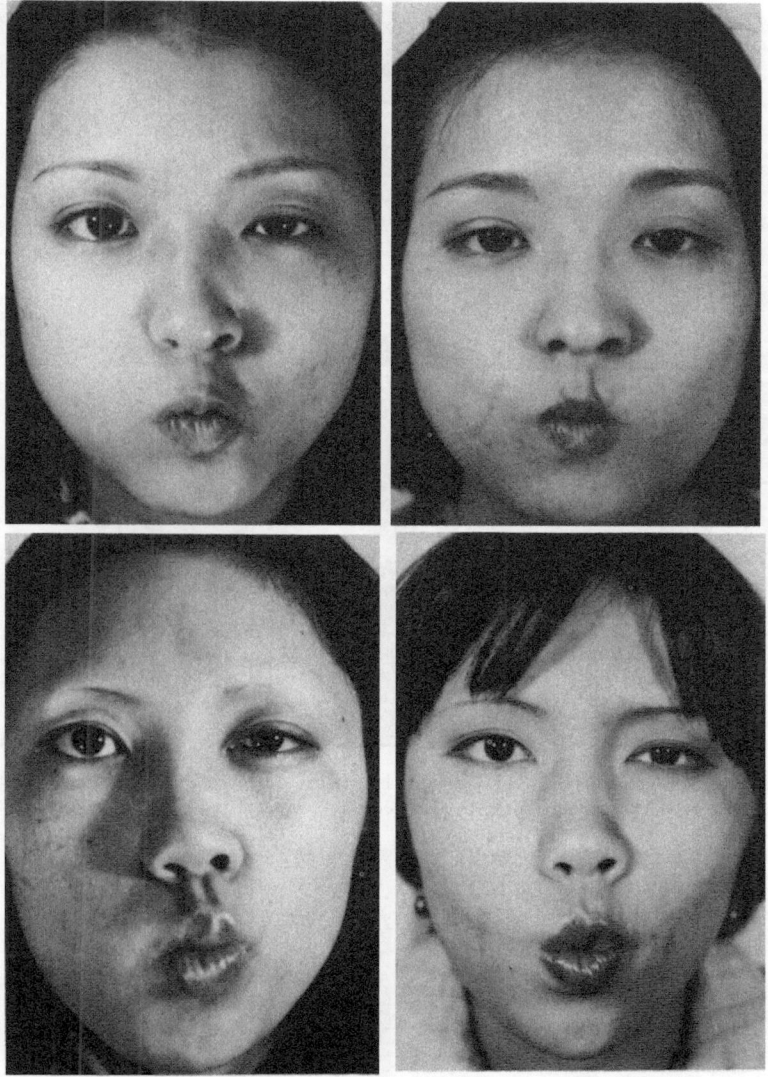

Fig. 4. Case 3 (above) and Case 4 (below); Left—before the operation. Right—after the operation. The drooped corner of the mouth is elevated when the mouth is pursed

## Conclusion

In spite of long hospitalization and many operative scars, most patients seem satisfied with this operation, and there is no doubt about its efficacy as to eyelid closure.

But sometimes even a simple operation can produce quite acceptable results in the case of the narrow almond-eyed Japanese, for instance, partial levator

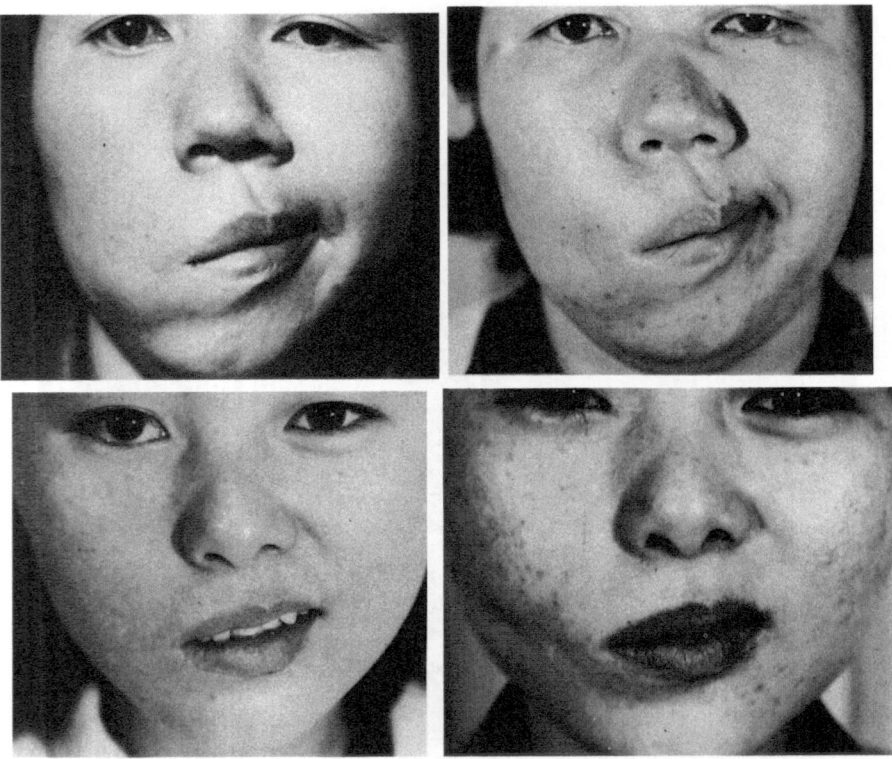

Fig. 5. Case 1 (above) and Case 8 (below); Left–before the operation. Right–after the operation. The drooping of the corner of the mouth became conspicuous at the time of laughing

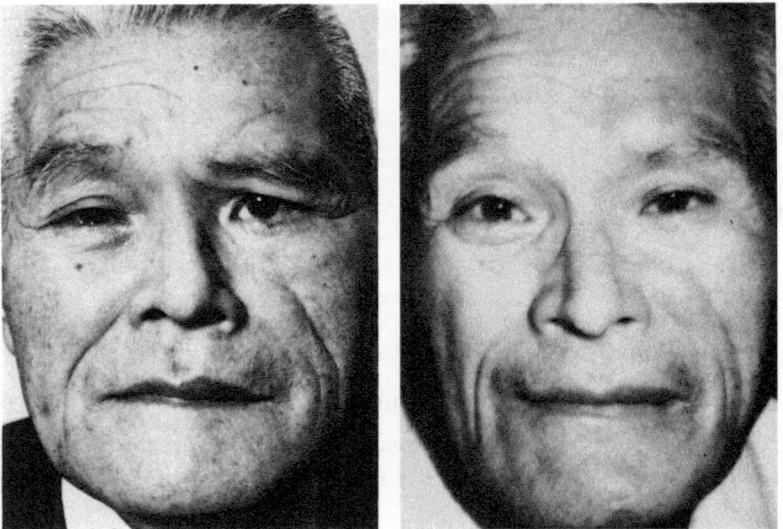

Fig. 6. The case with left facial nerve palsy; Left–before the operation. Right–after the operation. Partial levator muscle and redundant skin of the upper part of the eyebrow were resected

muscle excision for hyperretraction of the upper eyelids and resection of redundant skin just above the eyebrow, as shown in Fig. 6.

As to rehabilitation around the mouth, some other devices, such as free muscle grafts with microneurovascular anastomosis, seem mandatory.

## Summary

Thompson's free muscle grafts were performed on the eight cases of unilateral facial nerve palsy. The advantages and disadvantages of this method were discussed with some racial characteristics as Japanese being noted.

### Acknowledgement

I would like to thank Prof. I. Tange, Department of Plastic and Reconstructive Surgery, Juntendo University Hospital, for his helpful advice and Dr. B. Wakasugi and his staff of Pain Clinic, Kantoteisin Hospital, who kindly referred several patients to me.

### References

1. Thompson, N.: Autogenous free grafts of skeletal muscle. A preliminary experimental and clinical study. Plast. Reconstr. Surg. *48*, 11–27 (1971).
2. Thompson, N.: A review of autogeneous skeletal muscle grafts and their clinical applications. Clinics in Plast. Surg. *1*, 349–403 (1974).
3. Hakelius, L.: Transplantation of free autogenous muscle in the treatment of facial paralysis. A clinical study. Scand. J. Plast. Reconstr. Surg. *8*, 220–230 (1974).
4. Mazzola, R. F.: A contribution to the treatment of permanent facial paralysis by free muscle grafting based on 21 cases. Chir. Plastica (Berlin) *3*, 59–74 (1975).
5. Miyake, I.: Thompson's operation for unilateral facial paralysis. The Japanese J. Plast. Reconstr. Surg. *20*, 554–562 (1977).

Author's address: Dr. I. Miyake, Department of Plastic and Reconstructive Surgery, Juntendo University Hospital, 3-1-3 Hongo, Bunkyo-ku, Tokyo, Japan, 113.

# The Treatment of Facial Palsy With Free Revascularised and Reinnervated Muscle Grafts

## D. E. Tolhurst

University Hospital,
Rotterdam, The Netherlands

With 6 Figures

The large number of operations described for the correction of facial palsy has not made the treatment of this deformity any easier. Besides the use of a static fascia sling, both muscle transpositions and free grafts have been employed, to say nothing of the rerouting of nerves, the use of cross facial nerve grafts and even combinations of some of these ideas. No doubt a good case can be made for each of these techniques but in the long run it should be possible to adhere to precise indications for each procedure based on logical and accumulated experience.

Although Thompson (1974, 1976) and Hakelius (1974) have reported good results with free denervated muscle grafts, my own experience and that of several other workers (Watson, 1976; Miller, 1978) with this technique have convinced us that it was desirable to find a more physiological and reliable method of restoring movement to the paralysed face. A free denervated muscle graft whose motor nerve is sutured to a cross facial graft can hardly be expected to fare any better than the classical Thompson graft so it seemed logical to attempt to revascularise the grafts immediately with microsurgical techniques.

As a preparatory stage a cross facial nerve graft was used to bring 7th nerve fibres from the normal side of the face as close to the muscle graft as possible.

## Indications

Not all cases of long-standing facial palsy should be treated in the same way for the residual muscle activity and resultant deformity can vary considerably. The indications for a free revascularised muscle graft which is to be reinnervated by a cross facial nerve graft are as follows:

1. There should be minimal or no activity of the elevators of the upper lip, corner of the mouth and zygomatic muscles causing marked facial imbalance on talking and smiling.

2. The muscles should be atrophic or incapable of becoming reinnervated.

3. The facial nerve lesion should be of more than one year's standing and/or central to the stylomastoid foramen.

At present it is still not certain, despite EMG examinations, how long denervated fascial musculature retains the ability to become reinnervated, but many put the upper limit at 18 months. The ability of a neurone to propel axons distally from the site of a lesion probably differs in motor and sensory nerves. Experimentally it has been shown by Holmes and Young (1942) that this property is retained for at least a year, but in man it is uncertain if the degree of atrophy in the motor nerve cell one year after a peripheral lesion precludes axon sprouting. For this reason a cross facial nerve graft should be used as the source of reinnervation for a muscle graft if the lesion is of more than one year's standing.

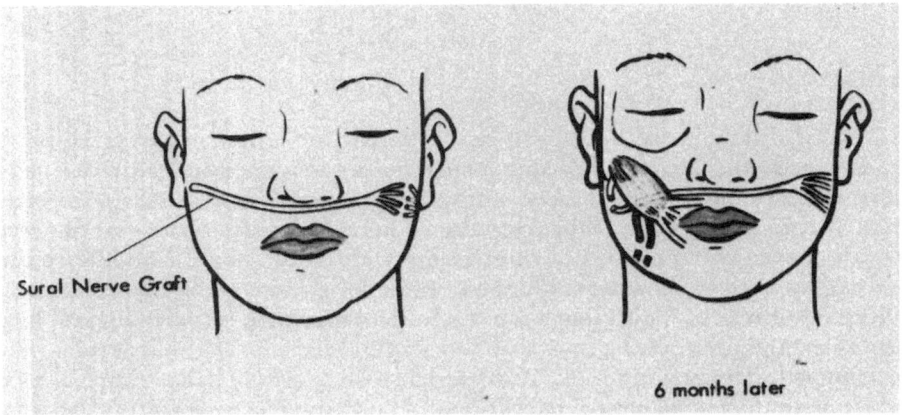

Fig. 1. Plan of 2 stage operation; note position of muscle graft (extensor digitorum brevis) in relation to facial vessels

## The Operation

A 2-stage procedure is required and a schematic representation of this is shown in Fig. 1.

### First Stage: Cross-Facial Nerve Graft (C.F.N.G.)

Our dissatisfaction with the exposure and scars resulting from the incision described by Smith (1971) and later by Anderl (1973) have lead us to use a modified parotid incision. The scar is scarcely visible, but even more important, the exposure of the facial nerve branches is in all respects better. By following the parotid fascia anteriorly one comes into the region of the peripheral branches of the 7th nerve as they leave the parotid gland. With the help of a nerve stimulator the largest buccal branches are isolated and may be used as the donor nerves without fear of paralysing the normal side of the face.

A tunnel is made across the upper part of the upper lip from the anterior limit of the dissection and connected to a tunnel across the paralysed cheek which is in turn made from a small preauricular incision.

Whilst the facial dissection is in progress a second team removes a sural nerve graft of at least 25 cms. Which is reversed and passed through the tunnel. One end is attached by a nylon suture through the epineurium to the dermis on the paralysed side as there is a tendency for this end to retract.

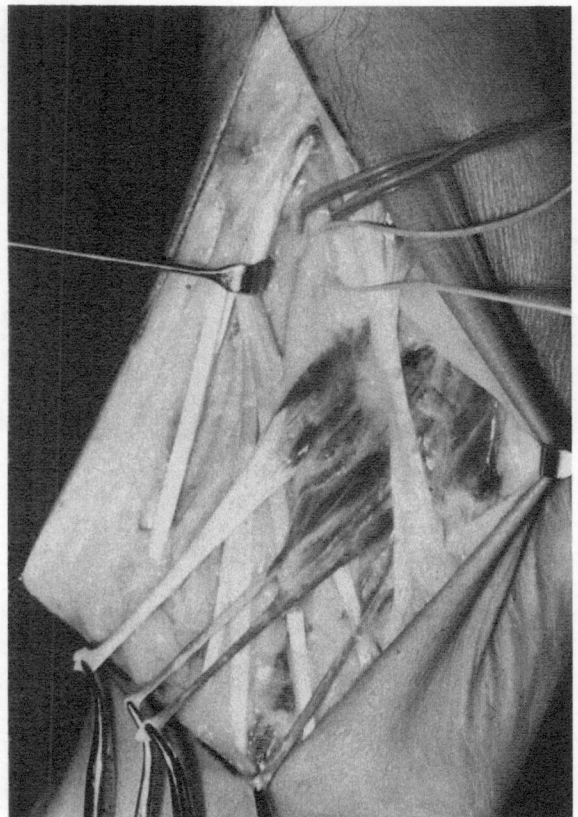

Fig. 2. Extensor digitorum brevis muscle and neurovascular bundle being removed from foot

The other end is trimmed, cleaned and the fascicles freed and sutured in the routine manner with one or two 10/0 nylon sutures to the divided buccal branches of the facial nerve, using the operating microscope. The wound is closed with drainage.

### Through-Growth of the 7th Nerve

It is usually assumed that axons proceed at the rate of about 1 mm. per day but they may grow much faster. The Hoffmann-Tinel sign indicates the extent

13*

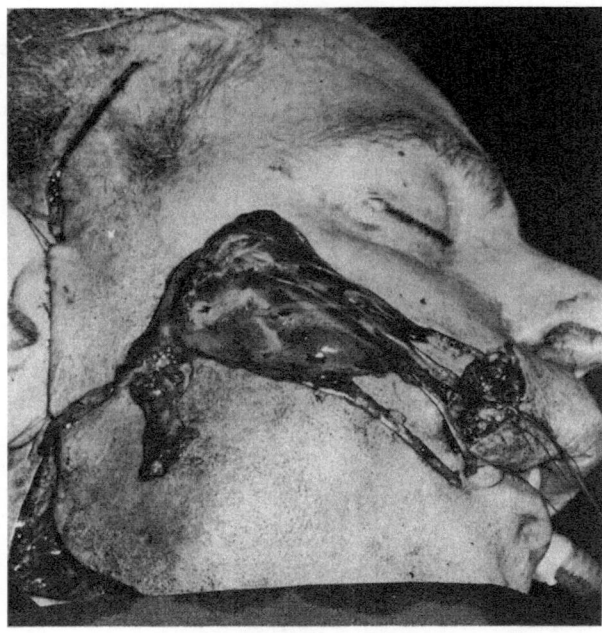

Fig. 3. Disposition of muscle graft. Artery and vein inferior to muscle and deep peroneal nerve posterior to vessels

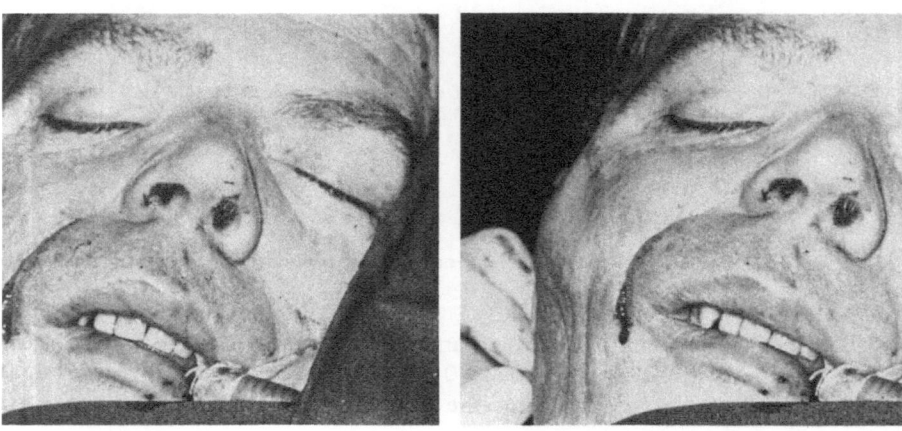

Fig. 4. Motor nerve stimulation prior to nerve suture. Compare exposure of canine tooth

of the proliferation. When one taps lightly along the course of the cross facial graft the patient will suddenly indicate a point at which pain or tingling can be located in the contralateral side of the face.

Since it is always stated that the peripheral branches of the 7th nerve are purely motor in quality this sign is somewhat difficult to explain. Facial musculature contains no muscle spindles, and proprioception is said to be mediated via 5th nerve branches from the overlying skin. Those who have experienced pain from spasm of the occipito-frontalis muscle during a prolonged grimace or sycophantic smile may wonder how such a sensation is mediated. I believe it may well be conducted via small 5th nerve branches, which intermingle with 7th nerve branches in the cheek and could well proceed with the latter to the facial muscles.

When the neuroma can be located well laterally in the cheek or if there is no progress after 6 months the time is ripe for the second stage.

### Second Stage: Free Muscle Graft

Two teams are employed, one of which dissects out the extensor digitorum brevis (E.D.B.) muscle and its neurovascular bundle (Fig. 2) and the other to prepare the paralysed side of the face for the free muscle graft.

The facial vessels are carefully isolated and freed superiorly and the neuroma of the C.F.N.G. trimmed until fascicles pout from the cut end. If one is in doubt as to the through-growth of axons a frozen section can be sent for examination to confirm the presence of nerve tissue.

The free muscle graft with its feeding vessels and motor nerve is now transfered to the face and placed as shown in Fig. 3. This manoeuvre is left until the last possible moment to reduce the ischaemia time. Thus anchoring sutures around corner of the mouth for the tendons and over the zygoma for the muscle belly are placed first.

Microvascular anastomosis of the dorsalis pedis vessels to the facial vessels is now carried out and the motor nerve fascicles sutured to suitable fascicles of the C.F.N.G. The terminal cutaneous branch of the deep peroneal nerve is implanted in the muscle.

Before carrying out the vessel and nerve suture, we stimulate the motor nerve to the graft to gain an idea of the contraction and facial movement which can be expected (Fig. 4). If necessary the tendons can be tightened, but this adjustment is rarely required if the muscle and tendons are attached under good tension.

Both the foot and face are drained with 2 suction drains for about 48 hours.

### Clinical Results (Table 1)

The only way to demonstrate a convincing success after this type of operation is to see the range of movement achieved in the patient himself or in a cinefilm. All of our cases were filmed pre- and postoperatively with a video camera and it was thus possible to compare various attempted movements fairly objectively.

Table 1. *Clinical results*

| Patient | Age | Duration palsy | Aetiology | Positive Hoffmann-Tinel sign after CFNG | Duration of operation | First movement postop. | End result |
|---|---|---|---|---|---|---|---|
| 1. S.-B. | 58 | 43 years | Bell's palsy | − | 9 hrs | 7 months | Poor. Mouth almost symmetrical at rest and fair elevation of upper lip present. Muscle contracture visible. |
| 2. B. | 25 | 19 years | Fracture base | − | 8 hrs | 10 months | Poor. Mouth symmetrical at rest. No movement except for minimal twitch lower lip. |
| 3. T. | 31 | 31 years | Congenital | + | 6 hrs 50 min | 7 months | Fair. Mouth symmetrical at rest. Good active movement visible in upper and lower lip both voluntary and involuntary. |
| 4. J.-V. | 42 | 42 years | Congenital | + | 7 hrs 20 min | 8 months | Poor. Mouth symmetrical at rest and almost so when smiling. Practically no movement. |
| 5. M.-P. | 33 | 33 years | Middle ear infection | + | 5 hrs 45 min | 6 months | Good. Mouth symmetrical at rest. Patient can elevate corner of mouth well. Clear muscle movement visible. |
| 6. G. | 41 | 40 years | Middle ear infection | + | 5 hrs 25 min | 5 months | Very good. Mouth symmetrical at rest and moves when patient laughs. Very good elevation of upper lip and muscle contracture clearly visible. |
| 7. D. | 34 | 32 years | Poliomyelitis | + | 5 hrs 35 min | 5 months | Good. Clear muscle contraction visible. Can elevate upper lip and voluntary movement of corner of mouth and alar possible. |

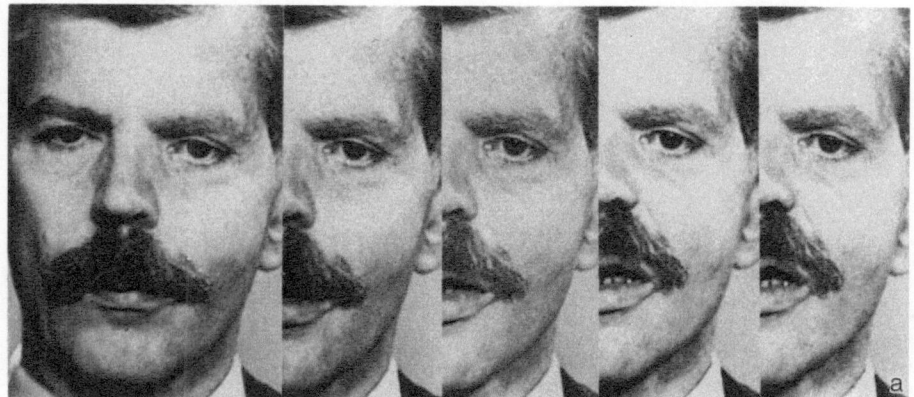

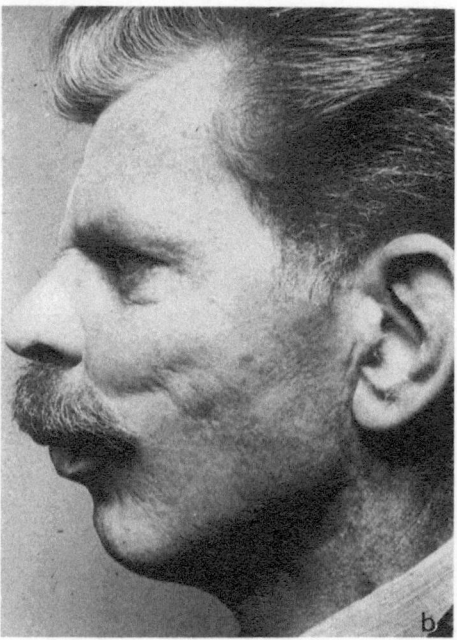

Fig. 5. *a* Post-operative result in a good case; note elevation of upper lip and development of nasolabial crese. *b* The same case showing involuntary muscle contraction on smiling

Results were classified into the following categories according to the criteria listed:

*1. Good* (Fig. 5): There was clear strong, voluntary movement visible with elevation of the corner of the mouth. Involuntary movement was sometimes present and the symmetry of the mouth on smiling and laughing was much improved though never perfect.

*2. Fair:* Voluntary movement was clearly visible but far from strong. No involuntary movement was present.

D. E. Tolhurst:

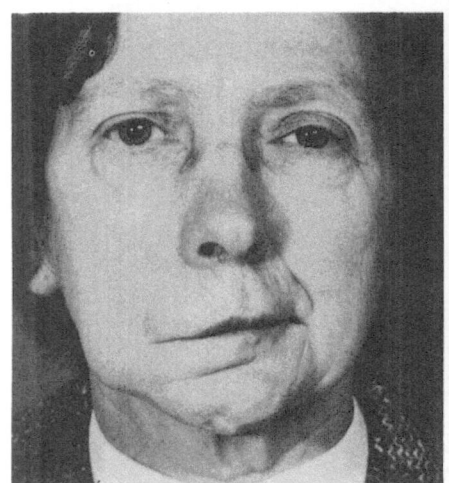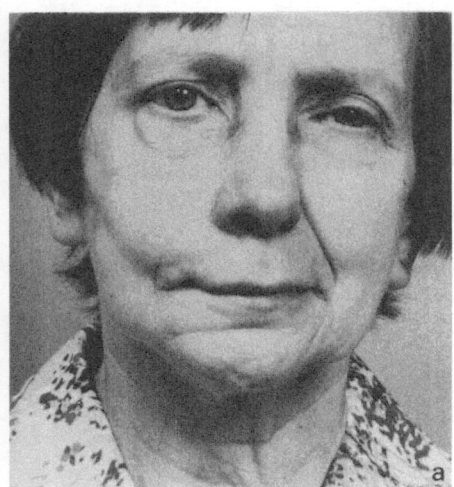

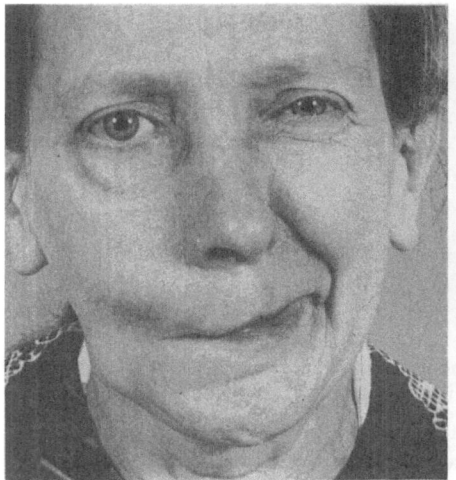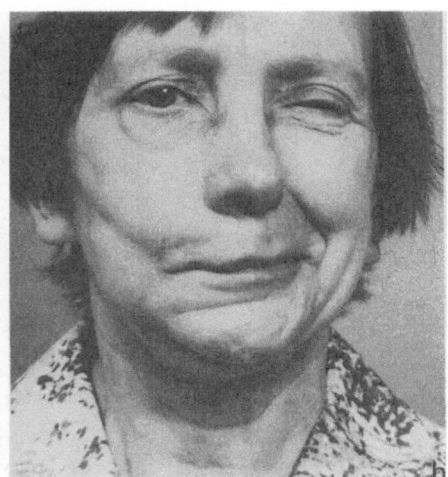

Fig. 6. Pre- and post-operative photos of a poor result. *a* At rest, *b* smiling

*3. Poor:* These cases were little better than failures with only minimal movement visible. Reinnervation via the C.F.N.G. was proved by EMG and the muscle twitch though feeble was present when the C.F.N.G. was stimulated and when the patient attempted to contract the graft.

In all 3 groups of patients there was virtual symmetry of the mouth at rest, which was superior to the usual result seen following a fascial sling. Even in the poor cases, where the results were little more than failures as far as movement was concerned, this symmetry was of some help to the patient (Fig. 6).

The video frames shown in fig. 5 do not do justice to the degree of movement achieved and a casual glance at the photos of a poor result (Fig. 6) would suggest that the operation had been a success in this case. Thus pre- and post-operative still photos are to our mind unreliable.

Objectivity is difficult for both the surgeon and the patient after 2 operations and many months of anxiety and therapy, but we nevertheless believe our assessment is honest, as will perhaps be better understood upon reading the conclusions we have drawn from our examinations.

## Electromyography Results (Table 2)

As a routine all of our patients were sent for a preoperative EMG examination and in all 7 cases total or subtotal unilateral paralysis was confirmed. EMG was also performed 6 and 12 months after the free revascularised graft and the examinations and results are shown in table 2.

It can be seen that it was possible to confirm reinnervation of the muscle by the C.F.N.G. in all cases after an interval 12 months. With a recording electrode in the grafted muscle the C.F.N.G. was stimulated in the contralateral cheek and the patient also asked to contract the muscle graft. The results varied from patient to patient, and besides being of different amplitude the wave forms of the poorer results were polyphasic which indicates that the muscle tissue is not of such good quality.

By and large the EMG findings correlated well with the clinical results. The absence of fibrillations in cases 5 and 6 after 12 months suggests that the graft had become well reinnervated, whilst in cases 1 and 2 the absence of fibrillations suggests atrophy of the graft. In fact in the latter case the muscle looked pale and thin at the time of operation and the clinical result was poor with only slight activity of the upper part of the graft.

Fibrillations, as registered after the insertion of a needle, are a sign that denervated muscle is present. Moreover the fibrillations reflect the state of a few muscle fibres in the vicinity of the needle and do not give anything more than presumptive evidence that the rest of the muscle is in a similar state. Thus EMG examination, although the best adjunct to clinical examination of muscle tissue, does have its limitations.

Our neurologist expects continued improvement in the function of reinnervated muscle for up to 2 years but it seems reasonable to suppose that the maximum improvement occurs within the first 12 months.

Table 2. *EMG results*

| | Insertion activity | | Fibrillations | | Reinnervation CFNG | | Electrical activity when attempting to contract muscle graft | Muscle twitch after stimulation contralateral facial nerve | Clinical result |
|---|---|---|---|---|---|---|---|---|---|
| | 6 mths | 12 mths | 6 mths | 12 mths | 6 mths | 12 mths | | | |
| 1. S.-B. | + | ± | + | − | − | ± | − | − | Poor |
| 2. B. | + | + | + | − | − | + | + | 100 Micro V | Poor |
| 3. T. | + | + | + | + | − | + | ++ | 700 Micro V | Fair |
| 4. J.-V. | + | + | + | + | − | + | + | 75 Micro V | Poor |
| 5. M.-P. | + | + | + | − | − | + | + | 150 Micro V | Good |
| 6. G. | + | + | + | − | + | + | ++++ | 3500 Micro V | Very good |
| 7. D. | + | + | + | + | + | + | +++ | 800 Micro V | Good |

## Discussion

It will have been clear by now that the technique described has been used to restore movement in the regions of the corner of the mouth, lips and alar base. Where the eyelids are incapable of providing adequate corneal protection a lateral tarsorrhaphy coupled with the implantation of magnets or a simple free muscle graft are indicated as a separate procedure.

The earliest sign of muscle function was 5 months post-operatively, but in most cases it can be seen that recovery took even longer. Since the C.F.N.G. axons must traverse the motor nerve of E.D.B., a distance which never exceeded 9 cm., one would expect an earlier return of function but it must not be forgotten that new motor end plates must form, myelination will increase and the muscle fibres themselves will improve in quality. Added to this the patient must learn to recognise and make use of his new abilities so that it is perhaps not surprising that the recovery phase takes so long.

The best results to date have been in the last 3 patients operated upon and when one considers that the duration of the operation has been steadily reduced from 9 hours to 5½ hours, this is not surprising. The worst results were seen in 3 of the first 4 patients treated but some specific problems account for these disappointments.

In the first case, the Extensor Digitorum Brevis muscle looked very pale and thin, and as we gained experience this remained the poorest muscle specimen. This patient was also the oldest in the series (58 years) and it is known that E.D.B. tends to become atrophic with age.

The second case probably failed because of difficulties with the C.F.N.G. This was found to have retracted or to have become so short, that the neuroma lay medial to the nasolabial crease. It was lengthened with a second sural graft but the 3 anastomoses probably caused some obstruction to the axonal growth although frozen section at the time of the muscle graft confirmed a through growth of axons.

In the other 5 cases no special difficulties were encountered. The improving results give one some confidence for the future but it is hoped that earlier referral of patients will make this type of operation unnecessary.

Since only about half of the patients treated with E.D.B. have demonstrated good function of the graft, the question arises as to whether gracilis would not be a more suitable muscle. Harii (1977) and O'Brien (1980) favour the gracilis, and in all honesty I would prefer to see more movement in those cases classified as good so that in the future we plan to use gracilis in a series of patients.

## Conclusions

It has been clearly shown that the technique does work, but the inconsistent results obtained with E.D.B. lead us to believe that a more powerful muscle would be preferable.

## Summary

7 cases of long-standing facial palsy were treated with a 2-stage operative procedure. In the first stage a cross-facial nerve graft was inserted and in the

second this was sutured to the motor nerve of a free muscle graft, revascularised by microsurgical anastomosis of its vessels to the facial vessels. In 3 cases good functional activity is present 12 months after the second operation.

### References

1. Anderl, H.: Reconstruction of the face through cross-facial nerve transplantation in facial paralysis. Chir. Plast. 2, 17–46 (1973).
2. Hakelius, L.: Transplantation of free autogenous muscle in the treatment of facial paralysis. A clinical study. Scand. J. Plast. Reconstr. Surg. 8, 220–230 (1974).
3. Harii, K.: Free gracilis muscle transplantation, with microneurovascular anastomoses for the treatment of facial paralysis. Plast. Reconstr. Surg. 57, 133–143 (1976).
4. Holmes, W., Young, J. Z.: Nerve regeneration after immediate and delayed suture. J. Anat. 77, 63–68 (1942).
5. Miller, T. A., Korn, H. N., Wheeler, E. S.: Can one muscle reinnervate another? A preliminary study of muscular neurotonisation in the rabbit. Plast. Reconstr. Surg. 61, 50–57 (1978).
6. O'Brien, B., Franklin, J., Morrison, W.: Cross-facial nerve grafts and microneurovascular free muscle transfer for long established facial palsy. Brit. J. Plast. Surg. 33, 202–215 (1980).
7. Smith, J. W.: A new technique of facial animation. Transactions of the 5th International Congress of Plastic and Reconstructive Surgery, pp. 83–84, 1971.
8. Thompson, N.: A review of autogenous skeletal muscle grafts and their clinical applications. Clin. Plast. Surg. 1, 349–357 (1974).
9. Thompson, N., Gustavson, E. H.: The use of neuromuscular free autografts with microneural anastomosis to restore elevation to the paralysed angle of mouth in cases of unilateral paralysis, with an analysis of late results of muscle grafts in the treatment of 103 cases of facial hemiparesis. Chir. Plast. 3, 165–174 (1976).
10. Watson, A. C. H., Muir, A. R.: Failure of free muscle grafts in dogs. Brit. J. Plast. Surg. 29, 27–33 (1976).

Author's address: Dr. D. E. Tolhurst, Department of Plastic Surgery, University Hospital, Rotterdam, The Netherlands.

## Discussion

*Freilinger:* Don't you think that by using a bigger muscle, like the gracilis muscle, you get a better functional result than with the short extensor muscle? Even the results, you have shown us, are very nice.

*Tolhurst:* I must say, I am not terribly convinced of this.

# Muscular Neurotisation in Ophthalmology –
# A New Method to Treat Pareses of Extraocular Muscles

## H. Aichmair

Second Ophthalmological University Clinic of Vienna, Austria

With 2 Figures

In modern reconstructive surgery, the treatment of paretic muscles gains more and more importance. The surgeon tries to reestablish the original physiological conditions, to reconstruct the original innervation as exactly as possible. In some groups of muscles only the method of muscular neurotisation offers the possibility to recover the initial functional and reflex unity of the paralysed muscle. Muscular neurotisation is the growth of preterminal nerve fibers from an implanted healthy muscle into the paretic host muscle which induces the development of medullated nerve fibers and motor end plates.

As regards the eyes, the paresis of one single extraocular muscle is enough to disturb markedly the muscle balance of both eyes by annoying diplopia. Every ophthalmic surgeon is well aware of the difficulties involved in the reestablishment of normal binocularity in cases of the extraocular muscle paresis. All operations could only bring the eyes into a parallel position without achievement of functional restoration.

Therefore, the application of muscular neurotisation seemed to be a new way to treat extraocular muscle pareses. Since we had first proved experimentally that muscular neurotisation is possible in extraocular muscles [1], we began to transpose in patients with abducens paresis the healthy inferior oblique muscle to the paretic lateral rectus muscle (Fig. 1) in order to induce a reinnervation of the paretic muscle [2]. We have now operated on about 30 patients; the results of the first 20 are given in Table 1. The following patients showed similar results. Our first patient operated on by this method in 1975 is shown in Fig. 2; the good result has not changed up to now.

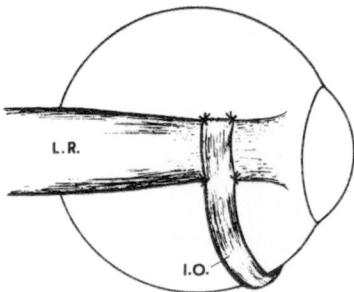

Fig. 1. Schematic diagram of the transposition procedure. *L. R.* lateral rectus muscle, *I. O.* inferior oblique muscle

*Table 1*

| Improvement of abduction and squint angle | after | | Total |
|---|---|---|---|
| | first | second | |
| | transposition | | |
| back to normal | 4 | – | 4 |
| almost normal | 2 | 2 | 4 |
| good | 9 | – | 9 |
| slight improvement | 2 | 1 | 3 |
| Total number of patients | 17 | 3 | 20 |

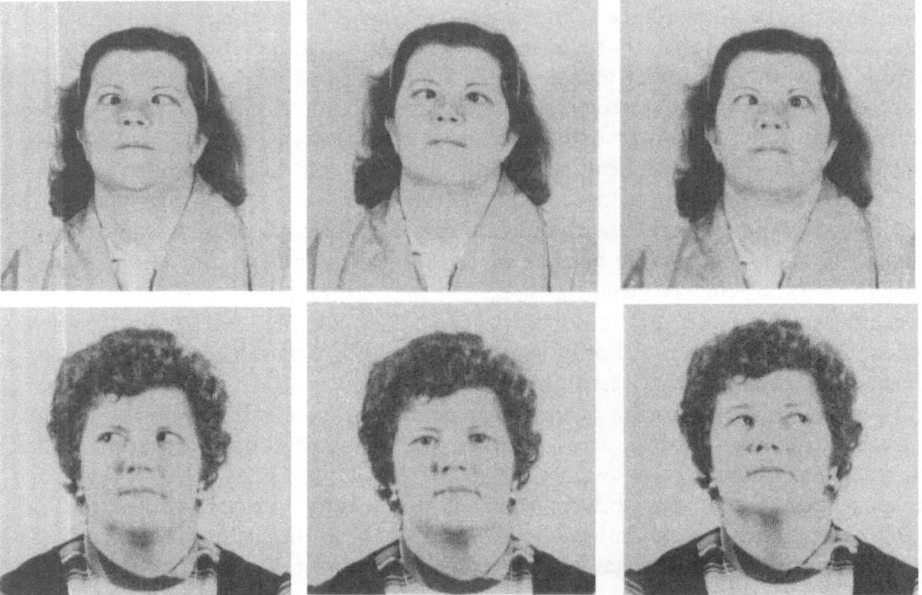

Fig. 2. Patient with traumatic bilateral abducens paresis. Gaze to the right, straight ahead and to the left before and after the transposition

## Discussion

The muscular neurotisation of extraocular muscles is indicated in cases where a spontaneous reinnervation may not be expected any more. The loss of the inferior oblique muscle causes no considerable restriction of the gaze upwards.

Before the transposition, a recession of the medial rectus muscle should be done to relieve any contraction of it, after having ascertained before, of course, that secondary contractions are existent in this muscle. The extent of recession should be generous (between 4 and 8 mm). Sometimes the recession operation allows the lateral muscle to spontaneously resume its function. Having waited about six months without observation of any sign of function of the lateral rectus muscle, the transposition operation should be carried out. The inferior oblique muscle must be placed near the bulbar muscular zone of the lateral rectus muscle because otherwise the expected success is prevented as the inferior oblique muscle is united with the tendon of the lateral rectus muscle where a muscular neurotisation is impossible.

The best results can be expected in cases where the transposition is timed according to the above mentioned guidelines. However, good results are possible at later times. In our cases the longest interval between accident and successfully treated abducens paresis was almost eight years [3].

If the transposition does not induce the expected success in time, a second transposition may still possibly render a good result. In this case, the inferior oblique is cut from the lateral rectus muscle which is recessed 5 to 6 mm, then both muscles are united again.

It often takes months until the effect of muscular neurotisation is evident; nevertheless, even on the second day after the operation, muscle exercises should be started. If the esotropia is not too great, diplopia should be eliminated by press-on prisms. Should vertical deviations occur after the transposition, no immediate therapy is necessary because often they adjust themselves of their own account after some months. All patients had the subjective feeling of an improvement immediately after the transposition.

*Summing up* all facts, one can say that the utilization of muscular neurotisation is a new and promising method of therapy for traumatic abducens pareses. The operation is technically simple, may be repeated at any time and will not interfere with other surgical techniques.

### References

1. Aichmair, H., Freilinger, G., Holle, J., Mandl, H., Mayr, R.: Muskuläre Neurotisation bei traumatischer Abduzensparese. Ein neuer Weg der operativen Behandlung. Klin. Mbl. Augenheilk. *167*, 580–583 (1975).
2. Aichmair, H.: Muscular neurotisation in surgery of traumatic abducens paresis. Jpn. J. Ophthal. *21*, 477–487 (1977).
3. Aichmair, H.: Auswirkungen operativer Eingriffe am Musculus obliquus inferior auf die Motilität des Bulbus. In: Augenbewegungsstörungen; Neurophysiologie und Klinik (Kommerell, G., ed.), pp. 105–110. München: J. F. Bergmann Verlag. 1978.

Author's address: Prof. Dr. H. Aichmair, II. Universitäts-Augenklinik, Alser Strasse 4, A-1090 Wien, Austria.

# Negative Experiences With Free Muscle Grafts to the Cheek in Patients With Facial Paralysis

## J.-P. A. Nicolai and P. H. Robinson

Department of Plastic Surgery,
St. Radboud University Hospital, Nijmegen, and
Department of Plastic Surgery, University Hospital,
Groningen, The Netherlands

With 1 Figure

To reanimate paralyzed elevators of the corner of the mouth with free muscle grafts several variations are possible. Over the past 100 years many operations for correction of facial paralysis have been described (Nicolai, 1979), and in the past ten years free grafting of skeletal muscle has been developed.

In the paralyzed cheek, muscular neurotisation is not possible and nerve impulses must be derived from elsewhere, preferably from the normal facial nerve through a cross-face nerve graft (Scaramella, 1975). This graft can be implanted at the same time as the muscle graft (Fig. 1A, C, E) or some months earlier so that reinnervation of the muscle graft occurs sooner (Fig. 1B, D, F). It has been maintained that predenervation some two weeks prior to transplantation is a prerequisite for muscle graft survival (Fig. 1A, B). Denervation lowers the metabolic rate, helps survival during the period of ischaemia after transplantation and possibly elicits production of a nerve growth factor (Murphy et al., 1977).

The technique in Fig. 1A has been described by Thompson and Gustavson (1976) and applied by Clodius (1979) and ourselves. Varying degrees of restoration of the voluntary movement of elevation to the angle of the mouth were reported in a minority of the patients treated. In neither series were duration, extent or cause of the facial paralysis mentioned.

The technique in 1B was used by Freilinger (1975), Rijnders (1978) and in principle in an animal experiment by Holle et al. (1974). All reported reinnervation of the graft, although actual function was minimal. The technique in D was applied in principle in two patients by Harii et al. (1976), by Tolhurst and Bos (1979) and by O'Brien et al. (1980). A certain degree of reanimation

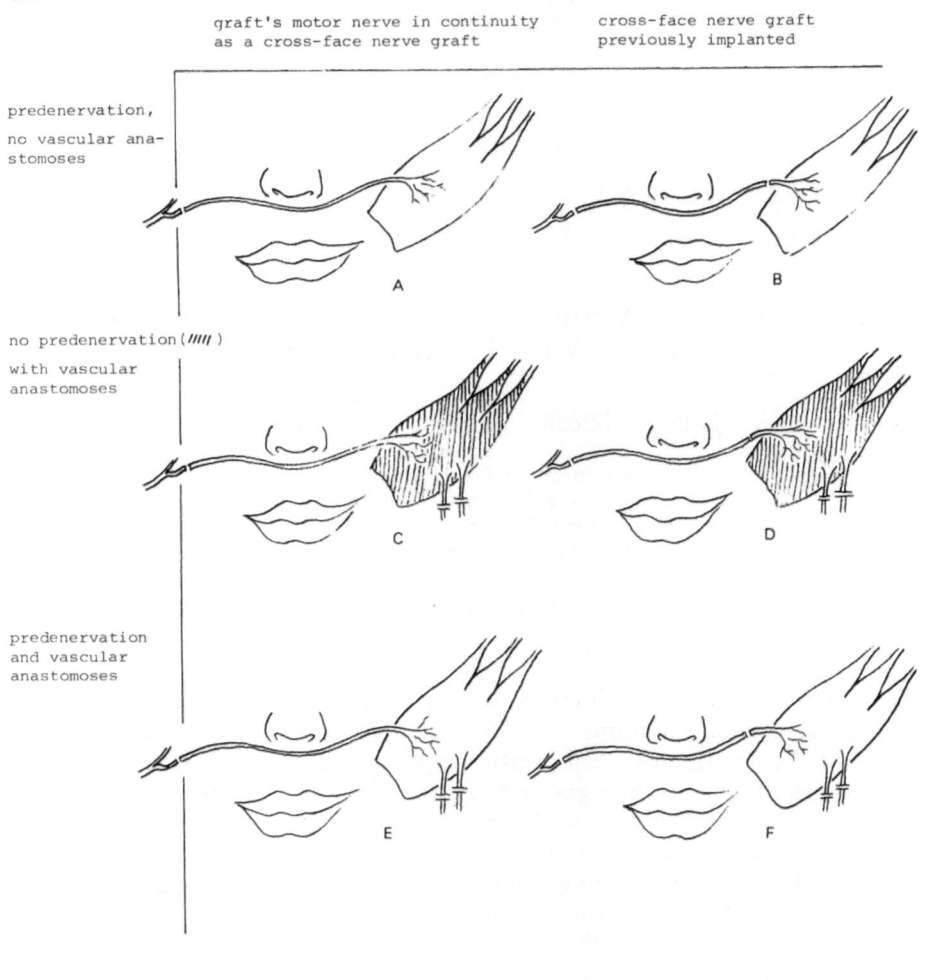

graft's motor nerve in continuity        cross-face nerve graft
as a cross-face nerve graft              previously implanted

predenervation,
no vascular ana-
stomoses

no predenervation (////)
with vascular
anastomoses

predenervation
and vascular
anastomoses

Number of operations required:
A: 2, B: 3, C: 1, D: 2, E: 2 and F: 3.

Fig. 1. Six variations of muscle and nerve grafting to the cheek in facial paralysis

resulted, although unconscious synchronous smiling was not stressed by the authors.

The technique in E was employed in ten patients by Mayou *et al.* (1978). Electromyographically the muscle grafts appeared to function, but the clinical results were disappointing. To our knowledge, the techniques C and F have not been reported in the literature. We report our experiences with technique A.

Eight patients with unilateral facial paralysis were treated as proposed by Thompson and Gustavson (1976) (Table 1). The facial musculature was electromyographically studied in all patients before operation. In all cases the extensor digitorum brevis muscle was grafted; the muscle was electromyographically studied before denervation, two weeks later on the day

*Table 1. Patients with unilateral facial paralysis treated according to the method described*

| Number | Sex | Age at operation | Cause of paralysis | Duration of paralysis (years) |
|--------|-----|------------------|--------------------|-------------------------------|
| 1. | f | 37 | extirpation of neurinoma in cerebellopontine angle | 8 |
| 2. | m | 22 | temporal bone trauma | 5 |
| 3. | m | 14 | congenital | 14 |
| 4. | f | 22 | congenital | 22 |
| 5. | m | 27 | poliomyelitis | 26 |
| 6. | f | 17 | congenital | 17 |
| 7. | f | 28 | extirpation of meningeoma in cerebellopontine angle | 7 |
| 8. | m | 29 | temporal bone trauma | 9 |

before transplantation and 3, 6, and 12 months after transplantation to the cheek. A standard series of six photographs of the patient's face was taken before and 3, 6 and 12 months after muscle-nerve transplantation.

The extensor hallucis and digitorum brevis muscles were denervated by cutting the deep peroneal nerve about 12 cm. proximal to the ankle joint in a bloodless field under pneumatic tourniquet. Two weeks later the muscle bellies with their tendons and the deep peroneal nerve in continuity were removed, again under tourniquet control. The sensory branch of the nerve was cut and its proximal stump implanted in the muscle graft. The fascia was meticulously removed from the muscle graft. A pocket was then made in the paralyzed cheek. The graft's tendons were fixed around the zygomatic arch and the other end was sutured to deep layers of the nasolabial fold. The nerve from the graft was tunnelled through the upper lip and microscopically sutured to branches of the facial nerve in the nasolabial region of the healthy side.

After operation the patients were given a liquid diet for four days and a soft diet for another four days.

Seven of the eight patients had a total unilateral facial paralysis without electromyographically recordable potentials. One (nr. 3) had a congenital paresis with some minimal movement in the cheek. In all patients the extensor digitorum brevis muscle appeared normal on clinical and electromyographical examination before denervation and paralysed afterwards.

The wounds in the donor area of the lower limb and in the face generally healed without problems. After transplantation, symmetry of the mouth at rest was improved in all patients. Yet, seven of the patients could never produce any movement with their grafts, and after a year electromyography could not show any surviving muscle tissue. Only the patient with the congenital paresis had some dynamic benefit. After a year he is even able to draw a dimple in his cheek. However, electromyography showed that his muscle graft was reinnervated from the ipsilateral paretic side and not through the nerve graft.

We believe that our technique of removal of muscle fascia and of suturing the muscle under proper tension was correct, as well as our nerve suturing. After the operation the patients showed a Hoffman-Tinel-like phenomenon in the upper lip, progressing in the direction of the muscle graft. But reinnervation probably took too long and the muscle grafts fibrosed before axons reached their destination. Implanting a cross-face nerve graft some months prior to muscle transplantation offers possibilities of earlier reinnervation.

The extensor digitorum brevis muscle has an amplitude of some 15 mm. at the most. Even under optimal conditions muscle grafts lose at least 50 % of their original working capacity (Terzis *et al.*, 1978; Benatar, Terzis, and Williams, 1981). After the techniques described, movement of the angle of the mouth would range 7 mm at best. The least loss of amplitude seems to be expected with the variation depicted in F. We conclude that the method we used (variation A), should no longer be applied.

## Acknowledgements

We wish to thank Prof. Dr. A. J. C. Huffstadt, Department of Plastic Surgery, and Dr. T. W. van Weerden, Department of Electromyography and Electro-encephalography of the University Hospital in Groningen, the Netherlands, where this work was performed.

## References

Clodius, L.: Facial animation with nonvascularized muscle transplantation. In: Microsurgical Composite Tissue Transplantation (Serafin, D., Buncke, H. J., eds.), ch. 32, p. 460. London: Mosby. 1979.

Freilinger, G.: A new technique to correct facial paralysis. Plast. Reconstr. Surg. *56,* 44 (1975).

Harii, K., Ohmori, K., Torii, S.: Free gracilis muscle transplantation, with microneurovascular anastomoses for the treatment of facial paralysis. Plast. Reconstr. Surg. *57,* 133 (1976).

Holle, J., Freilinger, G., Lischka, A.: Muscular and nerval neurotisation of muscle free grafts in pigs, in: Abstracts 9th Congress of the European Society for experimental surgery (Boeckl, O., Hell, E., Zimmerman, G., eds.), p. 21. Boltzmann-Institut für Experimentelle Chirurgie, Salzburg. 1974.

Mayou, B.: Free vascularized muscle transplants in the correction of facial paralysis. Winter Meeting of the British Association of Plastic Surgery, London, December 1978. Not published (1978).

Murphy, R. A., Singer, R. H., Saide, J. D., Pantazis, N. J., Blanchard, M. H., Byron, K. S., Arnason, B. G. W., Young, M.: Synthesis and secretion of a high molecular weight form of nerve growth factor by skeletal muscle cells in culture. Proc. Nat. Acad. Sci. USA *74,* 4496 (1977).

Nicolai, J. P. A.: Facial paralysis–100 years of treatment. Archivum Chirurgicum Neerlandicum *31,* 159 (1979).

O'Brien, B. M., Franklin, J. D., Morrison, W. A.: Crossfacial nerve grafts and microneurovascular free muscle transfer for long established facial palsy. Brit. J. Plast. Surg. *33,* 202 (1980).

Rijnders, W.: Behandeling van facialis paralyse met behulp van spierzenuwtransplantaties. Meeting of the Collegium Chirurgicum Neerlandicum, Nijmegen, May 6. Not published (1978).

Scaramella, L. F.: Anastomosis between the two facial nerves. Laryngoscope *85,* 1359 (1975).

Terzis, J. K., Sweet, R. C., Dykes, R. W., Williams, H. B.: Recovery of function in free muscle transplants using microneurovascular anastomoses. J. Hand Surg. *3,* 37 (1978).

Benatar, D., Terzis, J., Williams, B.: The Relevance of Preliminary Denervation in Muscle transplantation. This volume, p. 91. 1981.

Thompson, N., Gustavson, E. H.: The use of neuromuscular free autografts with microneural anastomosis to restore elevation to the paralysed angle of the mouth in cases of unilateral facial paralysis. Chir. Plast. *3,* 165 (1976).

Tolhurst, D. E., Bos, K.: Dynamic correction of facial paralysis, panel discussion. Meeting of the Collegium Chirurgicum Neerlandicum, Utrecht, May 12. Not published (1979).

## Appendix

*Film.* "Temporal muscle transposition after cross-face nerve grafting" by J.-P. A. Nicolai (Department of Plastic Surgery, St. Radboud University Hospital, Nijmegen, the Netherlands).

## Summary

The operative technique is shown of a combination originally published by Freilinger (1975). A temporal muscle flap is denervated and transposed to the nasolabial area according to principles described by Lexer (1931) and modified by Rubin (1978).

Then, fascicles at the end of a previously implanted crossface nerve graft are dissected out and buried between fibers of the muscle flap.

Since it is too soon to assess final results, these were not shown.

### References

1. Freilinger, G.: A new technique to correct facial paralysis. Plast. Reconstr. Surg. *56*, 44 (1975).
2. Lexer, E.: Die gesamte Wiederherstellungschirurgie, p. 755. Leipzig: J. A. Barth. 1931.
3. Rubin, L. R.: Temporalis muscle transposition technique for late permanent facial paralysis, in: Symposium on the neurologic aspects of plastic surgery, Vol. 17 (Fredericks, S., Brody, G. S., eds.), ch. 36, p. 289. St. Louis: C. V. Mosby. 1978.

Author's address: Dr. J.-P. A. Nicolai, Department of Plastic Surgery, St. Radboud University Hospital, 6525 GA Nijmegen, The Netherlands.

# Treatment of Facial Paralysis With Free Autogenous Muscle Transplants*

## L. Hakelius

Department of Plastic Surgery,
University Hospital, Uppsala, Sweden

Since 1972 I have used free muscle transplantation according to Thompson in cases of unilateral facial paralysis. The operative techniques are slightly modified from those developed by Thompson. I have used the method mainly for improving three important functions of the facial muscles.

1. To improve eye-lid closure. The muscle used in these cases is the extensor digitorum brevis of the foot. In my first cases I used two muscle bellies, one in the upper and one in the lower eye-lid on the healthy side. Later in the series I have used only one belly in the lower eye-lid with its tendon running through the nose and in a bow in the upper eye-lid on the paralyzed side. As lining of the tunnel through the nose I have used a vein graft except in the first 7 cases where a silastic sheet was used. 2. The second indication for free grafting has been to restore the sphincteric control of the oral commissure, the reinnervation of the graft is then coming from the healthy part of the orbicularis oris muscle. At the same time one can make a static support of the angle of the mouth with the tendon of the graft. In these cases I usually used the palmaris longus muscle split into two halves including the tendon. In a few cases I have used a part of the sartorius muscle. 3. The third indicion of muscle transplants has been to strenghten partially paralysed elevators of the angle of the mouth. The graft is then placed in contact with these muscles. A prerequisite is of course that the elevators are not totally paralysed and we believe that if the elevators have about 10–15 % left of the motor function compared with the healthy side there is a possibility for reinnervation of the graft.

* This paper is based on the following papers: Hakelius, L.: Transplantation of free autogenous muscle in the treatment of facial paralysis. Scand. J. Plast. Reconstr. Surg. 8, 220 (1974). Hakelius, L., Stålberg, E.: Electromyographical studies of free autogenous muscle transplants in man. Scand. J. Plast. Reconstr. Surg. 8, 211 (1974); Hakelius, L.: Free muscle grafting. Clinics in Plast. Surg. 6, 301 (1979).

Between the years 1972 and 1978 I have made 107 transplants to 89 patients. Etiologically the largest group was patients with intracranial tumours, mostly operated acoustic neurinomas, which includes 33 patients. 12 patients had a congenital palsy and 11 sequelae after a Bell's palsy. I have made transplantations to the eye-lid only in 44 cases, to both the eyelid and the orbicularis oris muscle in 17 cases, to the orbicularis oris muscle only in 10 cases, to the orbicularis oris muscle and to strengthen the partially paralysed muscle in 1 case, and to strengthen partially paralysed muscles only in 17 cases. The first clinical and electromyographical signs of reinnervation occurred 4 to 6 weeks after transplantation. I have divided the material in three groups when evaluating the results. The first group consists of the transplantations made for improving eye-lid closure. It consists of 61 cases, the patients were between 12 and 74 years of age at surgery with an average of 44 years. The greatest problem in these cases have been the connective tissue synechiaes that develop at both ends of the nasal tunnel during the period before reinnervation of the graft as during this period the grafts do not move. Because of that and the necessity to correct the length of the tendon in some cases, minor corrective operations are required, for example tenolysis at the ends of the nasal tunnel or correction of the tendon tension at the lateral margin of the orbit. The need for secondary procedures can be determined when reinnervation has occurred, usually three months after grafting. 79 such operations have been performed all in local anaesthesia and on an out-patient basis. In some cases more than one operation has been necessary. Secondary operations for paralytic ectropion has been made in 7 patients. In a trial to analyze the results objectively as regards transplant function I have divided the patients in three groups "good", "fair" and "unimproved". In the "good" group the patients have to fulfil these three criteria: Good palpable muscle contraction of the graft, a rima of the affect side of the same size as on the normal when the patient is looking straight forward and a persisting lagophtalmus of maximum 2 mm on eye-lid closure. In the "fair"-group the patients have to fulfil these three criteria: Good muscle contraction of the graft, a rima of the affected side big enough not to reduce the field of vision when the patient is looking straight forward, and a persisting lagophtalmus of maximum 3 mm on eye-lid closure. The results according to the criteria I have chosen are estimated good in 28 cases, fair in 19 cases and unimproved in 13 cases. The follow-up time has been between 5 and 68 months (average 24 months). The two groups good and fair constitute together about 78 % of the material. Included in the unimproved group are the 7 patients which I operated early in the series and instead of a vein graft as lining of the nasal tunnel a silastic sheath was used; this silastic sheath had to be removed later in all cases. The results on eye-lid closure are relatively easy to estimate compared with the other two groups where you have to inspect the muscle function and ask for the opinion of the patients of the results. The group where the muscle transplants have been used to improve the sphincteric function of the orbicularis oris muscle consisted of 28 patients. 19 of them were improved, 9 unimproved. That means that about 68 % of these cases were improved and had benefit from the operation. The observation time was here 8 to 67 months with an average of 24.5 months. In the third group, consisting of 16 patients in whom the transplant was used to improve the strength of the muscles lifting the angle of the mouth, 12 were improved and 4 unimproved, which means a percentage of improved patients of about 75 %. The follow-up time here was 5 to 52 months, with an average of 14.8 months.

Author's address: Prof. Dr. L. Hakelius, Department of Plastic Surgery, University Hospital, S-750 14 Uppsala 14, Sweden.

# Use of Muscle in Head and Neck Reconstruction

**R. F. Mazzola**

Department of Plastic Surgery,
Milan University School of Medicine,
Milano, Italy

With 7 Figures

Those who are familiar with head and neck surgery know the difficulties related to this type of operation, due to local and systemic factors such as saliva, irradiated tissue, scars from ablative procedures, age, malnutrition and poor defense mechanisms.

Infection and subsequent wound breakdown represent a major hazard. An uneventful postoperative follow-up is contingent upon awareness of many factors, neglect of which may lead to complications: e.g. care to maintain the skin and mucous membranes clean, intraoral hygiene, choice of the proper antibiotic, adequate nutritional support, and the correct surgical approach.

Surgery should be based on:

1. complete excision of irradiated tissue;

2. meticulous reconstruction of the lining without producing tension of the mucosal flaps;

3. use of safe viable flaps for coverage, transferred in one stage and outlined far from radiated fields;

4. the presence of a muscular layer between the lining and the covering, which provides a good blood supply for both.

This report is aimed at emphasizing the importance of the role played by muscle in achieving a higher rate of success in the reconstructive procedure: when transposed alone, or with the overlying skin, as a musculocutaneous unit, it provides the surgeon with a safe and effective method for one-stage operations in head and neck surgery.

## Muscle Flap Transposition

In certain head and neck reconstructions, particularly when the wound margins of the lining are traumatized and devascularized as a result of previous

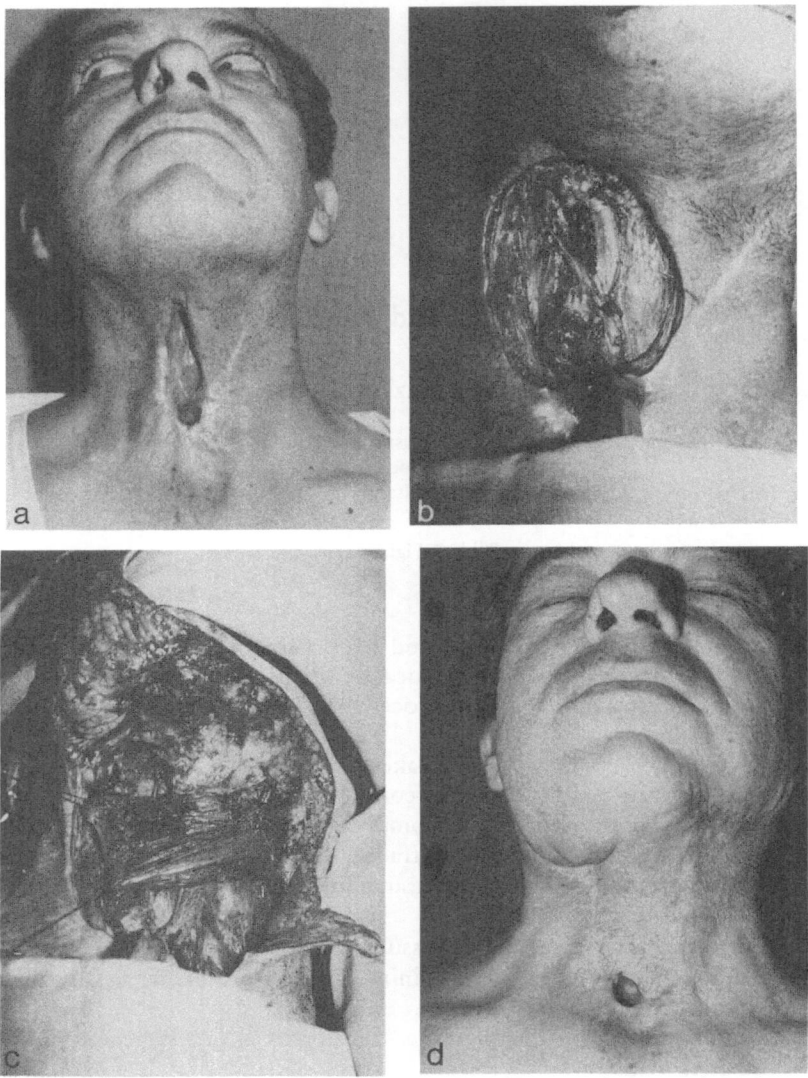

Fig. 1. Muscle flap transposition. *a* Large pharyngostome highly radiated. Preoperative view. *b* Closure of the pharyngeal layer in the midline. *c* The left sterno-mastoid muscle has been transposed between the lining and skin covering. *d* Result, 2 months postoperatively. A submandibular flap has been rotated down for covering

Fig. 2. Muscle flap transposition. *a* Large pharyngostome highly radiated. *b* Result 8 months postoperatively after closure with acromio-pectoral flap. *c* Intraoperative view. The pharyngeal tube has been reconstructed mobilizing the mucosa by wide undermining. *d* A superiorly based flap of left sterno-mastoid muscle, transposed onto the defect, enhances the blood supply to the lining. *e* A left acromio-pectoral skin flap is outlined for cover and *f* sutured in place with primary closure of the donor area. The flap is passed under the intervening bipedicled flap (visible in Fig. e) to collapse any dead space

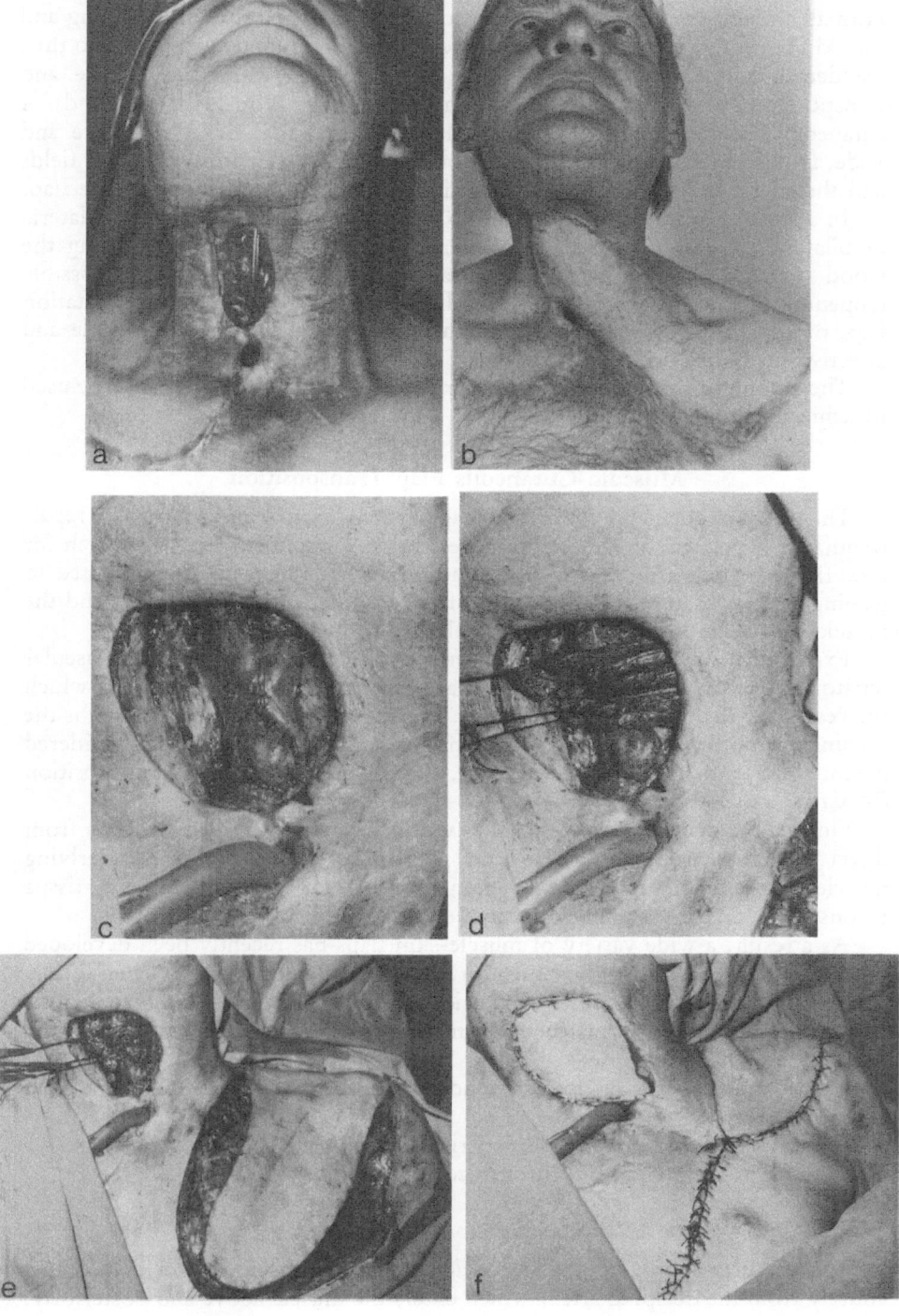

radiation treatment, affording an inadequate basis for satisfactory closure, we normally insert one or two sterno-mastoid muscle flaps between the lining and the skin covering, thus introducing tissue with a good blood supply. To do this, we detach and elevate the lower end of the muscle from the clavicle and transpose it onto the carefully sutured pharyngeal layer (Fig. 1b, c and 2c, d). A cutaneous flap provides the covering. It is essential that this flap is safe and wide, that it can easily rotate, that it is outlined in areas far from radiation fields and that the suture lines on the lining do not coincide with those on the flap.

In another report (Mazzola et al., 1979a) we emphasized how the unilateral or bilateral transfer of a portion of sterno-mastoid muscle, by enhancing the blood supply to the pharyngeal mucosa, represents a barrier against possible reopening of the pharyngostome. We also recommended the use of a rotation flap, outlined in the suprahyoid area, the submandibular flap, as a simple and effective procedure for skin covering (Fig. 1).

The acromio-pectoral flap (Fig. 2), or the delto-pectoral flap can also be used to achieve the same purpose.

### Musculo-Cutaneous Flap Transposition

The constant demand for single-stage reconstructive procedures to repair traumatic, neoplastic or radiation injuries, has prompted surgeons to search for new flaps. In the last decade, greater attention has therefore been devoted to gaining precise anatomical knowledge of the vascularization of muscles and the muscle-skin relationships in terms of blood supply.

Experimental and clinical studies have led to the identification of the vascular territories of each muscle and to the exact determination of the point at which the vessels enter the muscles, how many branches they produce and which is the dominant branch. On this basis certain non-essential muscles may be considered potential flaps of predictable viability, which are suitable for transposition (McCraw and Dibbell, 1977; McCraw et al., 1977).

Finally, the demonstration that skin vascularization is derived not only from direct cutaneous arteries, but also from perforating vessels from the underlying muscle, represented the starting point for a new concept in soft tissue reconstruction: the outlining of composite flaps.

As a result, a wide variety of muscle-skin flaps has recently been developed in different parts of the body, based on a specific vascular pedicle. When locally rotated or transferred to other territories as free flaps, they can repair defects that were virtually unreconstructable in the past, in one stage with safety and relative ease.

Myocutaneous flaps have also found revolutionary applications in the head and neck area.

The present paper reports our experience with some myocutaneous flaps we are familiar with in head and neck reconstruction.

### The Sternocleidomastoid Myocutaneous Flap

The vascular supply to the sternocleidomastoid muscle is provided almost entirely from the occipital artery which enters the muscle above and posteriorly, beneath the posterior belly of the digastric muscle. The superior thyroid artery and the transverse cervical artery also participate in vascularization of the muscle in its middle and inferior portion, but their contribution is not essential for the survival of the compound flap, when transposed. The flap is elevated distally. The muscle is detached from the sternal and clavicular attachments together with the overlying portion of platysma and skin. Where the carotid bifurcates, the dissection should be performed with the occipital artery in direct view to avoid any injury to it.

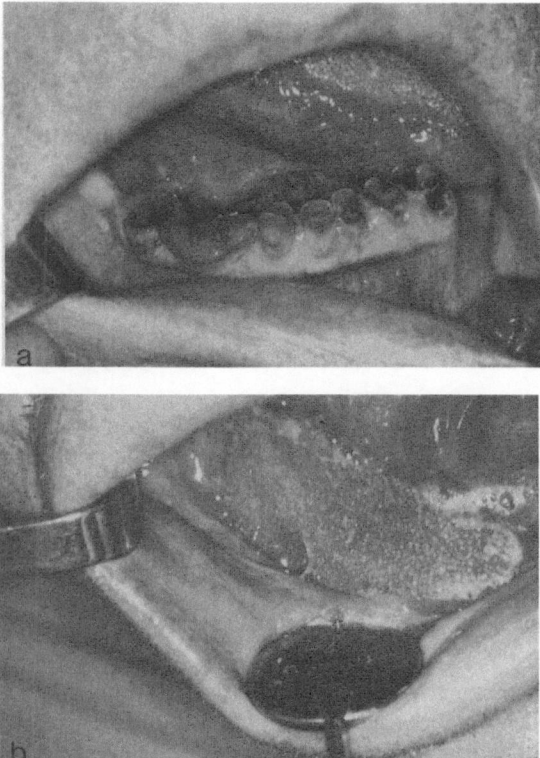

Fig. 3. Sterno-mastoid myocutaneous flap. *a* Squamous cell carcinoma of the floor of the mouth. *b* The repair of the defect created by the ablation is by rotation of sterno-mastoid myocutaneous flap

The flap may be elevated either with the skin attached along the entire length of the muscle or with only an island of skin attached over the distal portion, depending on the size of the defect.

Normally the donor area is closed primarily. The flap is well vascularized and has a good arc of rotation allowing it to reach the temporal area, the tonsillar fossa, the floor of the mouth, the palate, the mastoid region and the neck. It has been used to repair facial defects (Owens, 1955), the cheek and lips (O'Brien, 1970), to line the palate after maxillectomy (Bakamjian, 1963), and to resurface the floor of the mouth after excision due to cancer (Fig. 3).

The sterno-mastoid myocutaneous flap provides a satisfactory means of covering defects of reasonably limited size, in the head and neck area. It is well vascularized and supplies a hairless supple skin with minimal fat.

However, if previous radiation or ligation of the superior vascular pedicle has been carried out, other methods should be used.

## The Trapezius Myocutaneous Flap

The dominant vascular pedicle for the trapezius muscle is the transverse cervical artery which enters the anterior margin of the muscle at the base of the neck, normally giving off an ascending and a descending branch. The ascending branch, which sometimes originates from the thyrocervical trunk, supplies the superior trapezius muscle fibres, while the perforating musculocutaneous vessels supply the overlying skin territory in the nape of the neck. The descending branch runs between the deep portion of the trapezius and the levator scapulae parallel to the vertebral column. The perforating musculocutaneous vessels supply the skin between the scapula and the vertebral column. Finally, the inferolateral portion of the trapezius is supplied by the suprascapular artery, and the fibres located in the upper neck by the occipital artery.

The trapezius muscle is the source of two main compound flaps: a lateral and a posterior one.

The *lateral flap,* outlined over the anterior portion of the trapezius muscle and based either on the occipital artery or on the ascending branch of the transverse cervical artery, according to different authors, can easily cover the lower two thirds of the face and the anterior neck.

Donski and McCraw (1970) have described an extension of this flap over the deltoid muscle, while Mathes and Nahai (1979) have elevated the skin with the entire upper portion of the muscle down to the lateral surface of the upper arm.

The *posterior flap* is based on the descending branch of the transverse cervical artery. Before outlining this flap it is suggested that the transverse cervical artery be identified in the supraclavicular fossa and that its pedicle be followed while penetrating the deep aspect of the muscle. The "paddle" of skin is then elevated in the area located between the vertebral column and the scapula (Fig. 4 b). Undermining of the myocutaneous unit is accomplished bluntly by hand: the descending artery is identified on the undersurface of the muscle and its fibres may be safely divided medially and laterally to include this vessel (Fig. 4 c). The muscle should be freed as far as the anterior border of the trapezius, avoiding any injury to the spinal nerve, which runs at this level.

This myocutaneous unit, thanks to its wide arc of rotation, may then easily be used to cover defects located in the head, skull, mastoid region (Fig. 4), anterior and posterior neck, shoulder and upper thoracic region.

The posterior trapezius myocutaneous unit offers several advantages in head and neck reconstruction. It supplies a considerable amount of bulk muscular tissue for repairing major defects. The overlying skin is thick, frequently

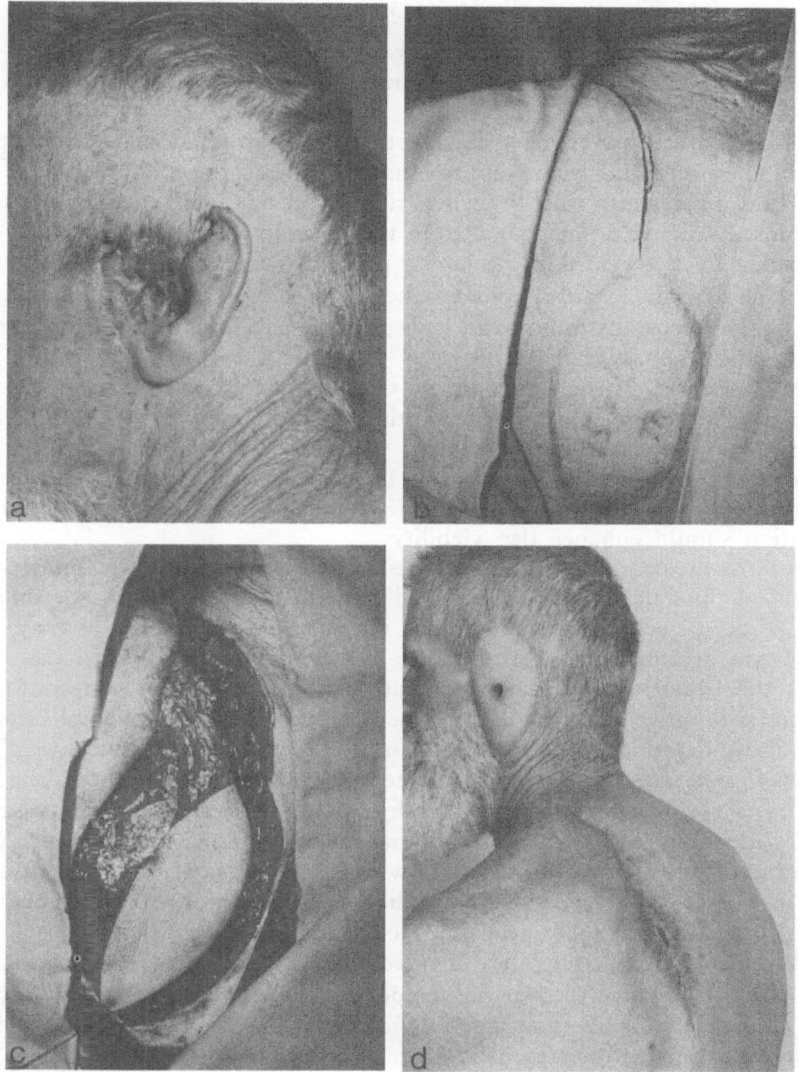

Fig. 4. Trapezius myocutaneous flap. *a* Baso-squamous cell carcinoma of the left auricle involving the superficial lobe of the parotid and temporalis muscle. *b, c* A posterior trapezius myocutaneous flap is outlined to cover the wide defect located in the temporal region. *d* Final result one month postoperatively. The donor area has been primarily closed

hairless, extremely viable and normally outside any previously radiated field. The donor area can be primarily closed (Fig. 4d).

On the contrary, its main limitation lies in the positioning of the patient, who has either to be turned on the operating table, or to be directly placed in a lateral position, thus complicating the ablative stage.

## The Pectoralis Major Myocutaneous Flap

The pectoralis major muscle derives its blood supply mainly from the thoracoacromial artery and the lateral thoracic artery, which are branches of the axillary artery.

The thoraco-acromial artery pierces the clavipectoral fascia at the upper border of the pectoralis minor (approximately beneath the middle third of the clavicle) and divides into four branches, the largest of these being the pectoral, which runs parallel to a line drawn from the acromion to the xiphoid, and it is accompanied by the vein and the lateral pectoral nerve.

The lateral thoracic artery pierces the clavipectoral fascia laterally to the tendon of the pectoralis minor and runs in a cephalo-caudal direction almost parallel to the thoraco-acromial artery.

Both arteries lie in the undersurface of the muscle, enclosed in its fascial component. As they give no branches to the pectoralis minor, the existing plane between these two muscles is avascular.

According to Freeman *et al.* (1981), the lateral thoracic artery also contributes significantly to the vascularity of the pectoralis major and its preservation should enhance flap viability.

As regards the *operative technique,* we follow the suggestions of Freeman *et al.* (1981). A "paddle" of skin is outlined over the anterior chest, according to the size of the defect to be covered. The incisions are carried out as far as the fascia of the pectoralis muscle is visible. Once the island of skin has been isolated, the supero-lateral incision round the "paddle" is prolonged to the acromion, without injuring the fascia. The skin over the whole pectoralis muscle is carefully undermined. The humeral insertion of the muscle is divided. This manoeuver gives access to the plane between the pectoralis major and minor, the two muscles are separated by hand with a blunt dissection and the vascular pedicle is identified and preserved. The medial costosternal insertions are then sectioned and the island of skin may now be gently elevated with the vascular pedicle in direct view (Fig. 5c and 6c). The pectoralis major myocutaneous flap is then positioned into the defect to be covered (Fig. 5d).

With the insertions completely divided, based only on the major vascular pedicle, the flap can easily cover the temporal bone (Aryian, 1979), the orbital region (Aryian, 1980), the pharyngoesophageal region (Theogaraj *et al.,* 1980), the floor of the mouth for resurfacing defects after hemiglossectomy (Fig. 5) or the anterior neck for closing pharyngostomes or wide skin losses (Fig. 6).

The pectoralis major myocutaneous flap has many advantages for head and neck reconstruction compared to other methods previously described in the literature (e.g. forehead, delto-pectoral flap, etc.) and to the two myocutaneous flaps discussed above. It possesses a wider arc of rotation and, thanks to its vascular pedicle, has predictable viability, allowing a large amount of thick skin

Fig. 5. Pectoralis major myocutaneous flap. *a* Ulcerated squamous cell carcinoma of the floor of the mouth. *b* The defect at the end of the ablative stage. *c* The left pectoralis major myocutaneous flap has been outlined. *d* The "paddle" of skin is positioned into the oral defect. *e* Result two months postoperatively. The myocutaneous flap is visible on the left side

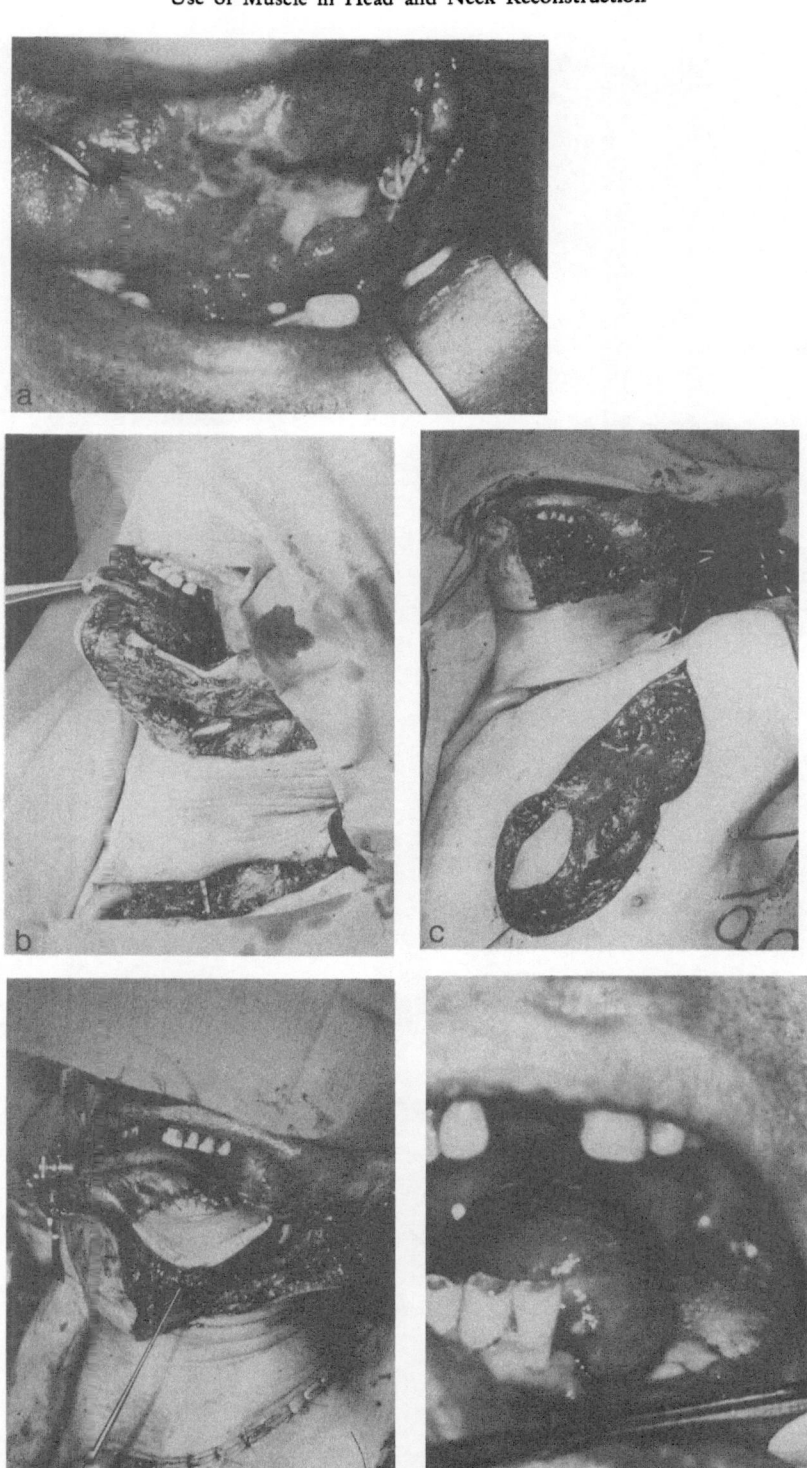

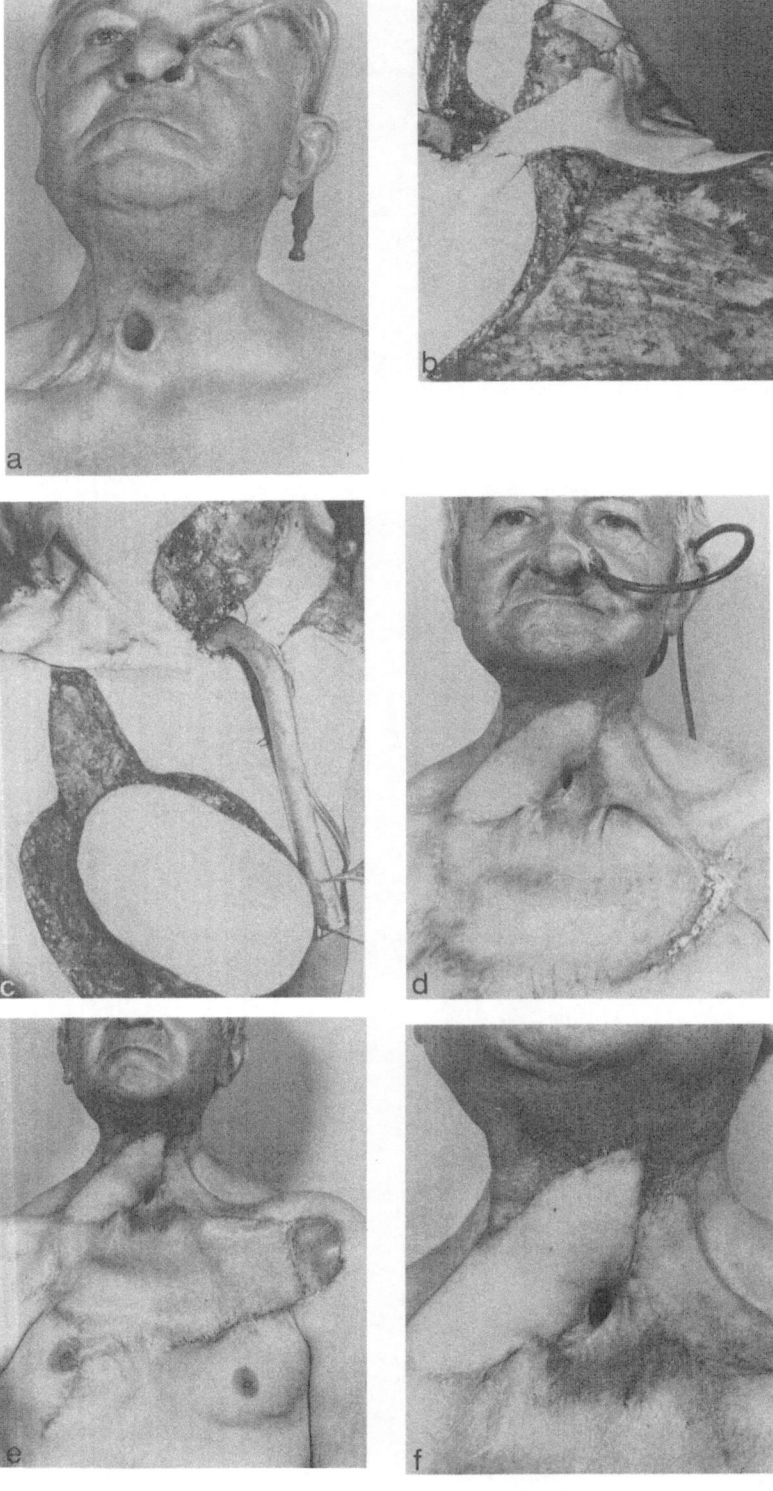

to be transferred. It is outlined far from radiated areas, and the muscle pedicle protects the large vessels of the neck, provided that radical dissection has been performed. It can also be used on patients in whom previous reconstructive procedures (e.g. delto-pectoral flaps) have failed, because the blood supply to the flap lies deep in the pectoralis muscle and therefore is very seldom interrupted. The donor area is closed primarily, leaving an acceptable scar (Fig. 6e).

In some cases the island of skin over the pectoralis major muscle is hairbearing. In our opinion this is the only disadvantage with this flap, when used for intraoral coverage (Fig. 7).

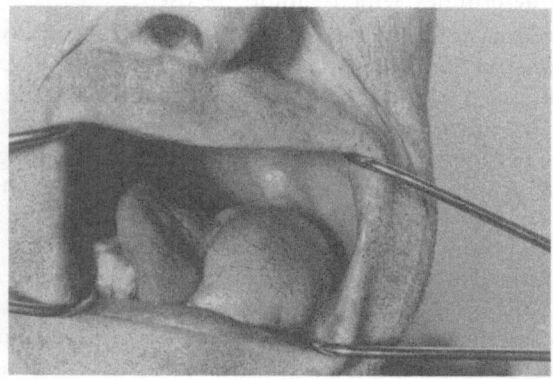

Fig. 7. Pectoralis major myocutaneous flap. Exemple of hair-bearing "paddle" of skin used for intraoral reconstruction

## Discussion

The modern concept of reconstructive surgery calls for single-stage operations to be performed.

In the present report we have sought to demonstrate the important role played by muscles in facilitating achievement of successful results.

*When transferred alone,* the muscle provides a vascular contribution which reinforces the mucosal suture, thereby improving healing.

We have presented cases of highly radiated pharyngostomes, in which the rotation of one or two flaps of sterno-mastoid muscle, interposed between the

---

Fig. 6. Pectoralis major myocutaneous flap. *a* Squamous cell carcinoma of the hypopharynx with cutaneous invasion. The ablation included removal of hypopharynx with wide excision of overlying skin. *b* Cervical esophageal reconstruction with a left delto-pectoral flap. *c* A pectoralis major myocutaneous flap with wide "paddle" of skin has been outlined for covering the defect in the anterior neck. *d* End of the first stage of cervical esophageal reconstruction. Observe the temporary fistula on the left side, and the myocutaneous flap in place. The donor area has been primarily closed. *e* Final result one month postoperatively with the unused portion of the delto-pectoral flap returned to the original position. *f* Closer view of the pectoralis major myocutaneous flap

lining and the covering, by including highly vascularized tissue, prevents the mucosal suture from reopening (Fig. 1 and 2).

*When transferred with the overlying skin* and subcutaneous tissue, based on a specific vascular pedicle, the muscle offers an important step forward in head and neck reconstruction, since with a single manoeuver it satisfies two of the essential prerequisites for successful surgery mentioned at the outset. It provides a good blood supply to the lining and deep structures and at the same time feeds the island of thick skin needed for a safe covering, with perforating vessels.

We have reported our experience with the use of sternocleidomastoid, trapezius and pectoralis major musculo-cutaneous units. Each of these flaps has its advantages and disadvantages, but the site and particularly the size of the defect ultimately determines which should be used.

The sternocleidomastoid myocutaneous flap has been employed with success for intraoral reconstruction when the defect created by the ablation does not require a large amount of skin for coverage (Fig. 3). However, flap viability may be compromised by previous radiation or neck dissection.

The trapezius myocutaneous flap, based on the descending branch of the transverse cervical artery, supplies a good amount of viable, thick skin, which may usefully be employed, for instance, to close large defects in the temporal region (Fig. 4). Its main disadvantage is the position of the patient on the operating table during surgery, which may interfere with the ablative stage.

The pectoralis major myocutaneous flap is extremely versatile and reliable, and represents a significant advance over other available techniques.

The delto-pectoral flap has been the mainstay in head and neck reconstruction for many years, but its use involves a two-stage procedure, and the donor area requires skin grafting (Bakamjian, 1965; Mazzola *et al.*, 1979b).

The pectoralis major myocutaneous flap provides a thin, well vascularized skin with a single-stage operation, and the donor area is closed primarily, leaving an acceptable scar on the patient's anterior chest wall (Fig. 6e).

Although the island of skin over the pectoralis major muscle may be hair-bearing when used intraorally, this minimal discomfort involved is greatly outweighed by the advantages of the operation (Fig. 7).

Moreover, the pectoralis muscle, when transferred to the neck, gives the large vessels adequate coverage.

Its morbidity is negligible. Indeed, there was no failure in our series of 14 pectoralis major myocutaneous flaps used to effect intraoral repairs after ablative procedures for cancer, and the closure of pharyngostomes and defects in the anterior neck.

We agree with Magee *et al.* (1980), that the pectoralis major myocutaneous flap may be the delto-pectoral of the future.

## Summary

The author emphasizes the importance of the role played by muscle achieving a higher rate of success in reconstructive procedure in the head and neck area.

To repair defects created by ablation due to cancer, the muscle may be transposed either alone, or with the overlying skin as a musculo-cutaneous unit, thus giving the surgeon a safe, effective method for single-stage operations.

*When transposed alone,* the muscle provides a vascular contribution which reinforces the muscosal suture. The rotation of one or two flaps of sterno-mastoid muscle, interposed between the lining and skin covering, thus prevents the mucosal suture from reopening.

*When transferred with the overlying skin,* and based on a specific vascular pedicle, the muscle represents a revolutionary advance in head and neck reconstruction.

The author reports technical details and his clinical experience on the use of sternocleidomastoid, trapezius and pectoralis major myocutaneous flaps to cover various types of defect.

### References

Aryian, S.: Further experiences with the pectoralis major myocutaneous flap for immediate repair of defects from excision of head and neck cancer. Plast. Reconstr. Surg. *64*, 605–612 (1979).

Aryian, S.: Pectoralis major, sternomastoid and other musculocutaneous flaps for head and neck reconstruction. Clin. Plast. Surg. *7*, 89–109 (1980).

Bakamjian, V. Y.: A technique for primary reconstruction of the palate after radical maxillectomy for cancer. Plast. Reconstr. Surg. *31*, 103–117 (1963).

Bakamjian, V. Y.: A Two-stage method for pharyngoesophageal reconstruction with a primary pectoral skin flap. Plast. Reconstr. Surg. *36*, 173–184 (1965).

Donski, P., McCraw, J. B.: Myocutaneous flaps in head and neck reconstruction. Chir. Plast. (Berl.) *4*, 255–261 (1979).

Freeman, J. L., Walker, P. E., Wilson, J. S. P., Shaw, H. J.: The vascular anatomy of the pectoralis major myocutaneous flap. Brit. J. Plast. Surg. *34*, 3–10 (1981).

Magee, W. P., Gilbert, D. A., McInnis, W. D.: Extended muscle and musculocutaneous flaps. Clin. Plast. Surg. *7*, 57–70 (1980).

Mathes, S. J., Nahai, F.: Clinical atlas of muscle and musculocutaneous flaps. St. Louis: Mosby. 1979.

Mazzola, R. F., Oldini, C., Sambataro, G.: Use of submandibular flap to close pharyrgostomes and other defects of lower anterior neck region. Plast. Reconstr. Surg. *64*, 340–346 (1979a).

Mazzola, R. F., Sambataro, G., Oldini, C.: Our experience with pharyngoesophageal reconstruction. Ann. Plast. Surg. *2*, 219–228 (1979b).

McCraw, J. B., Dibbell, D. G.: Experimental definition of independent myocutaneous vascular territories. Plast. Reconstr. Surg. *60*, 212–220 (1977).

McCraw, J. B., Dibbell, D. G., Canaway, J. H.: Clinical definition of independent myocutaneous vascular territories. Plast. Reconstr. Surg. *60*, 341–352 (1977).

O'Brien, B.: A muscle-skin pedicle for total reconstruction of the lower lip. Plast. Reconstr. Surg. *45*, 395–399 (1970).

Owens, N. A.: A compound neck pedicle designed for the repair of massive facial defects: formation, development and application. Plast. Reconstr. Surg. *15*, 369–389 (1955).

Theogaraj, S. D., Merritt, W. H., Acharya, G., Cohen, I. K.: The pectoralis major musculocutaneous island flap in a single-stage reconstruction of the pharyngoesophageal region. Plast. Reconstr. Surg. *65*, 267–276 (1980).

Author's address: Prof. Dr. R. F. Mazzola, Via Marchiondi 7, I-20122 Milano, Italy.

### Discussion

*Nicolai:* Do you have troubles with contraction of your muscle flaps?

*Mazzola:* No, I don't have troubles. They of course contract but this is more a cosmetic problem and not a problem from the reconstructive point of view. It is very important to preserve the nerve; otherwise the muscle atrophies with consequent troubles in the early postoperative period.

*Bruck:* If you keep the nerve and vessels of the myocutaneous flap you lose about 30% of the muscle because of inactivity.

*Hakelius:* Did you ever see reinnervation of the transposed myocutaneous flap by the underlying host-muscles?

*Mazzola:* Yes, I saw such a phenomen in a reconstruction of a facial cheek with a myocutaneous flap, where I got muscle contraction several months later.

*Tolhurst:* Dr. Hakelius' question was rather interesting, because wasn't it showed once that when a muscle is supplied by a nerve, unless you divide this nerve, it can never accept a second nerve supply?

*Hakelius:* I think they can do it if the muscle is only partially denervated. Then some fibres can receive reinnervation by muscular neurotisation.

*Harii:* I don't think that innervation of the myocutaneous flap is of any importance. I always denervate the muscle and so I have less complication than with an innervated transposed muscle, which always gives some unpleasant impressions to the patient. Only if transposed to the face, I try to anastomose the motor nerve of the muscle with the facial stump to get reinnervation of the muscle with fibres of the facial nerve.

# Summary

*Harii:* Much superb experimental work has been shown yesterday and many critical clinical communications have been given this morning. We are now very happy to have different ways to transplant a skeletal muscle. And I think, in a free muscle transplantation, once the muscle is detatched, the muscle loses very quickly its original excursion and contraction. And many muscles after the transfer cannot gain the original amplitude. But though it is my opinion that this fact is completely proved and therefore I believe, we must transplant a larger amount of muscle, because it is losing its amplitude after the transfer. And if we applied this free muscle graft to the face, there are a lot of difficult problems. The first one are the two different motions in the face, for instance the emotional motion and the balance motion. Most patients are only able to innervate their balance muscles and do not innervate during emotional activity. The healthy muscles on the healthy side are very strong compared with the muscles on the paralyzed side, and I therefore believe in transplanting powerful muscles to come up with the powerful healthy muscle on the opposite side. Also when these muscles are transferred to the hand, it is important to transport bigger muscles to gain a good amplitude of the transferred muscle.

# Myoplastic Operations for Sphincter Reconstruction, Upper Extremity and Other Regions

# Treatment of Anal and Urinary Incontinence With Free Muscle Transplants*

## L. Hakelius

Department of Plastic Surgery,
University Hospital, Uppsala, Sweden

## Anal Incontinence

The human anal sphincter system is composed of three muscles. The smooth internal sphincter, the striated external sphincter and the striated puborectalis muscle. The internal sphincter appears to contribute to the tonic closure of the anus at rest and plays no part in maintaining continence when the rectum is distended with faeces. The external sphincter contracts when the pressure in the rectum increases, but it can maintain the contraction only for about 1 minute and plays a relatively minor part in the mechanism of continence. Stephens, a pediatric surgeon interested in anal atresia, pointed out the dominant role of the pubo-rectalis muscle in maintaining continence. The pubo-rectalis muscle is the caudal and medial portion of the muscular floor of the pelvis. The muscle is formed as a U-shaped sling, arising at the back of the pubic bone near the symphysis, and corresponding fibres from both sides unite into a sling behind the rectum at the ano-rectal junction. The pubo-rectalis contracts as soon as increased intrarectal pressure endangers continence. The shortening of the muscle sling pushes the ano-rectal junction forward and upward, making the angle between the rectum and the anal canal more acute, thereby preventing passage of the contents. Stephens has demonstrated that after surgery for imperforate anus, continence could be achieved by use of the puborectalis muscle alone. When the pubo-rectalis muscle is damaged, atrophic or lacking, anal continence is disturbed. In such cases the incontinence can be treated by free muscle transplantation. The aim of the operation is to place a muscle graft as a sling around the rectum, imitating the position and function of the

* This paper is partially based on the following papers: Hakelius, L.: Free autogenous muscle transplantation in two cases of total anal incontinence. Acta Chir. Scand. *141*, 69 (1975); Hakelius, L., Gierup, J., Grotte, G., Jorulf H.: A new treatment of anal incontinence in children: Free autogenous muscle transplantation. J. Ped. Surg. *13*, 77 (1978); Gierup, J., Hakelius, L.: Free autogenous muscle transplantation in the treatment of urinary incontinence in children: Background, surgical technique and preliminary results. J. Urol. *120*, 223 (1978).

pubo-rectalis muscle. The transplant must be in contact with normally innervated levator ani muscles to permit reinnervation.

## Operative Technique

Two weeks after denervation the whole muscle intended as graft is dissected free and extirpated. The recipient area is exposed through a vertical incision in crena ani behind the anus. From this incision a tunnel is created in the levator ani plane on both sides of the rectum to the inferior ramus of the pubic bone. The muscle transplant is then placed around the rectum with the tendinous ends pulled through the tunnels on both sides of the rectum. The ends of the transplant are sutured to the periosteum of the pubic bone, with the graft under slight tension.

## Material and Results

I would like to report the results of this operation in two groups of patients. One group of grown-up patients and one of children born with anal malformations. The first material consists of 38 grown-up patients, 33 females and 5 males. Age at surgery was between 23 and 72 years (average 48.4 years). The etiology of the incontinence was tear at delivery in 15 cases, operated anal fistulas in 6, congenital ano-rectal agenesis in 6, surgery for hemorrhoids in 5, pull-through-operation for rectal cancer in 1 and unknown cause in 5 cases. The duration of incontinence before surgery was at least 2 years and in most of the cases the incontinence was much older, up to 50 years in one case. All the patients had pronounced incontinence which means that they had no possibility to keep the stools and they all used napkins in the underwear. It seems reasonable to regard these patients as highly socially disabled. In 29 of the cases the palmaris longus muscle was used as transplant and in 9 cases the sartorius muscle. The sartorius muscle was used when the palmaris longus was lacking or was very small. The results of the operations have been judged through palpation of the transplant, anographies and the patients' estimation. The normal course of the postoperative period has been that during the first three months after transplantation there was no improvement. The transplants were palpable but they had no contractile function. Between the third and the sixth month an improvement was registered. As the first sign the patients reported that they could feel the presence of faeces in rectum but they could not keep the stools; this rectal sensation gradually developed. Later the ability to keep the stools increased and the improvement continued up to one year postoperatively.

The follow-up time is 1 to 7 years with an average of 40 months. 16 of the patients were totally cured from the incontinence; 12 were markedly improved and needed no more napkins in the underwear, and they can keep the stools for a minimum of 5 minutes. These 12 patients can live a practically normal social life. In 10 cases the transplantation had no effect.

The second material consists of 13 children with anal incontinence due to congenital malformations. They are 11 boys and 2 girls. Age at surgery 8 to 15 years (average 11.5 years). The primary diagnosis was anorectal agenesis in 11 cases, congenital megacolon in 1 case and ano-rectal diaphragm in 1 case. In the

11 cases with ano-rectal agenesis the previous surgery was a pull-through operation according to Rhoads in 3 cases, pull-through operation and later a Stephens operation in 4 cases. In one case there was a pull-through operation and later an ano-rectal plasty and in 3 cases the only previous surgery was a Stephens procedure. Preoperatively all patients had a severe incontinence and were in need of napkins. Their degree of incontinence was estimated by means of the Kelly score and cine-X-ray-studies of anus and rectum. The Kelly score takes three parameters into account. The continence for solid faeces, the degree of soiling, and the voluntary sphincter activity judged by palpation. There is a scale from 0–2 points for each parameter. A total score of 0–2 points is a "poor" result, a score of 3–4 points significes a "fair" result and 5–6 points significes a "good" result. The 13 patients have been followed 1 to 5 years postoperatively with an average of 35 months. The scheme of improvement was the same as in the grown up patients with the first signs of functioning transplant about 3 months after transplantation. All of the cases had 0–1 point according to Kelly preoperatively and all except one have improved. 11 have reached 3 points or more which means that they have achieved social continence and do not need napkins any more.

As a conclusion you can say that these two series, with a relatively long follow-up period, show that free muscle transplantation is a method that can be used with success as a treatment for anal incontinence caused by damage to the pubo-rectal muscle.

### Urinary Incontinence

The normal sphincter mechanism of the urethra is a complex function not yet fully understood, and a great number of surgical techniques are being used for the correction of urinary incontinence. Perhaps most common are the methods of putting a dacron sling or a fascia-lata-sling around the urethra in order to angulate it and in such a way try to improve the continence. In comparison with these methods it seems that a free muscle transplant would be a better solution because no foreign material will be deposed in the body, and a dynamic function with tonus, contractility and relaxation of the transplant is obtained, and there may be a positive effect from training.

### Operative Technique

After denervation 2 weeks before grafting the graft, usually one of the bellies of the extensor digitorum brevis muscle of the foot, was placed as a U-sling around the posterior urethra with the graft in contact with the urogenital membrane and the muscles of the pelvic floor. The tendinous ends of the transplant were sutured to the back of the symphysis. In girls it was possible to place the transplant in correct position through a suprapubic approach. In boys both a perineal and a suprapubic approach were needed.

### Material and Results

In co-operation with the pediatric surgeons we have used the method in 9 children with urinary incontinence. In 5 of them the postoperative follow-up is long enough to permit some evaluation of the results. The material comprises 2 girls and 3 boys, all but one being between 5 and 6 years of age at the time of transplantation. One patient was incontinent after transurethral resection of a posterior urethral valve. The others had epispadia or bladder extrophy and were operated upon several times before in an effort to create continence. Preoperatively none of these patients displayed any functional bladder capacity, which means that urine dribbled from the bladder as it arrived there from the ureters. In all patients there was an improvement 2–5 months postoperatively, with an increase of bladder capacity. The ability of complete continence during day time is so good in three cases that they don't need a napkin any more, but two cases have still to wear napkins during the day time. Postoperative follow-up with cinemicturation studies showed that all patients could contract their transplanted sling and in this way completely disrupt the urinary stream at will. The estimation of urinary flow rate showed normal values in all patients, which means that there were no signs of infravesical obstruction.

Even if this series is small and the observation time short, the results are promising. The method with free muscle transplantation is not of course intended to imitate the complex normal sphincteric function but it should at least theoretically have certain advantages in comparison with other methods, and I hope it will be possible to report later the results from a larger series with a longer observation time.

Author's address: Prof. Dr. L. Hakelius, Department of Plastic Surgery, University Hospital, S-750 14 Uppsala 14, Sweden.

## Discussion

*Freilinger:* How do you train your patients after the operation?

*Hakelius:* Yes, I always start the training about 6 weeks after the operation, not before that time.

*Holle:* Do you use a free muscle transplantation for anal sphincter reconstruction in old patients with a relaxation of the pelvic floor musculature and anal incontinence caused by that? And second question: Do you think that by reconstructing only half of the circumference of the anal sphincter with a muscle graft, you get sufficient continence? It is my opinion, that continence can only be achieved by reconstructing a muscle ring around the anal canal.

*Hakelius:* Even in old patients with pelvic floor relaxation we do muscle grafting to reconstruct continence, but if an anal prolapse exists, this is treated by general surgeons before we do our grafting. And to the second question, my opinion: The important point of reconstruction of the anal sphincter is to reconstruct the ano-rectal angle with the muscle graft.

*Thompson:* It seems to me, that a muscle graft should be the solution for the reconstruction of anal incontinence. There are three important points to be kept in mind: the first factor is the ano-rectal angle, the second factor is the flatter vealve in the ano-rectal function–so, when intraabdominal pressure rises as for instance in coughing, you don't become incontinent, because the intraabdominal pressure compresses the slit; the third factor is the external sphincter, which I am told by rectal surgeons, can only maintain adequate tension for a period of about four minutes. To reconstruct the ano-rectal angle, I do in addition to putting muscle around, I put a tendon around and screw holes into the pubic symphysis, on each side and put the tendon on maximum tension entirely to increase the ano-rectal angle to the maximum. And that was a static sling. I also repaired the pubo-rectalis loop with one palmaris longus muscle, and in addition to that I repaired the external voluntary sphincter with a further graft from the palmaris longus.

*Hohlschneider:* One important point is that one has to make an exact diagnosis, and I think all the different methods we have heard in this afternoon, would not be good for every kind of incontinence. So I think you have to choose. We have now made about 12 patients with the method. Dr. Hakelius, about 8 with the palmaris longus and the other ones with the Sartorius muscle and we unfortunately don't have as good results as you seem to have. I think we have to choose, whether we will do a gracilis plastic, when the puborectalis sling is functioning preoperatively.

# Myoplastic Operations for Anal Sphincter Reconstruction

J. Holle

Department for Plastic and Reconstructive Surgery
of the Second Surgical University Clinic of Vienna, Austria

With 6 Figures

The anal sphincter is a complex organ consisting of the ampulla recti, the corpora cavernosi recti, the internal smooth sphincter muscle, the puborectalis sling, the external striated sphincter muscle and the rectal and anal mucosa (Stelzner, 1965).

The maintenance of continence is a complex and poorly understood phenomenon relying largely on reflex mechanisms. Warning signals from the anal receptors allow voluntary contractions of the external sphincter muscle (Schuster, 1968).

The external sphincter consists of three bundles of striated muscles, which are deep, superficial and subcutaneous. The two deeper bundles surround the internal sphincter throughout its length, while the subcutaneous portion lies caudal to the internal sphincter and encircles the terminal portion of the anal canal. Combined manometric and electromyographic recordings from the external sphincter muscle are unique compared with other skeletal muscles in that: 1. The discharges are constantly present even during the resting state, in amplitude and duration and 2. the action potentials are much smaller than those of other skeletal muscles.

Up to now all attempts undertaken to treat anal incontinence were directed into the reconstruction of an only voluntary contracting muscle ring (Pickrell, 1951). The last most impressive technique for sphincter reconstruction was published by Pickrell 25 years ago using the gracilis muscle as a dynamic sling. Besides all the impressive comments (Hartl, 1972) about the good results, a limb muscle, such as the gracilis, transposed into the sphincter region with its original nerve supply, will remain a limb muscle consisting predominantly of rapidly contracting muscle fibres. This muscle is not able to maintain a continuous tonus, has no connections to recto-sphincteric and anal reflex mechanism, and contracts by voluntary intention only.

The reconstruction of a reflexly contracting sphincter or of a smooth muscle ring seemed to be impossible (Reichmann, 1970).

The aim of our experimental and clinical work was therefore to reconstruct in the most physiologically possible way a reflexly contracting anal sphincter muscle.

The new sphincter muscle should be integrated into the anal and rectal reflex mechanism and should have some degree of constant tonus like the original sphincter.

The first *experimental series* was theoretically based on the findings of Thompson (1971). Thompson found in his animal experiments that a muscle could be transplanted successfully if it had been denervated for 2–3 weeks previously. Reinnervation could be gained during a period of several weeks by close contact with a functioning host muscle over muscular neurotisation. To examine the value of free muscle transplantation for anal sphincter reconstruction, a series of animal experiments was performed in 15 Vietnamese pigs. A partly destroyed external anal sphincter muscle was reconstructed in 2 series of 10 and 5 animals. In the first series a 1.5 cm resection and in the second series a semi circumferential resection of the muscle sphincter was replaced by muscle grafts from the front leg of the pig. These muscle grafts have been denervated 14 days before the transplantation. 6 months after the sphincter reconstruction all transplants were examined. In 7 cases of the first series a perfect muscle quality morphologically and functionally could be found. The muscle grafts had become a real part of the original sphincter with similar reflex and functional properties.

In the second series the area of muscles that was not in contact with underlying sphincter muscles showed a marked fibrotic change (Freilinger, 1974).

In another experimental model we could demonstrate on rats, that 7 weeks after transplantation of a limb muscle onto the surface of a well innervated intercostal muscle, reinnervation of the graft by muscular neurotisation was found. In this experimental model, besides old degenerating end plates, newly formed motor end-plates could be identified on one single muscle fibre (Gruber, 1974).

Encouraged by our experimental results, we started using free muscle transplantation in clinical cases with anal incontinence (Holle, 1975, 1976). In cases, where parts of the original sphincter muscle could be identified by myographical and tensiometrical methods preoperatively, the indication for free muscle transplantation was given. To gain reinnervation of the muscle graft, it had to be brought in close contact with the remnant of the original sphincter (Holle, 1979). By collateral nerve sprouting of the nerves in the original sphincter muscle, the muscle graft could be reinnervated by nerve branches of the original motor sphincter nerve (Holle, 1978). Free muscle transplantation was used in 8 clinical cases with a partial defect of the external anal sphincter muscle. This partial defect of the otherwise well functioning muscle had been identificated by electromyographic, electromanometric and clinical methods. The age of the 8 patients was between 18 and 57 years. The cause of the incontinence was in 1 case an impalement lesion, in 3 cases periproctitic infections, in 2 cases the result of a vaginoplastic, in another case a postparturitional rupture of the perineum and in the last case a prolapse of the rectum with unclear genesis.

## Operating Procedure

In 7 cases the short extensor muscles of the toes of one leg were denervated and 14 days later transplanted (Fig. 1). These short muscles were placed into

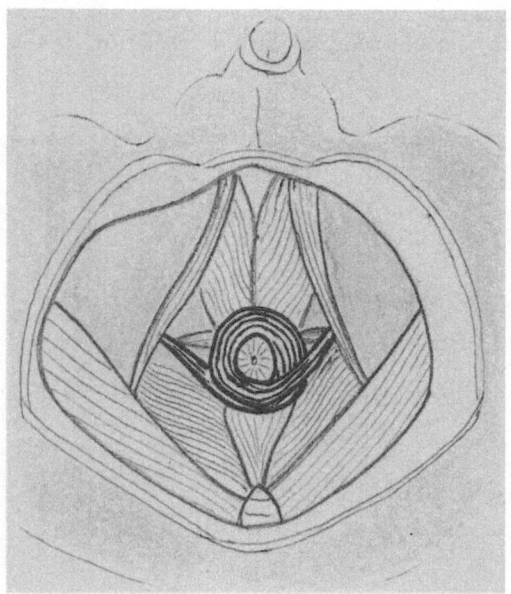

Fig. 1. Scheme of free muscle transplantation for reconstruction of a partly destroyed external sphincter muscle of the anus. The muscle graft is brought into close contact with the remaining functioning part of the sphincter muscle and the pelvic floor musculature

direct contact on the remaining original sphincter muscles bridging over the sphincter defect and encircling the whole anal canal. The tendons of the graft were fixed to both tuber ossi ischii. In one case a part of the Sartorius muscle of one leg was transplanted in a similar way. 3 weeks after the operation intensive physical therapy had been started and was continued for several months.

## Results

An improvement of anal continence could be recognized 6–9 months later. From this time a continuous improvement of the contractility of the new sphincter could be found, depending on the age, intelligence and the motivation of the patient.

All follow-up examinations were performed two years postoperatively at the earliest. To judge the results, the anamnestic data of the patients, digital

investigation of the sphincter tonus and the most possible active contraction of
the sphincter, were taken in account together with a X-ray of the sphincter
function, a myographic examination of the muscle and in several cases a
manometric functional examination.

In all 8 cases the patients showed to be continent for soft and firm faeces.
Digital examination of the anal ring indicated a well palpable tonus. The
electromyographic investigation with a concentric needle-electrode demonstrated active motor units in the transplants. In 4 cases a manometric
investigation showed a reflex contraction of the new sphincter muscle after distension of the rectum, simultaneously with a relaxation of the smooth internal
sphincter (Fig. 2).

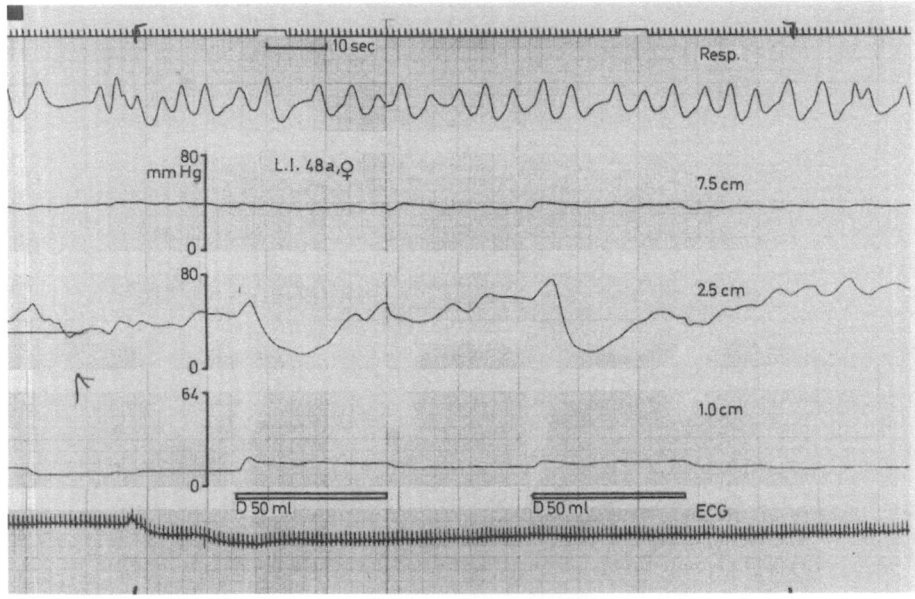

Fig. 2. Manometric investigation of a reconstructed external sphincter muscle by a muscle graft 2
years after surgery. Registration of the pressure in 1 cm, 2.5 cm, and 7 cm distance of the anus.
After an increase of the pressure in the ampulla recti by insufflation of 25 ml air, a reflex pressure
decrease in the region of the internal sphincter muscle and a reflex increase in the region of the
reconstructed external sphincter can be registred. Increase of all registred pressure values after
contraction of the sphincter by voluntary intention

*In another experimental* series on 7 pigs anal sphincter reconstruction was
investigated by transposition of a vascularized, but denervated limb muscle
corresponding to the human gracilis muscle. The limb muscle was denervated
and transposed onto the surface of the pelvic floor musculature of the pig
following total excision of the original sphincter muscle. Reinnervation of the
vascularized limb muscle was to occur by collateral nerve sprouting from the
pelvic floor musculature. By that way the denervated limb muscle should be
reinnervated with nerve fibres of original sphincter muscles (N. pudendus). By

electromyographic, histochemical and clinical investigations we could demonstrate that a muscle transposed and reinnervated in this manner functioned like an original sphincter muscle 3 months later. It acts not only like a reflex sphincter muscle, but also has changed its enzyme structure to some degree from a fast twitch limb muscle to a slowly contracting pelvic floor muscle (Holle, 1975). Being afraid that free transplantation of a large muscle for total sphincter reconstruction in clinical cases might result with a fibrotic muscle because of retarded regeneration in large muscles, we decided to use a denervated but vascularized muscle, if the entire anal sphincter had to be reconstructed (Holle, 1977).

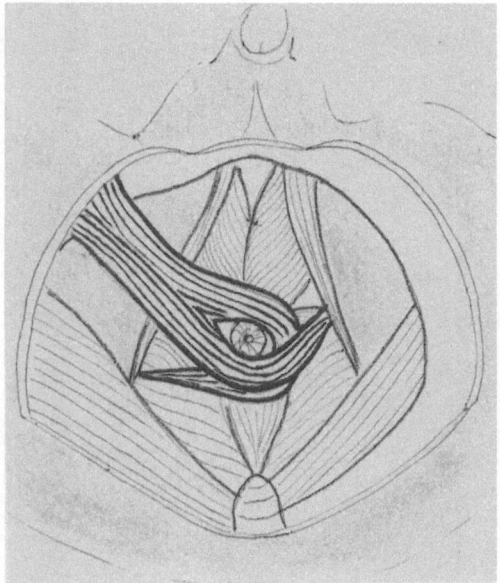

Fig. 3. Scheme of anal sphincter reconstruction with a vascularised, denervated gracilis muscle, transposed onto the surface of the pelvic floor musculature

## Clinical Application of Muscle Transposition

The indication for muscle transposition was in 7 cases incontinence after a pull-through operation following congenital anal atrophy and, in one case, an impalement lesion. In all these patients the whole sphincter reconstruction was done with a denervated, but vascularized transposed gracilis muscle.

### Operating Procedure

After exact dissection of the levator ani muscles, a gracilis muscle from one leg was denervated and split in its distal part into two pieces. Both pieces were transposed around the anus, each on one side, and brought into close contact with the pelvic floor musculature. The ends of the muscle parts were fixed on each tuber ossi ischii (Fig. 3). The age of the 8 patients was between 6 and 40 years.

## Results

Again about 9 months after the operation, an improvement of continence could be registered. The follow up examinations of all cases was done 2 years after the operation and the same investigating parameters were used as in the group with the muscle transplantation. Except in one case all patients were able to control firm faeces. 2 patients were able to control fluid bowel content.

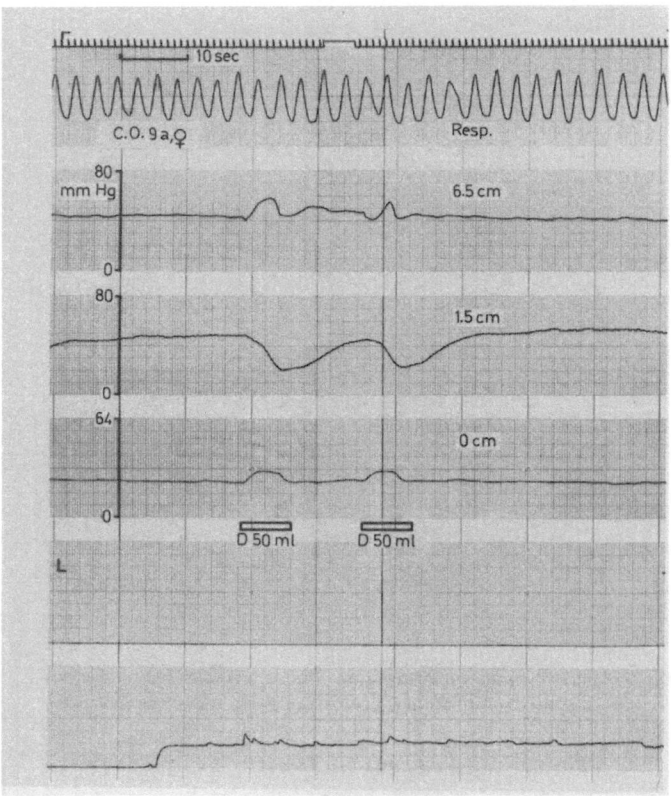

Fig. 4. Electromanometric investigation of a reconstructed anal sphincter by transposition of a denervated gracilis muscle 2 years after surgery. Reinnervation by muscular neurotisation. Pressure registration in the anal region, 1.5 cm and 6.5 cm proximal. Reflex decrease of the pressure in the region of the internal sphincter and simultaneous pressure increase in the region of the reconstructed sphincter after insufflation of 50 ml air into the ampulla recti

In 3 cases a manometric investigation demonstrated a reflex response of the transposed gracilis muscle in place of the anal sphincter after distension of the ampulla recti (Fig. 4). Electromyographically an increase of activity was found during coughing. In one case the transposed gracilis could be inspected 2 years

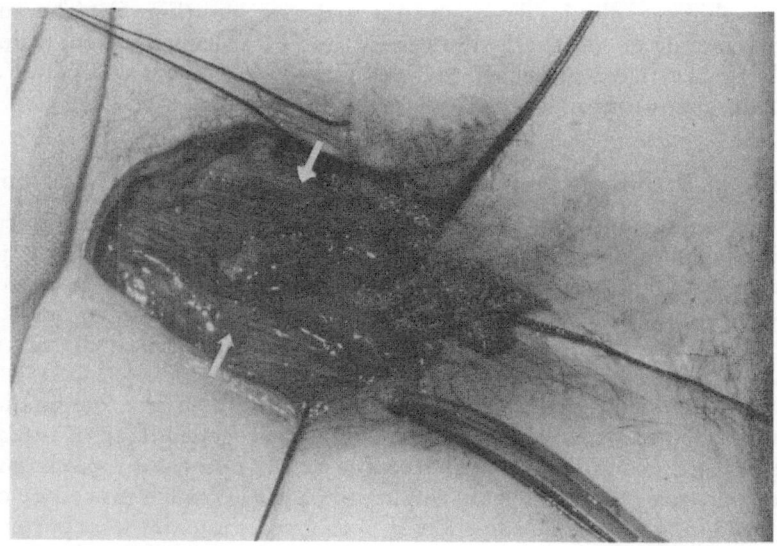

Fig. 5. Identification of the transposed and reinnervated gracilis muscle two years after sphincter reconstruction during surgery of a prolapse of the anal mucosa

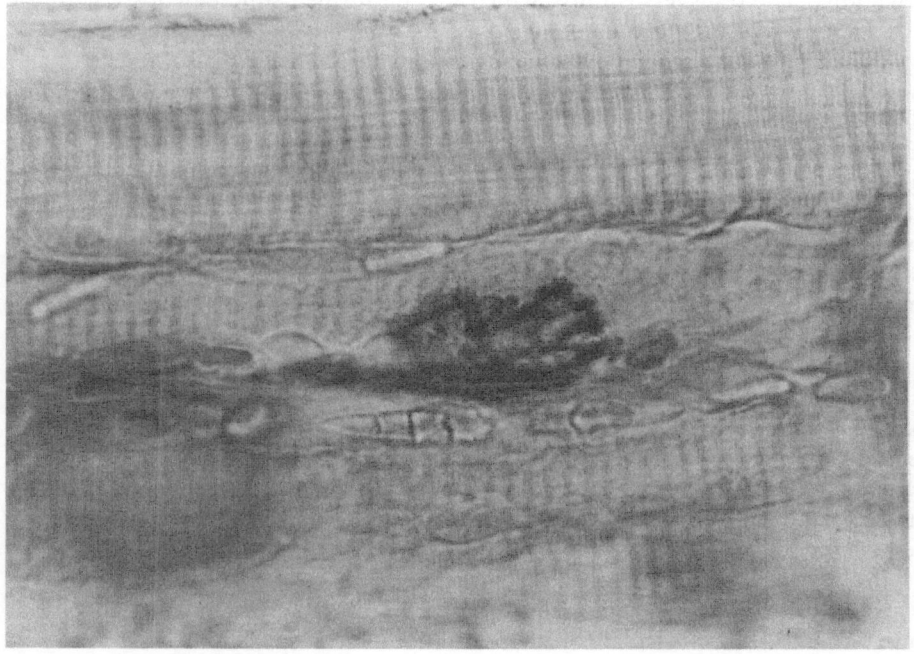

Fig. 6. Motor endplate (staining of acetylcholinesterase) on striated muscle fibres taken from the reconstructed sphincter (reinnervated gracilis muscle) two years after surgery

after the sphincter plastic during a mucosal revision (Fig. 5). The muscle
contracted by direct electrical stimulation and in specimen taken from this
muscle, normal striated muscle fibres with functioning motor end-plates could
be detected (Fig. 6) (Holle, 1980).

## Sphincter Reconstruction After Excision of the Whole Pelvic Floor

If an anal sphincter has to be reconstructed after a typical amputatio recti, no
muscle is available to supply muscular neurotisation because the whole pelvic
floor musculature has been removed together with the recto-anus. In this case a
transposed limb muscle can be reinnervated by neural neurotisation only. Neural neurotisation can be achieved by a nerve anastomosis or by nerve
implantation into the muscle.

In 3 cases sphincter reconstruction had been performed after amputation of
the rectum together with the spincter and the whole pelvic floor musculature.
The reason for the amputation of the rectum was in all 3 cases a carcinoma. In
the same operating session after the amputation a pull-through procedure of the
sigmoid combined with a transposition of both gracilis muscles were performed.
1 of the 2 gracilis muscles was denervated and nerve branches from the pudendal
nerve, which had been dissected by blunt dissection prior to amputation, were
connected with the denervated gracilis. The second gracilis muscle was placed
around the new anal canal without being denervated. All 3 patients underwent
postoperative physical therapy during 1 year and were trained with fluid
irrigations. The transversostomy, which was performed simultaneously with the
amputation, was in every case closed 12 months later.

2 years later all 3 patients were able to control firm faeces to some degree and
they have adjusted their lives to the situation of not being totally safe in control
of the faeces. A big problem of these patients is the lack of a reservoir function
of the rectum and the peristaltic of the pulled through sigmoid is always in
direction of the anus and still without control. No internal sphincter can
support the new reconstructed external one, and therefore the continence of
these new reconstructed sphincters can never be perfect. But all 3 patients are
most satisfied with the result and would never change with their situation before
the sphincter reconstruction, when they had their transversostomy.

*Summarizing* our myoplastic sphincter reconstructions, I would say that the
transplantation of the muscle is indicated, when some degree of defect of the
external sphincter muscle has to be bridged. The results 2 years after
reconstruction were satisfying; firm and soft faeces could be controlled by all 8
patients. The integration of the new muscle into rectosphincteric reflex
mechanism could be myographically and manometrically, as well as clinically
demonstrated.

If the whole external sphincter muscle has to be replaced, we prefer the
transposition of a denervated gracilis muscle onto the surface of the pelvic floor
musculature. By muscular neurotisation the transposed muscle will be
reinnervated after 9–24 months. This muscle changes not only its reflex
properties, but also its histochemical structure, which we demonstrated in our

animal experiments. By muscular neurotisation from pelvic floor muscles, the transposed gracilis muscle has changed into a sphincter muscle with reflex properties.

Anal sphincter reconstruction following the amputation of the whole rectum after carcinoma is characterized by complex difficulties. The sigma, forming the new rectal canal, has no reservoir function and there is a constant peristaltic wave to the anus. Sensory and reflex receptors are absent. The continence after such a sphincter reconstruction can by only of limitated success. But even these results in selected cases can be of great benefit for the patient.

Until sensitivity receptors in the anal canal, the function of the ampulla recti and the internal sphincter can not be reconstructed, the sphincter reconstructions are limited to the structure of the external sphincter muscles and the pubo-rectalis sling. The results of a sphincter reconstruction are better the closer the new reconstructed sphincter comes to physiological conditions. The possibility of transforming a limb muscle to a sphincter- or pelvic floor muscle by transplantation or transposition is a new important possibility in the physiological reconstruction of the anal sphincter muscle.

### References

1. Freilinger, G., Holle, J., Mamoli, B.: Free muscle transplants for anal sphincter reconstruction in pigs. Chir. plastica (Berl.) 2, 133–141 (1974).
2. Gruber, H., Freilinger, G., Holle, J., Mayr, R.: Motor endplates in autologous muscle transplants. Experientia 30, 1191–1192 (1974).
3. Hartl, H.: Modifizierte Gracilisplastik. Pädiatrie u. Pädologie, Suppl. 2, pp. 99–107. Wien-New York: Springer. 1972.
4. Holle, J., Freilinger, G.: Funktionsgerechte Rekonstruktion des quergestreiften Sphinktermuskels bei Inkontinentia ani. Langenbecks Arch. Chir. 351, 133–144 (1980).
5. Holle, J.: Can one muscle innervate another? J. Plast. and Reconstr. Surg. 1979.
6. Holle, J., Freilinger, G., Mamoli, B., Spängler, H. P., Braun, F., Krenn, R.: Neue Wege zur chirurgischen Rekonstruktion der analen Sphinktermuskulatur. Wien. med. Wschr. 125, 735–743 (1975).
7. Holle, J.: Die muskuläre Neurotisation in der rekonstruktiven Chirurgie. Wien. klin. Wschr. 88, Suppl. 48 (1976).
8. Holle, J., Freilinger, G., Lischka, A., Braun, F.: Die Bedeutung der Innervation und Funktion für die freie Muskeltransplantation. Plast. Chir. 2, 181–189 (1978).
9. Holle, J., Freilinger, G., Mandl, H.: Neue myoplastische Operationsverfahren. Acta Chir. Austr., Sondersuppl. 1976–77, 476–478.
10. Pickrell, K.: Construction of a rectal sphincter and restoration of anal continence by transplanting the gracilis muscle. Ann. Surg. 135, 853–862 (1951).
11. Reichmann, W., Stücker, F. J.: Chirurgische Behandlungsverfahren der Sphinkterinsuffizienz. Der Chirurg 11, 159–162 (1970).
12. Schuster, M. M.: Handbook of physiology–alimentary canal IV, Ch. 103, pp. 2121–2146. Baltimore: Williams & Wilkins. 1968.
13. Stelzner, F.: Kontinenz, Superkontinenz und Inkontinenz im Anorektalbereich. Dtsch. med. Wschr. 51, 2275–2281 (1965).
14. Thompson, N.: Investigation of autogenous skeletal muscle free grafts in the dog. Transplantation 12, 353–363 (1971).

Author's address: Doz. Dr. J. Holle, Abteilung für Plastische und Wiederherstellungschirurgie, II. Chirurgische Universitätsklinik, Spitalgasse 23, A-1090 Wien, Austria.

## Discussion

*Miller:* What is your incision for sphincter reconstruction after post-carcinoma excision and do you use the same design of your gracilis muscle in cases of recreation of a sphincter and do you have any trouble finding the pudendal nerve fibres in your dissections? Please tell us a little bit more about the technical aspect.

*Holle:* The first question can be answered very simply—the reconstruction is done in the same stage as the amputation of the rectum, so we have a big hole to put our muscle transpositions for sphincter reconstruction, there is no problem of incision. Secondly we use the same design of our gracilis plastic as in other sphincter reconstruction procedures. The nerve fibres of the pudendal nerve are really difficult to find and we have been training this by cadaver dissections.

*Grim:* Do you have some experience with the human anal muscle? Are there really static resistant muscle fibres present? I have not found in my experiments muscle fibres rich with succinodehydrogenase activity. Have you seen some preparations of human patients?

*Holle:* We have not done human preparations of the anal sphincter succinodehydrogenase activity staining, but we have found this in our animal experiments on pigs.

*Grim:* If you divide the gracilis in two portions and put it around the anal canal, do you think, the contraction of this two parts of the muscle fibres in this position is able to compress the anal canal?

*Holle:* In our opinion the position of the muscle is more physiologic than any other way of positioning the transposed muscle around the anal canal and it is quite similar to the natural position of the anal sphincter. This position of the two parts of the gracilis muscle encircling the anal canal and crossing on the back side of the canal gives us the possibility to keep the muscle on tension during the resting state, which improves the possibility of contraction.

Question: Does your sphincter reconstruction give any possibility of a reservoir above the sphincter and do you think that an only voluntary sphincter is enough to gain continence in these patients?

*Holle:* To reconstruct a voluntary sphincter with reflex properties is the only way to gain some sphincter function in this region. Up to now we are not able to reconstruct a smooth internal sphincter and other compartments of the pelvic floor musculature, and I told in my paper that we are far away from restoring a normal sphincter function by that technique as described. But all three patients who have had this sort of sphincter reconstruction are very pleased with the result.

# Free Smooth Muscle Transplantation

E. Schmidt, H.-P. Bruch, A. Rothhammer, and W. Skrobek

Department of Surgery, Würzburg University,
Federal Republic of Germany

With 3 Figures

Sphincter incontinence, ileostomies, colostomies and other corporal deficiencies may be remedied by means of plastic smooth muscle reconstructions. This has been postulated because of its suitability for free transplantation, its tendency to undergo secondary vascularization and innervation, and the retention of its ability to contract and its histological integrity.

In contrast to highly differentiated skeletal muscle, smooth muscle with its energy economy, is able to maintain a continuous state of contraction for long periods of time. Smooth muscle is trophically unexacting and does not atrophy after denervation. The important sphincters of the body are smooth muscles. The internal anal sphincter is the direct anatomic continuation of rectal circular muscle. Intestinal muscle therefore, seems to be especially suited for plastic sphincter reconstructions.

Studies on isolated human intestinal muscle strips have shown the maximum contractile force of circular muscle to be 60 g/mm² and that of longitudinal smooth muscle to be 40 g/mm². This is equivalent to the tension developed in a biceps muscle. This contractile force can only be obtained with maximal muscle tension, i. e. with optimal pre-stretching. When removed from adjacent tissue, isolated muscle contracts to its resting length. Further contraction in this state is virtually impossible. For this reason, the muscle must be brought to peak contractility by stretching during the operative suturing of the sphincteroplasty. This pre-stretching is necessary; it guarantees maximum contractility and optimal sphincter function. The intestinal mucosa, with its mucus secretion, high metabolic activity and contaminating bacteria, must be removed from the transplant. Even at a pre-stretching greater than 100 %, there is no danger of strangulation of mesenteric vessels in the cuffed intestine. The flat course of its length-tension curve and plastic and visco-elastic properties of intestinal muscle account for this. In animal experimental and clinical studies in more than 130

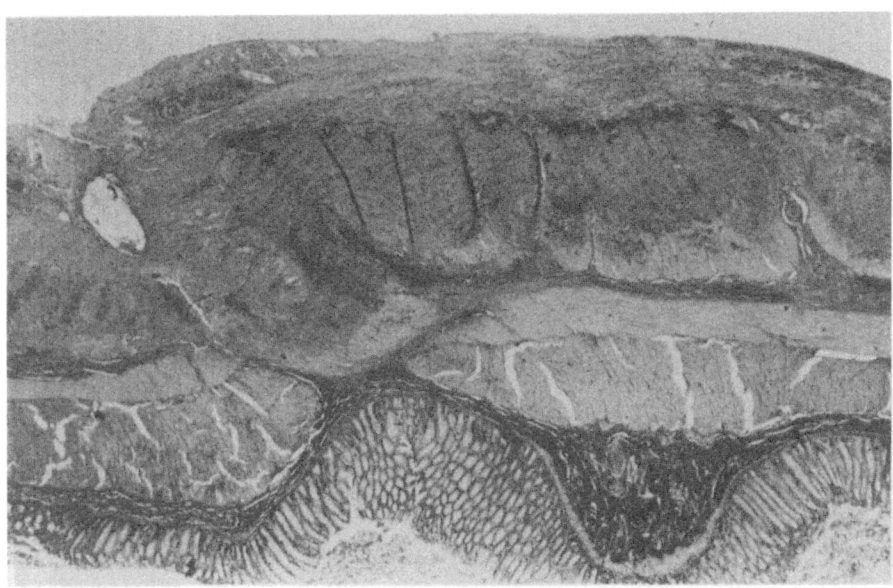

Fig. 1. Histology of the transplant (4 months postoperatively-dog) with hypertrophy and hyperplasia of smooth muscle cells

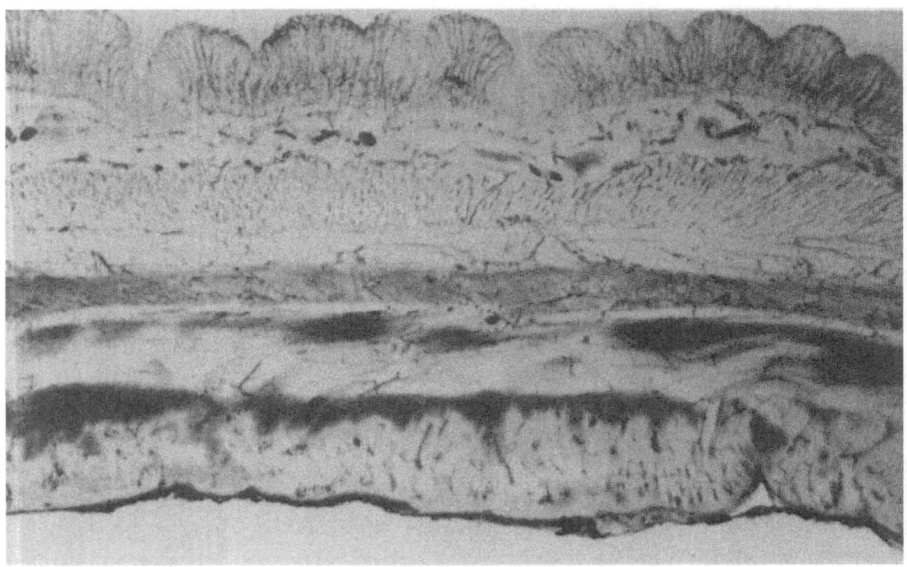

Fig. 2. India ink microangiography (48 hour postoperatively)

patients at Würzburg University Hospital, necrosis of the preternatural anus after sphincteroplasty was never observed.

Animal experiments have shown, that the transplanted muscle freed of mucosa, undergoes no significant histological changes. In many specimens, profuse hypertrophy and hyperplasia of smooth muscle cells were observed

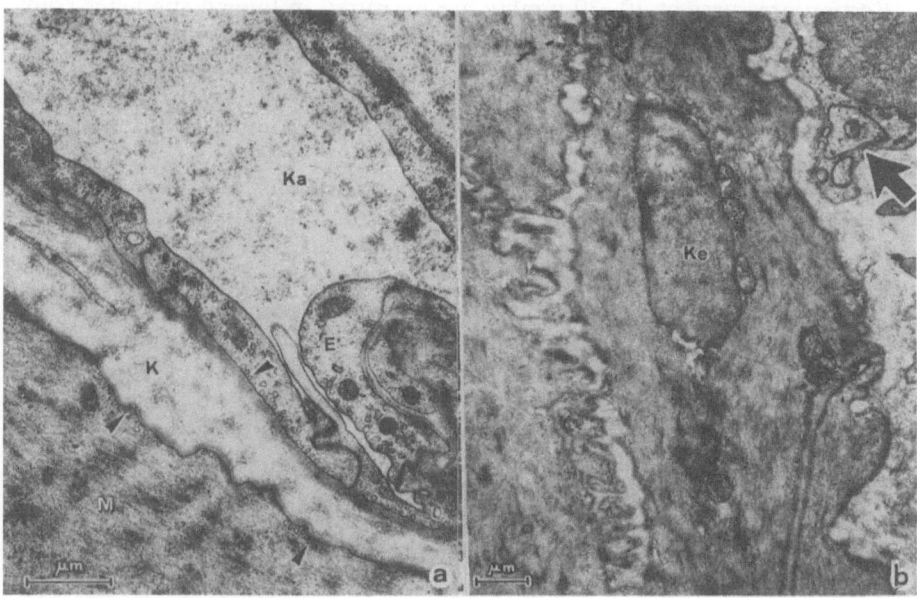

Fig. 3. Electron microscopy (18 months postoperatively). *Ka* Capillary, *E* Endothel, *K* Collagen, *M* Myocyt, *Ke* Nucleus. *a* Cytopempsis small black arrows, *b* nerve fibre, large black arrow

(Fig. 1). The pre-stretching may be responsible for this. The transplants are nourished by means of secondary vascularization, which can be made visible using India ink microangiography. After 48 hours, sprouting blood vessels appear in the free smooth muscle transplants (Fig. 2). Secondary vascularization and transplant nutrition are only possible after pre-stretching. This opens the tissue meshwork so that sprouting vessels can join with the existing vascular system of the transplant. This was shown to be true in full-thickness skin grafts by Zoltan in 1957.

Electron micrographs of the transplants taken 18 months postoperatively, reveal active metabolic transport via cytopempsis from the capillary to a myocyte (Fig. 3a).

Surprisingly, after 4 months ganglion cells of both Auerbach's and Meissner's plexus are still present in the transplants and occasionally show signs of hypertrophy; their function is unclear.

After several months, there is also development of poorly myelinated vegetative nerve fibers with a sheath of Schwann (Fig. 3b). These fibers appear to be irrelevant for continence, since the latter is already present one week postoperatively – at a time when sprouting nerve fibers are definitely absent.

Histological investigations of the completely preserved continent sphincteroplasty of a 54-year old female, which had to be removed 16 months postoperatively due to the growth of a second ovarian carcinoma, verified these histological findings in the human being.

Resting pressures of 10–20 mmHg are measured in human sphincter colostomies with balloon and perfusion manometry. Spontaneous intermittent contractions with pressures of up to 100 mmHg are observed. Dilation of the sphincter induces contractions with peak pressures of 80–100 mmHg. To paraphrase, the transplant responds to stretch stimuli with myogenic contractions.

Free autologous intestinal smooth muscle transplants for sphincter reconstruction, have the important advantage, that they are independent of 1. the location of the oriface, 2. the constitution of the abdominal wall and 3. its thickness. The transplant assumes a sphincter function in maintaining a continuous 24 hour tonus. It is not known if voluntary and reflex relaxation of these sphincters is possible. Prior to defecation, the constant sphincter tonus must be overcome by means of a small clyster to stimulate bowel movement. After defecation the sphincter closes again by an active myogenic smooth muscle contraction. During the rest of the day and at night, the wearing of a colostomy bag is unnecessary.

In addition to the restoration of continence in stomas and gastric fistulas, free smooth muscle transplants would seem to be applicable in urinary incontinence and in the high pressure region of the lower esophageal sphincter.

Author's address: Doz. Dr. E. Schmidt, Chirurgische Universitätsklinik, Josef-Schneider-Strasse 2, D-8700 Würzburg, Federal Republic of Germany.

## Discussion

*Hohlschneider:* I think I agree with you that beside the puborectalis sling, the internal sphincter is the most important point in anal continence. Did you find sympathic a-receptors in your reconstructed smooth sphincter?

*Schmidt:* No, we did not examine our new sphincter in that direction.

*Freilinger:* My question is, when you stretch the muscle tissue for 100%, is there not the danger of overstretching the muscle fibres?

*Schmidt:* No, there is no danger. We must stretch the smooth muscles so intensively, because the smooth muscle of the graft loses it's prestretching, which it has had in the original position, because the smooth muscles are physiologically prestretched. This prestretch is about 100% for a large intestine. All contractile tissues are prestretched in our body and this prestretch is quite different for a skeletal muscle, where it is only 10–20% and in the large bowel muscles it is about 100% – so have to give it back to the graft, when we place it into the new position.

*Hakelius:* Don't you think the sphincter is like an elastic band and does not relax by itself? You have to overcome the elasticity to get defaecation.

*Schmidt:* We don't know this exactly. Perhaps the sphincter can relax itself too. We have a lot of patients who can defaecate without a clysma or irrigation, and this clysma or irrigation introduces the beginning of the peristaltic waves of the bowel. And a lot of patients defaecate only by abdominal pressure.

*Hakelius:* Do you think, that your internal sphincter has any contact with the smooth muscle rest of the bowel?

*Schmidt:* I don't think there is a direct contact between the muscle graft and the smooth muscles of the bowel.

*Grim:* Have you observed some degenerating smooth muscle cells in your transplants?

*Schmidt:* Yes, we have found that, but most of the cells are alive.

*Benetar:* Have you done any histology examinations of the layers between the two serosas? Did you see, what was happening between the both layers?

*Schmidt:* Yes, we have done some histological examinations and there is some fibrotic and some collagenous material, and many vessels and nerve fibres. So there is no evidence of neurotisation from the bowel musculature.

*Grim:* How do these smooth muscle really contract?

*Schmidt:* Smooth muscles have their own automatism. They don't need any innervation. And smooth muscles do not degenerate after denervation.

*Faulkner:* Do you have evidence that this is an active tension of the smooth muscle in the graft, or only a passive tension?

*Schmidt:* We have done some manometric work on these sphincters and we have seen that the sphincter has a basal tone. This basal tone is about 20–30 mm of mercury and if the sphincter is dilated, we have peaks of pressure up to 100 mm of mercury. This means, that there is an active component in these sphincter plastics.

*Carlson:* Have you seen evidence of mitosis in these smooth muscle cells in the transplant?

*Schmidt:* We have seen hyperplasia of the muscle cells, but no evidence of mitosis.

# Sphincter Substitutes in Ostomies – Indications, Technique, Results

## H.-P. Bruch, E. Schmidt, and E. Kern

Department of Surgery, Würzburg University,
Federal Republic of Germany

With 6 Figures

## Indications and Contraindications

Sphincteroplasties can generally be applied to all colostomies, ileostomies, gastric fistulas, incontinent bladders, the incontinent anus, and the incompetent gastric cardia. There are only some contraindications for sphincteroplasty. In cases of ileus, where the distended bowel cannot be decompressed proximally (by means of manipulation and gastric tube suction), a sphincteroplasty should not be performed primarily. If a sphincteroplasty is desired by the patient, a second transforming operation should be performed. Extensive diverticulosis of the colon is not a contraindication, provided that the affected segment is resected. The sphincteroplasty itself can be taken from bowel affected with diverticulosis, since its muscle is especially well developed and therefore particularly suited for sphincter function.

In ileostomies, the smooth muscle transplant should not be taken from the affected intestine, since it will be destroyed by cells of the body's immune system.

## The Operative Technique (Using the Colostomy As an Example)

The vascular arcades of the aboral end of the colon are ligated and a 10 cm long segment is resected. This muscle sleeve is freed of mesenteric fat and inverted.

The mucosa is now on the outside. The muscle sleeve is placed in warm Ringer's solution and cleansed of feces. Using sharp dissection, the tela mucosa is removed from the submucosa (Fig. 1).

The seromuscular graft needed for transplantation is obtained by a longitudinal incision of the muscle cylinder. The transplant is soaked for 2–3 minutes in Neomycin® (Bacitracin) and Ringer's solution.

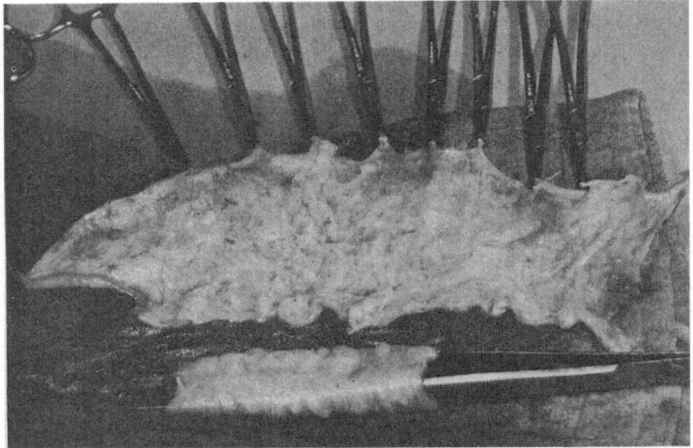

Fig. 1. Freeing the muscle sleeve of fat and mesentery

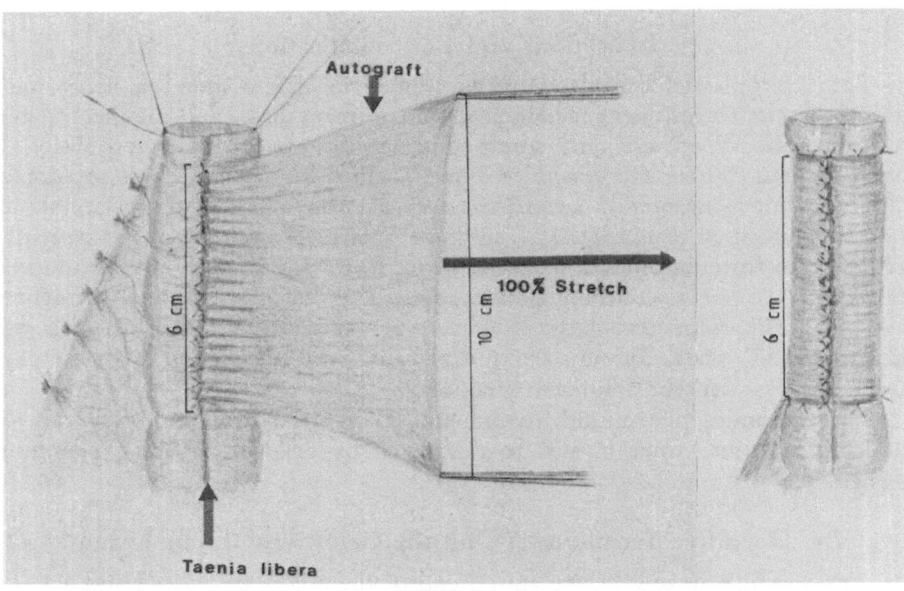

Fig. 2. The antimesocolically fixed transplant is prestretched

Interrupted sutures are used to fix the transplant to the colon 2–3 cm proximal of the aboral end. Sutures are placed antimesocolically near the tenia libera. Note that the transplant has been ruffled so that it is now only 6 cm wide instead of the original 10 cm. This results in a significant increase in circular muscle mass.

The muscle graft is stretched 100% and slung circularly around the colon. The colon's intact mesentery is folded over, and the transplant is antimesocolically fixed using interrupted sutures (Fig. 2).

Single sutures on the proximal and distal ends of the transplant prevent slipping of the sphincter. The plastic and viscoelastic properties of smooth muscle prevent a significant rise in rest tension at high degrees of prestretching. There is therefore no danger of mesenteric vessel strangulation (Fig. 3). The stoma is fixed to the skin without tension in the usual manner. This technique can also be used to transform a conventional stoma into a continent one (Schmidt, 1979).

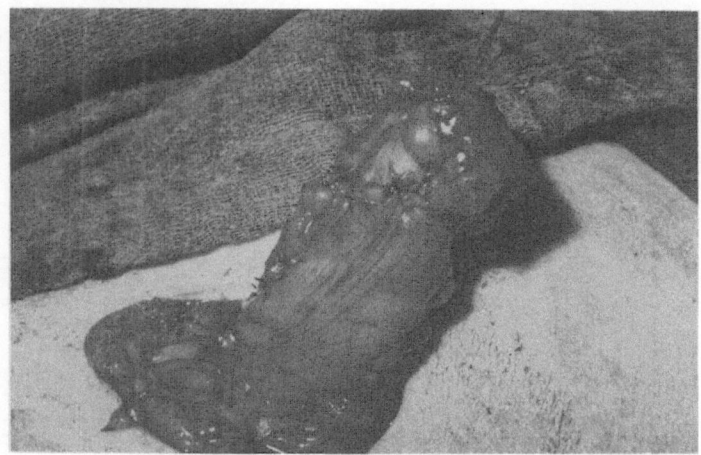

Fig. 3. Transplant in situ

## Perineal and Ileal Sphincteroplasty

Fecal incontinence due to anorectal agenesis or to secondary partial or total destruction of the natural sphincter apparatus can be improved or eliminated by a sphincteroplasty (Fig. 4). The necessary muscle is obtained from a sigmoid resection. If the sphincter is totally destroyed or absent, the rectum can be perineally mobilized and the muscle transplant fixed 2 cm proximally (Schmidt, 1978). The Mason procedure may be applicable in cases of partial incontinence. The sphincter and its innervation remain intact. The rectum would be mobilized cranially and the muscle transplant sutured above the sphincter apparatus (Bruch, 1980, unpubl.).

Due to the highly aggressive fluid content of the small intestine, a modification of our technique was necessary in creating a continent ileostomy. An 8 cm long muscle sleeve is used. An antimesenteric duplicature of the intestinal wall creates a pre-sphincter valve. The sphincter canal acts as a counterbalance.

Because of the rigidity of small intestinal muscle relative to that of the large intestine, a reservoir must be placed proximal to the sphincter valve. This is accomplished by an omega loop of handbreadth width and a Braun's entero-enterostomy (Fig. 5; Bruch, 1980).

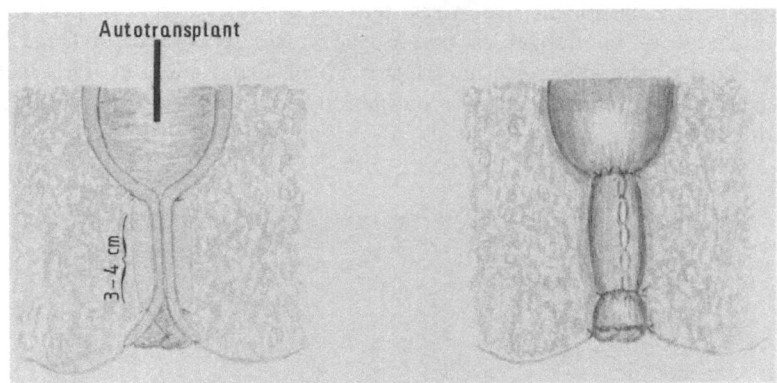

Fig. 4. Perineal sphincter plasty

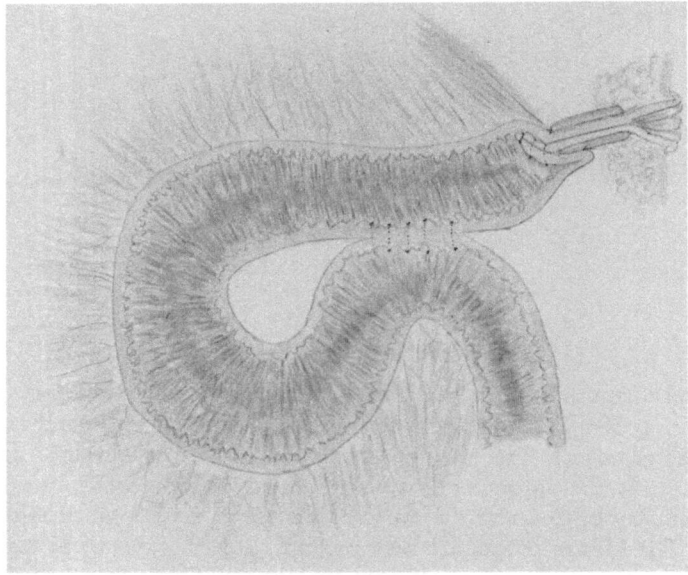

Fig. 5. Continent ileostomy

## Postoperative Care

Free muscle transplants adopt the function of a sphincter.

The transplanted muscle maintains a continuous tone and responds to stretch stimuli with contractions. A leakproof closure of the viscus is achieved.

Solid and fluid stools can be retained. Voluntary and reflex relaxation of the transplant is not possible. The continuous muscle tone must be overcome prior to defecation. In colostomies a clyster is administered on the morning starting on the third postoperative day. This stimulates peristalsis and liquifies the stool; with additional abdominal straining satisfactory intestinal voiding is achieved. In most cases a colostomy bag is not necessary during the rest of the day and at night. With the return of intestinal motility after perineal sphincteroplasty, patients are asked to defecate every four hours by straining. A virtually complete continence appears in a few weeks.

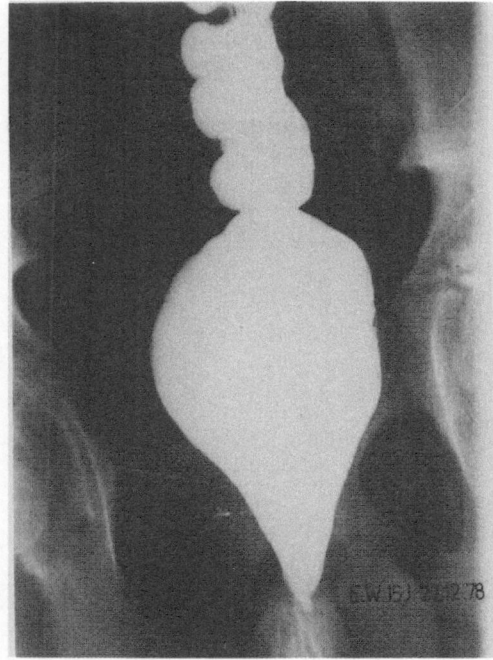

Fig. 6. Pseudoampulla 6 months postoperatively

A pseudoampulla could be demonstrated radiographically 6 months postoperatively in a patient with anorectal agenesis. The sphincter was continent for solid and semisolid stools (Fig. 6).

In ileostoma carriers, bougienage is primarily digital; the valve is pressed inward and the fluid content is emptied. In 14 days, when normal nutrition has been resumed, the ileal content acquires a firmer consistency.

Bougienage with a soft catheter is then necessary every 4 hours in order to eliminate feces.

## Results

Complications attributed to the sphincter, such as secondary cicatrization with stenosis of the preternatural anus or severe disturbances of intestinal motility, never occurred. Secondary incontinence appearing after hospital discharge was always caused by an inadequate diet or improper care of the stoma. Sphincteroplasties for helpless, senile, bed-ridden patients are a great time–and work–saver for nursing personnel.

In the meantime, more than 160 sphincteroplasties have been carried out in Würzburg. About 85 % of the patients are continent according to the above mentioned criteria. Over the past three years, the value of this simple and clinically efficient method has been substantiated in our hospital.

### References

1. Bruch, H.-P., Schmidt, E.: Unpubl. results (1980).
2. Bruch, H.-P., Schmidt, E., Rothhammer, A., Galandiuk, S.: ESR *12*, 4, 233–241 (1980).
3. Schmidt, E., Bruch, H.-P., Greulich, M., Rothhammer, A., Romen, W.: Chirurg *50*, 96–100 (1979).

Author's address: Dr. H.-P. Bruch, Chirurgische Universitätsklinik, Josef-Schneider-Strasse 2, D-8700 Würzburg, Federal Republic of Germany.

# Experimental and Anatomical Basis for Reconstruction of Anal Sphincter Musculature Employing Gracilis Muscle Grafts With Intact Neurovascular Supply

M. Grim, L. Dittertová, R. Vejsada, P. Hník, K. Smetana jr., and P. Haninec

Department of Anatomy, Faculty of Medicine,
Charles University, Prague,
Department of Pediatric Surgery, Faculty of Pediatrics, Prague,
and Institute of Physiology,
Czechoslovak Academy of Science,
Prague, Czechoslovakia

## Introduction

The surgical solution of anal incontinence by employing muscle grafting has already been attempted by many authors. Only a few of the procedures, however, have been based on experimental data (Freilinger *et al.*, 1974; Holle *et al.*, 1975; Hakelius, 1975; Hakelius *et al.*, 1978). These authors have substituted a predenervated free graft (Thompson, 1971), which subsequently becomes reinnervated *in situ* from neighbouring muscles, for the deficient sphincter musculature. The methods cannot, therefore, be employed in cases with missing or impaired innervation of the perianal region. Our report presents a procedure, based upon experimental and anatomical results, that is suitable even for patients with impaired muscle innervation in the perianal region.

## Muscle Grafting in Rats

Three series of experiments were performed in 2-to-3-month-old male rats (Wistar strain) in order to define the optimal conditions for transferring a skeletal muscle into the perianal region. We compared the results of free grafts (FG), grafts with intact innervation (IG) and muscles transposed with intact nerve and vascular supply (IVG) (Fig. 1). The gracilis anterior muscle (GA) was substituted for the levator ani muscle (LA). The LA muscle is in close contact with the terminal segment of the rectum in male rats. From developmental aspect, LA is homologous with the external sphincter ani muscle in man (Čihák, Gutmann and Hanzlíková, 1967). Functionally, it apparently plays no role in anal continence in the rat, but–as for its topographical relations–it is suitable for being substituted by heterotopic grafting. Furthermore, the arrangement of its muscle fibres and the pattern of its innervation (two zones of end-plates) is similar to the GA (Fig. 1).

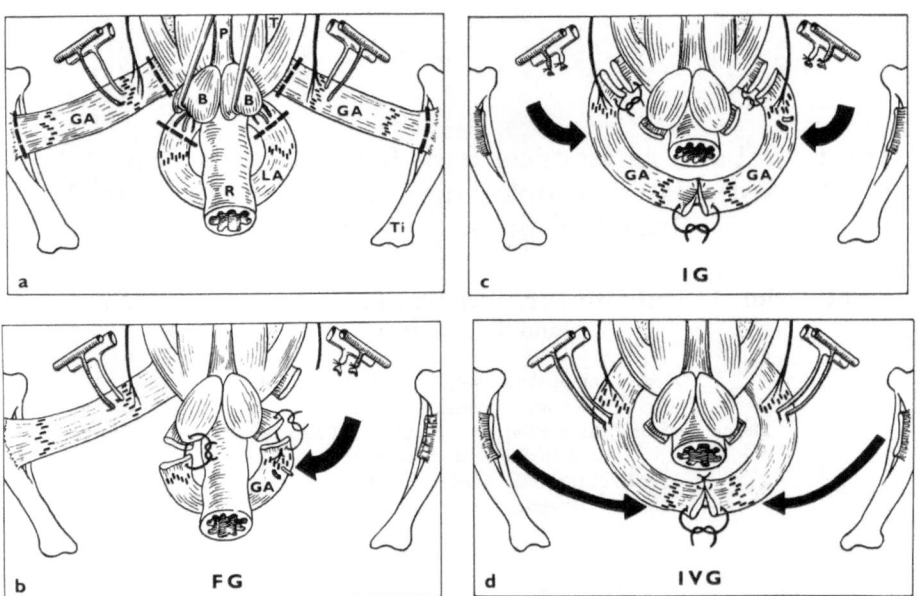

Fig. 1. Experimental procedure. *a* Scheme of the anatomical relations and extent of removal of the levator ani muscle *(LA)* and excision of the gracilis (dashed lines) in all experimental series. Black marks indicate the location of motor end-plates in the gracilis anterior muscle *(GA)* and LA muscle. *B* bulbocavernosus muscle, *P* penis, *R* rectum, *Ti* tibia, *T* cranially displaced testes. *b* Heterotopic transplantation of the GA as a free graft *(FG)*. Suturing of the graft to the edge of the bulbocavernosus muscle and to the stump of LA. *c* Heterotopic transplantation of the right and left GA with intact nerves *(IG)*. Dissection and subsequent suture also eliminates extra-hilar blood vessels. Both grafts are sutured together in the midline. *d* Transposition of the distal ends of the right and left GA. The neurovascular hilum is preserved *(IVG)*

The time sequence of regeneration and extent of necrosis and survival of original muscle fibres were studied in histological sections during the first month. The success of the operation was evaluated morphologically and functionally during the third month after transplantation, i. e. at a time when the graft is stabilized, both morphologically and physiologically (Gutmann and Carlson, 1976; Carlson, 1978; Carlson *et al.*, 1979). Stimulation electromyography (EMG) was performed using bipolar "fish-hook" electrodes (Basmajian and Stecko, 1962). The animals were under pentobarbital anaesthesia (Nembutal, 45–60 mg/kg body weight). Muscle contraction was evoked by indirect stimulation (via either the pudendal nerve–series FG, or the obturator nerve–series IG and IVG) employing rectangular pulses 0.2 ms in duration and of supramaximal intensity. The contractile properties of muscle grafts were measured *in vitro* using an automatic analyser (Rohlíček, 1968). We evaluated twitch tension (TwT), twitch tension per gram muscle weight (TwT/g), tetanic tension (TeT) and full contraction time (FCT). Each graft in series IG and IVG was evaluated individually. After this, the muscles were processed for histology. Experiments in series FG were performed on 19 rats, in series IG on 13 rats and in series IVG on 19 rats. Eleven rats of corresponding body weight served as controls.

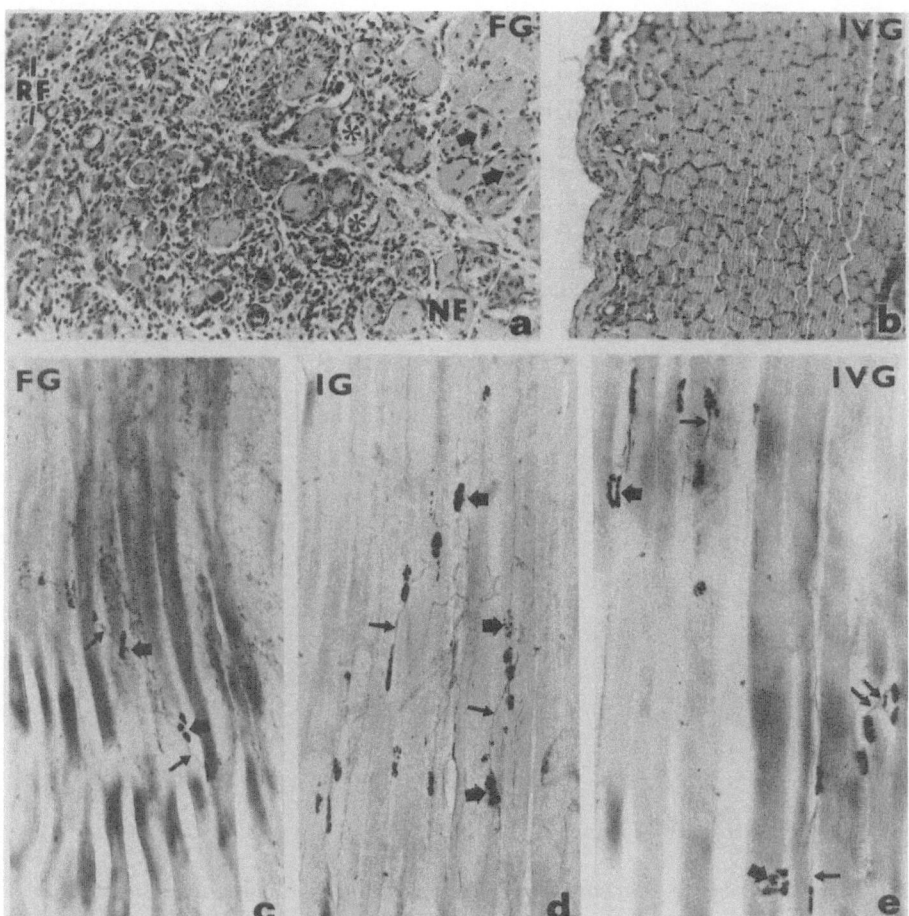

Fig. 2. Paraffin-embedded cross-section of the rat GA 6 days after transplantation (*a* and *b*) and longitudinal froze sections of the rat GA muscle during the third month after grafting (*c, d* and *e*). *a* Most muscle fibres in the free grafts *(FG)* are necrotic. Immature regenerating muscle fibres *(RF)* are present in the intermediate zone (on the left). More centrally placed are necrotic muscle fibres *(NF)*, being phagocytized by macrophages (on the right). Myoblasts lie inside the basal membrane of the original fragmented muscle fibres (asterisks). *b* Survival of all muscle fibres (series IVG). Muscle fibres are smaller in diameter. *c, d, e* Motor end-plates (larger arrows) with innervating nerve fibres (smaller arrows) in muscles the FG series are small and sparsely distributed. Muscles from the IG series contain more numerous end-plates and their size is variable. In the IVG series, their size and number correspond to end-plates in the control muscles. Magnification in *a* and *b* × 100, H & E stain, in *c, d, e* × 50, staining for AChE and silver impregnation

## Morphological and Contractile Properties of Gracilis Anterior Muscle Grafts in the Rat

Most muscle fibres in GA muscles transplanted into the perianal region as FG and IG grafts undergo ischaemic necrosis during the postoperative period (Fig. 2a), similarly as in other muscles of the rat transplanted orthotopically either with or without the nerve (Carlson and Gutmann, 1975; Carlson *et al.*, 1981). However, the removal of necrotic muscle fibres and the onset of regeneration was delayed in both these series by 1–2 days. Sparse adipose connective tissue in the perianal region did not, apparently provide optimal conditions for revascularization. On the contrary, muscle fibres in the graft from series IVG survived throughout the muscle. It was apparent, nevertheless, that even in this series a certain decrease in fibre diameter occurred in muscle fibres during the first week (Fig. 2b). Three months after transplantation, muscle grafts in all three series contained muscle fibres throughout the whole cross-sectional area. The surface of the muscle grafts was convered by a connective tissue sheath, which in places was thicker, than the original fascia.

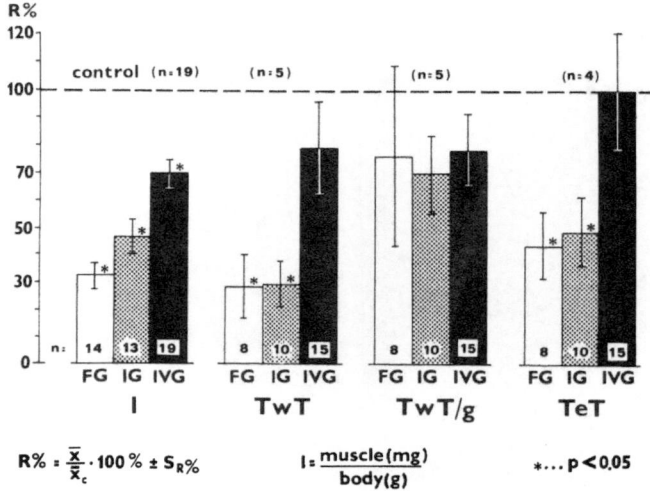

Fig. 3. Functional properties of 60-day grafts of rat gracilis anterior muscles transplanted either as free grafts *(FG)*, as grafts with an intact nerve *(IG)* or as grafts, the distal end of which was transposed and neurovascular hilum was preserved *(IVG)*. *I* muscle weight index, *TwT* twitch tension, *TwT/g* twitch tension per gram wet muscle weight, *TeT* tetanic tension. In order to compare the individual series the values are expressed as a percentage (R %) of the control group

The muscle cross-section was smallest in series FG and largest in series IVG. The profile of the grafts became altered from the original oval shape to a circular one. The muscle mass of the grafts, expressed as index I (wet muscle weight in mg/body weight in g) attained 33 % of the controls for series FG, 47 % for series IG and 70 % for series IVG (Fig. 3).

The staining of motor end-plates and of their nerve fibres has made it possible to demonstrate that the density of end-plates in free grafts was lower than in grafts with either intact nerve or intact nerve and blood supply. The subneural apparatus was less extensive in free grafts than in other groups (Fig. 2c, d, e). The distribution of end-plates correspondend to the original zones in all investigated muscles.

When the functional efficacy of these neuromuscular junctions was tested, we were able to demonstrate by stimulation EMG that neuromuscular transmission was present in all grafted muscles. Free grafts attained about $1/5$ of the control amplitude, while in grafts with an intact nerve, or an intact nerve plus vascular supply, the EMG response corresponded to $2/3$ of the controls. The difference compared with the controls was not significant for either series IG or IVG. The same applied to the difference between groups IG and IVG. The neuromuscular apparatus of groups IG and IVG thus had properties analogous to control muscles, while free grafts exhibited a markedly decreased functional capacity.

The results of measuring the contractile properties are shown in Fig. 3. Individual values were compared as percentage of control muscles. The IVG group exhibited optimal results not only as far as the weight index was concerned, but also with respect to TwT and TeT. When twitch tension was expressed per gram wet muscle weight, no significant differences were found between individual groups. Muscle tension, as measured *in vitro*, was thus found to be proportional to muscle mass. The contraction time values in the three experimental groups and the controls were grossly similar.

It may be stated from these experiments that, if the graft is required to attain at least 70% of the muscle mass and force of the control muscle, it should be transposed with its nerve and vascular supply intact. Vascularization will probably become more important, the larger the muscle. We have attempted to apply these findings to the surgical treatment of anal incontinence.

## Anatomical Considerations and Suggested Surgical Procedure

In man, the most important component of the anal sphincter musculature is apparently the puborectalis muscle (Stephens, 1953; Scharli and Kiesewetter, 1970; Stelzner, 1976). The muscle is V-shaped, compresses the anal canal and diminishes the angle of the perineal flexure (Fig. 4a). This anatomical arrangement can be achieved by muscle grafting, as had been first demonstrated by Hakelius (1975). This author employed the palmaris longus muscle as a free, pre-denervated graft.

The more caudally located external anal sphincter is circular in its external shape (Fig. 4b). It has a complicated internal structure due to the different origin and insertion of its muscle fibres. It is more difficult, therefore, to replace this structure by grafting of any single muscle. Furthermore, some authors do not consider the external anal sphincter to be critical for ensuring continence (Scharli and Kiesewetter, 1970; Stelzner, 1976). It is worth mentioning, that Shafik (1975) described the anal sphincter as a triple-loop system. He included the puborectalis muscle as an integral part into the top loop of the sphincter. However, the puborectalis muscle has a different developmental origin from the sphincter (Popowsky, 1899) and therefore, one ought to consider mutual relations of both muscles as a secondary fusion. Contrary to Shafik's (1975) description, Ayoub (1979) described the external sphincter muscle as a circumferentially arranged continuous muscle bundle. The solution of this question deserves further studies.

The muscle most usually employed for reconstruction of anal sphincter musculature is the gracilis muscle, which was invariably sutured around the anal

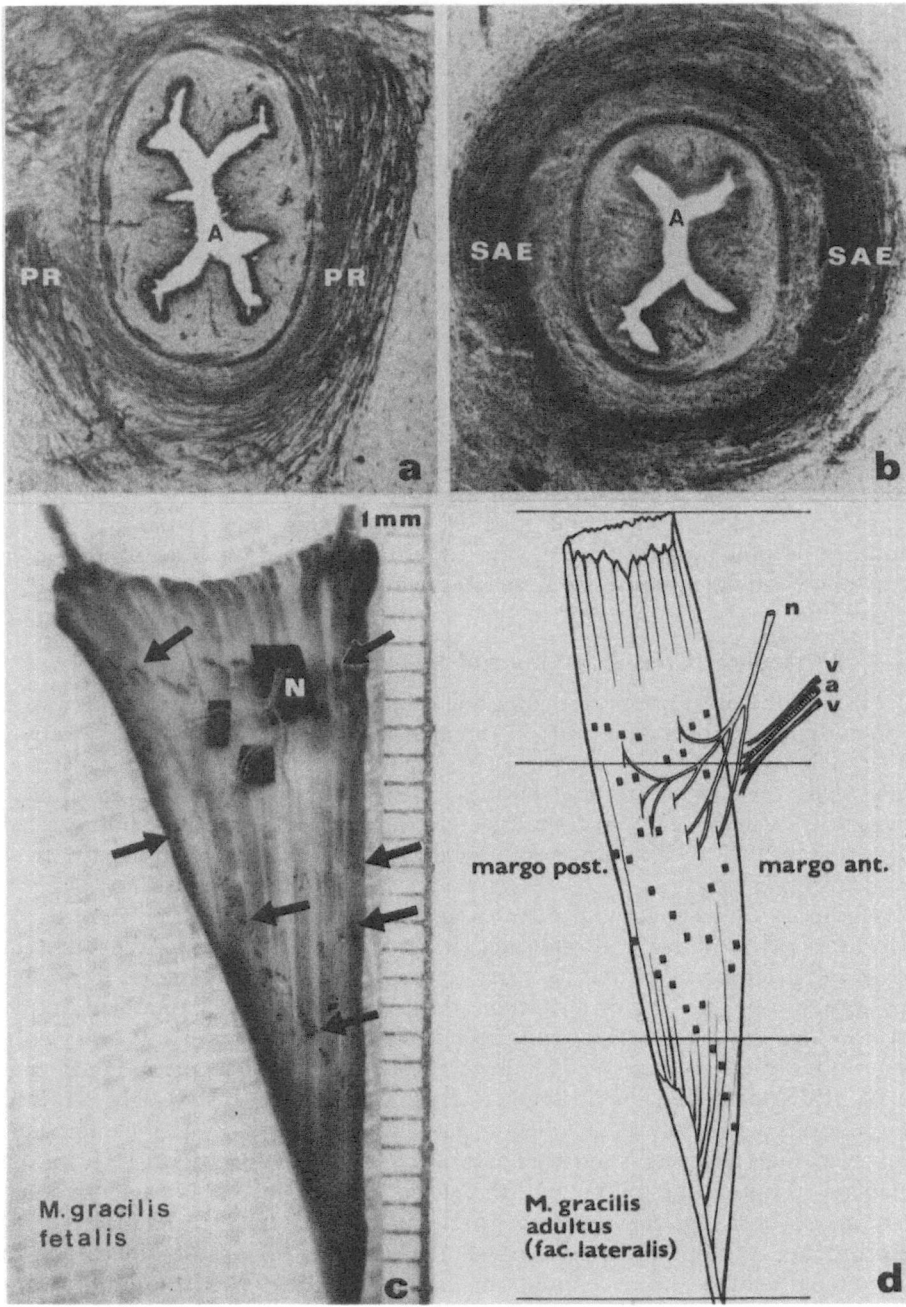

M. gracilis
fetalis

M. gracilis
adultus
(fac. lateralis)

canal (Pickrell *et al.*, 1952; modifications by Hartl, 1972; Corman, 1979). This procedure leads to considerable stretch of both the nerve and blood vessels, even to their traumatization by movements of the limb (Skácel *et al.*, 1978). Furthermore, the circular course of muscle fibres in such a graft does not seem to ensure physiological conditions for muscle contraction. It is not surprising that results of these operations are not always successful (Nixon, 1980). Nevertheless, the gracilis muscle, due to its topographical and nerve supply relations, seems to be suitable enough for being transposed into the perianal region with its nerve and blood vessels. Its nerve supply from segments $L_{2-4}$ remains intact even when sacral nerves, innervating the pelvic and perineal musculature, are impaired.

The possibility of employing the gracilis muscle in a new way for surgical treatment of anal incontinence was tested by anatomical preparations. On the basis of our experimental results we consider the muscle graft with intact nerve and blood supply the best solution of the problem. The principal condition for the graft, however, is to take the part of muscle containing end-plates, which are indispensable for the function of the grafted material.

The staining of motor end-plates in the gracilis muscle of six 3-to-5-month-old fetuses has shown that the end-plates in the human gracilis are distributed randomly (Fig. 4c, d). A group of end-plates always lies at the level of the neuro-vascular hilum. The hilum is located nearer to the muscle origin, 38 % of the length of the muscle belly in children (11 muscles, children aged one year, or less) and 27 % of the length in adults (12 muscles). For adults, Brash (1955) and Skácel *et al.* (1978) stated similar values. Additional nutrient vessels, entering variably the middle and distal thirds of the muscle, are not important since the entire muscle can be supplied by vessels of the hilum alone (Harii *et al.*, 1976).

The possibility of transferring a gracilis muscle graft into the perianal region was tested in cadavers of 12 adults and 4 children (up to one year of age). We ascertained, that if the proximal end of the gracilis muscle is transferred into the perianal region, a sufficiently long graft may be obtained without exerting undue stretch upon the nerve and blood vessels. If the proximal halves of the left and right gracilis muscles are used, a V-shaped graft imitating the anatomical course of the puborectalis muscle supporting the perineal flexure may be obtained. The right and left halves of the grafts are sutured in the midline dorsally to the anal canal. The distal ends of the graft are sutured to the pelvic arc (Fig. 5). It is possible that the functional recovery of patients with such grafts may be accelerated and enhanced by employing during the postoperative period the biofeedback method recently described by Ben-Hur *et al.* (1980).

---

Fig. 4. *a, b* Transverse sections of the anal sphincter musculature of a 10-week-old human foetus. *a* The Puborectalis muscle *(PR)* forms of V-shaped opening oriented ventrad. *b* Muscle fibres of the external sphincter *(SAE)* encircle the anal canal *(A)* along the whole circumference. Frozen sections, light green stain, magnification × 30. *c* Neurovascular hilum and motor end-plates in the fetal human gracilis muscle. End-plates (arrows) are stained for AChE. Their distribution is scattered. At the level of the hilum and in the vicinity of the inserting tendon, end-plates are more numerous. *d* Schematic representation of the distribution of end-plates and position of the neurovascular hilum in adult muscle. *N.a.v.* nerve, artery and veins of the hilum

For incontinent patients with intact sacral nerves, but damaged sphincter musculature, muscle reinnervation may be achieved by modification of this technique. It is possible e.g., to transfer the gracilis muscle with its blood supply intact, but its nerve severed, so that the graft would become reinnervated by neurotization from pelvic musculature (sacral nerve segments). This would facilitate functional reintegration of the grafted muscle into the motor pattern, ensuring continence.

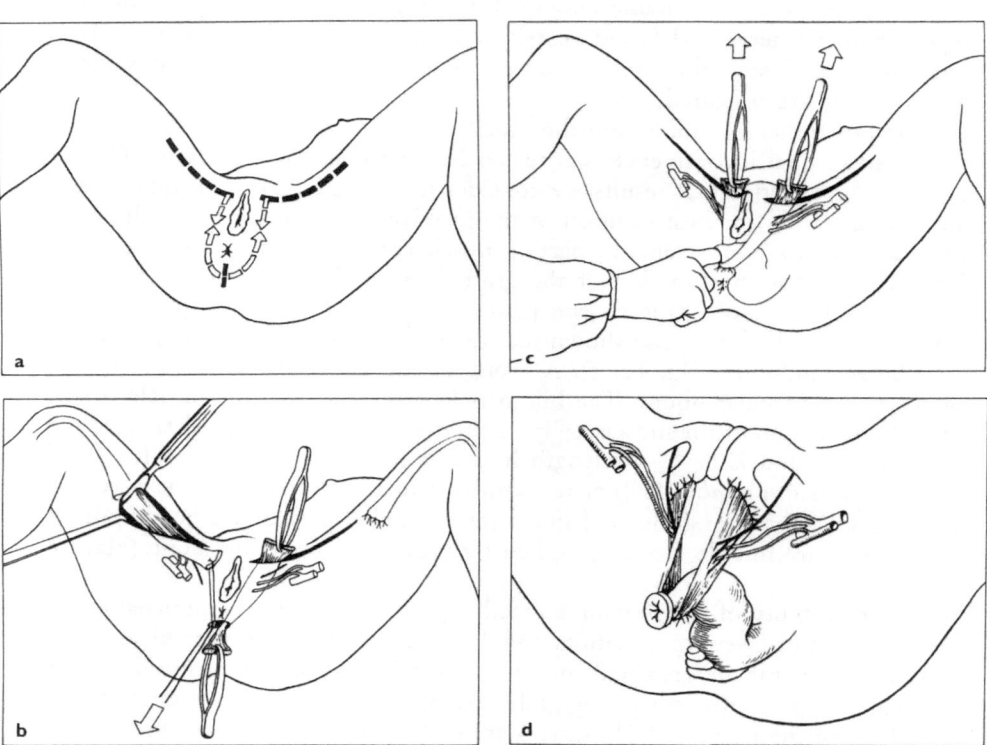

Fig. 5. The proposed surgical procedure for treatment of anal incontinence by muscle grafting of the right and left gracilis muscles, with the neurovascular hilum intact. *a* Thick broken lines – cutaneous incisions; arrows indicate the preparation of tunnels in the perineum. *b* On the left is indicated the length of the gracilis muscle graft and the manner in which its proximal end is transferred into the perineum. On the right – the situation after graft transposition. The unused distal portion of the gracilis muscle is sutured to the surrounding musculature. *c* The situation after suture of the right and left halves of the grafts dorsal to the anal canal. The length and tension of the muscle grafts are checked by digital control *per rectum*. *d* Scheme of the final stage of the surgical procedure. The V-shaped graft supports the perineal flexure of the anal canal

## Acknowledgments

The authors wish to express their gratitude to Mr. M. Med, artist and medical illustrator, for preparation of Fig. 1, 3, 4d and 5, and to Mrs. E. Jandová, Mrs. A. Herbrychová, and Mr. J. Škaloud for technical assistance throughout this work.

## References

Ayoub, S. F.: Anatomy of the external anal sphincter in man. Acta anat. *105*, 25–36 (1979).

Basmajian, J. V., Stecko, G. A.: A new bipolar indwelling electrode for electromyography. J. appl. Physiol. *17*, 849 (1962).

Ben-Hur, N., Gilai, A., Golan, J., Sagher, U., Issac, M.: Reconstruction of the anal sphincter by gracilis muscle transfer: the value of electromyography in the preoperative assessment and postoperative management of the patient. Brit. J. Plast. Surg. *33*, 156–160 (1980).

Brash, J. C.: Neuro-vascular hila of limb muscles, p. 75. Edinburgh-London: Livingstone. 1955.

Carlson, B. M.: A review of muscle transplantation in mammals. Physiol. Bohemoslov. *27*, 387–400 (1978).

Carlson, B. M., Gutmann, E.: Regeneration in free grafts of normal and denervated muscles in the rat: morphology and histochemistry. Anat. Rec. *183*, 47–62 (1975).

Carlson, B. M., Hansen-Smith, F. M., Magon, D. K.: The life history of a free muscle graft. In: Muscle Regeneration (Mauro, A., *et al.*, eds.), pp. 493–507. New York: Raven Press. 1979.

Carlson, B. M., Hník, P., Tuček, S., Vejsada, R., Bader, D. M.: Comparison between grafts with intact nerves and standard free grafts of the rat extensor digitorum longus muscle (1981, in press).

Corman, M. L.: Management of fecal incontinence by gracilis muscle transposition. Dis. Col. and Rect. *22*, 290–292 (1979).

Čihák, R., Gutmann, E., Hanzlíková, V.: Morphologische, physiologische Merkmale, Entwicklung und Homologie des M. „levator" in der Ratte. Anat. Anz. *120*, 492–506 (1967).

Freilinger, G., Holle, H., Mamoli, B.: Free muscle transplants for anal sphincter reconstruction in pigs. Chir. plast. (Berlin) *2*, 133–141 (1974).

Gutmann, E., Carlson, B. M.: Regeneration and transplantation of muscles in old rats and between young and old rats. Life Sci. *18*, 109–114 (1976).

Hakelius, L.: Free autogenous muscle transplantation in two cases of total anal incontinence. Acta Chir. Scand. *141*, 69–75 (1975).

Hakelius, L., Gierup, J., Grotte, G., Jorulf, H.: A new treatment of anal incontinence in children: free autogenous muscle transplantation. J. Pediatr. Surg. *13*, 77–82 (1978).

Harii, K., Ohmori, K., Torii, S.: Free gracilis muscle transplantation with microneurovascular anastomoses for the treatment of facial paralysis. Plast. Reconstr. Surg. *57*, 133–143 (1976).

Hartl, H.: Modifizierte Gracilisplastik. Pädiatrie und Pädologie, Suppl. 2, pp. 99–107. Wien-New York: Springer. 1972.

Holle, J., Freilinger, G., Mamoli, B., Spängler, H. P., Braun, F., Krenn, R.: Neue Wege zur chirurgischen Rekonstruktion der analen Sphinctermuskulatur. Wien. med. Wschr. *125*, 735–743 (1975).

Nixon, H. H.: In: Goligher, J. C.: Surgery of the Anus, Rectum and Colon, 4th ed., p. 275. London: Baillière, Tindall. 1980.

Pickrell, K. L., Broadbent, T. R., Masters, F. W., Metzger, J. T.: Construction of a rectal sphincter and restoration of anal continence by transplanting the gracilis muscle. Ann. Surg. *135*, 853–862 (1952).

Popowsky, J.: Entwicklungsgeschichte der Darmmuskulatur beim Menschen. Anat. Hefte *12*, 13–48 (1899).

Rohlíček, V.: An automatic analyser of muscle contraction. Tech. Digest *61*, 383–387 (1968).

Scharli, A. F., Kiesewetter, W. B.: Defecation and continence: some new concepts. Dis. Col. and Rect. *13*, 81–107 (1970).

Shafik, A.: A new concept of the anatomy of the anal sphincter mechanism and the physiology of defecation. I. The external anal sphincter: A triple-loop system. Invest. Urol. *13*, 412–419 (1975).

Skácel, V., Laichman, S., Gatěk, J.: Notes on replacement of the anal sphincter by muscle. Folia Morphol. (Prague) *26*, 61–64 (1978).

Stelzner, F.: The morphological principles of anorectal continence. Progress in Pediatr. Surg. *9*, 1–6 (1976).

Stephens, F. D. (1953) quoted by Hakelius (1975).

Thompson, N.: Autogenous free grafts of skeletal muscle. Plast. Reconstr. Surg. *48*, 11–27 (1971).

Author's address: Dr. M. Grim, Department of Anatomy, Faculty of Medicine, Charles University, U. nemocnice 3, 128 00 Prague 2, Czechoslovakia.

## Discussion

*Grim* (Summary): At least by this technique a stretch on the nerves and vessels of the transposed gracilis can be avoided and therefore the success of a gracilis transposition with it's original vascularity and innervation guarantees more success than the original method described by Pickrell.

# Transplantation of the Rectus femoris Muscle

## R. R. Schenck

Section of Hand Surgery, Departments of Plastic and Orthopedic Surgery,
Rush-Presbyterians-St. Luke's Medical Center,
Chicago, Illinois, U.S.A.

With 4 Figures

Pioneer work in muscle transplantation was carried out by Tamai, Kubo, Harii and Ikuta [1–4]. The first use of the rectus femoris muscle in a human was performed May 20, 1976, in a 49 year old man whose flexor aspect of the forearm was severely injured in an industrial accident. Prior reconstructive steps included initial debridement and coverage with a pedicle skin flap; with later sural nerve grafting to reconstruct the median and ulnar nerves.

McGraw [5] had earlier demonstrated that the rectus femoris muscle could be used for nonstaged direct rotation flap coverage (e.g. of an abdominal wall defect) and its overlying composite skin used as well. Surgical steps of importance were: use of an electrical stimulator to help identify residual motor functional portions of the median nerve, intraoperative fluorescein to aid in identification of viability of the composite skin, and relevant micro-arterio-venous anastomoses. Postoperatively early edema was evident, with later decrease in the size of the functioning muscle mass.

The use of the rectus femoris muscle was found to have the following potential advantages:

1. One arterial supply, providing safety and simplicity.

2. Adequate length of the donor nerve.

3. Adequate size and power of the muscle.

4. Correct intertendinous length–from median epicondyle to the digital flexor tendons at the wrist.

5. Composite skin coverage is available safely for all but the most distal portion of the muscle.

6. No donor leg disability.

Free transfer by microneurovascular anastomoses of the rectus femoris myocutaneous flap can now be added to the surgeon's choices of treatment for properly selected cases.

18*

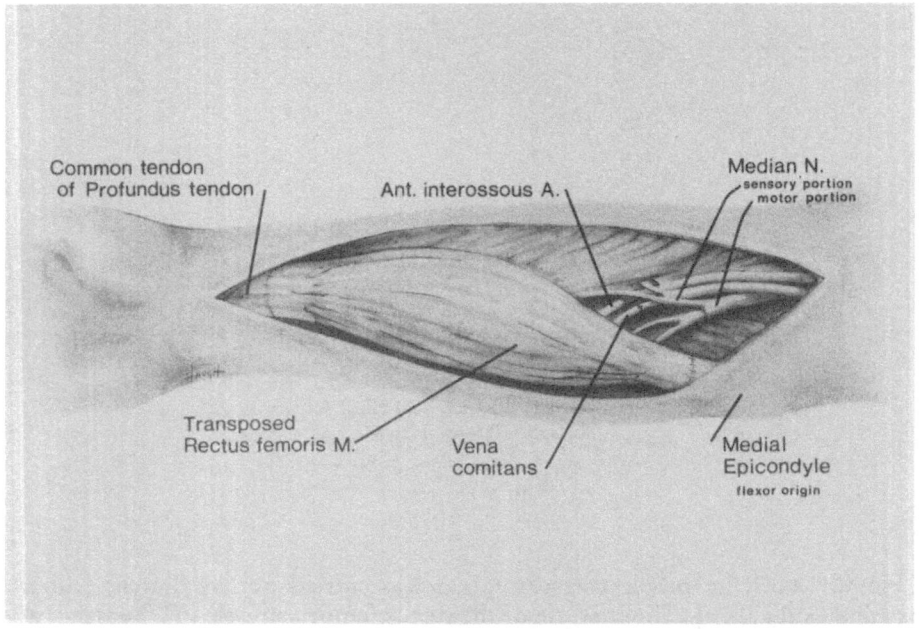

Fig. 1. The anatomy of the donor rectus femoris muscle is diagramed to show its tendinous origin and insertion and its easily obtained arterial supply from one source, in contrast to the gracilis muscle, which may have multiple arteries supplying it. The overlying composite skin to be transferred is not shown in this diagram

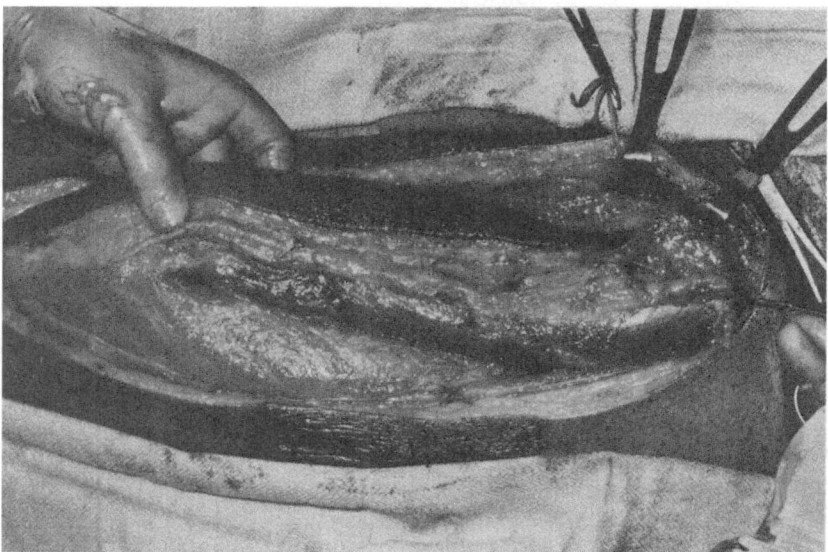

Fig. 2. The left rectus femoris is being dissected, the origin being from the inferior iliac crest on the right and the patellar tendon on the left. The elliptical composite skin flap is shown being taken carefully with the muscle, with its margins extending no farther than that of the muscle

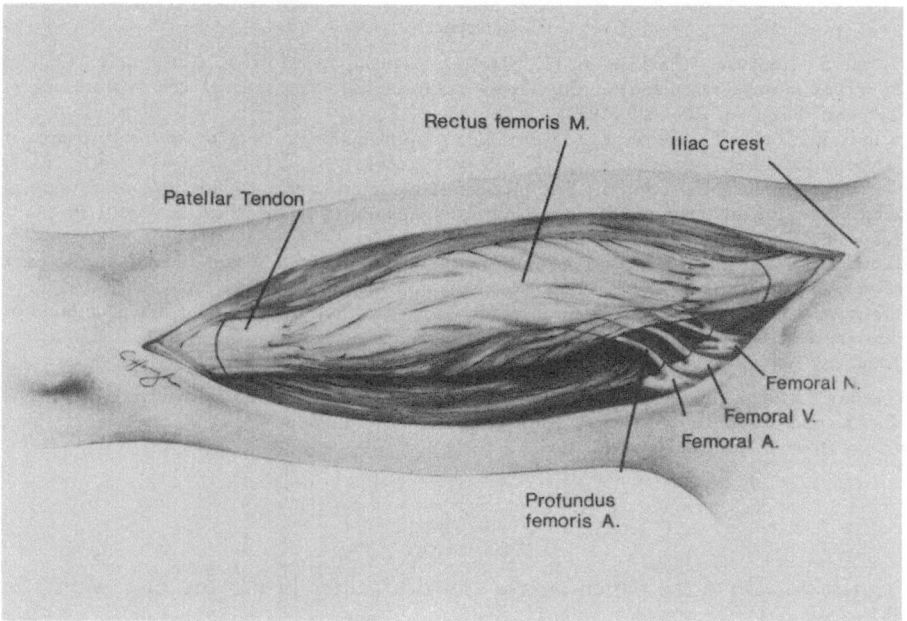

Fig. 3. The transferred rectus femoris muscle now lies in its new functional position, taking origin from the flexor origin at the median epicondyle and inserting into the common mass of the flexor profondus tendons just proximal to the partially divided transverse carpal ligament

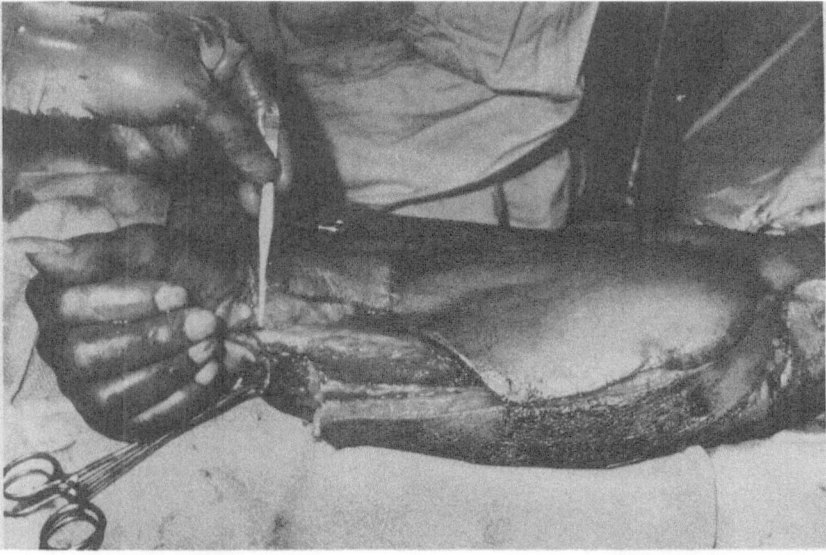

Fig. 4. The site of insertion of the transferred muscle can be seen, just prior to closure of all wound margins, using the composite skin. A small split thickness skin graft (not visible) is necessary on the most ulnar aspect

## References

1. Tamai, S., Komatsu, S., Sakamoto, H., Sano, S., Sasauchi, N., Hori, Y., Tatsumi, Y., Okuda, H.: Free muscle transplants in dogs, with microsurgical neurovascular anastomoses. Plast. Reconstr. Surg. *46*, 219–225 (1970).
2. Kubo, T., Ikuta, Y., Tsuge, K.: Free muscle transplantation in dogs by microneurovascular anastomoses. Plast. Reconstr. Surg. *57*, 495–501 (1976).
3. Harii, K., Ohmori, K., Torii, S.: Free gracilis muscle transplantation, with microneurovascular anastomoses for the treatment of facial paralysis: a preliminary report. Plast. Reconstr. Surg. *57*, 133–143 (1976).
4. Ikuta, Y., Kubo, T., Tsuge, K.: Free muscle transplantation by microsurgical technique to treat severe Volkmann's contracture. Plast. Reconstr. Surg. *58*, 407–411 (1976).
5. McGraw, J. B., Dibbel, D. G., Horton, C. E., Adamson, J. E., Carraway, J. H.: Definition of new arterialized myo-cutaneous vascular territories. Talk presented at the 55th Annual Meeting, American Association of Plastic Surgeons, Atlanta, Georgia, May 12, 1976.

Author's address: Dr. R. R. Schenck, Prof., Director, Section of Hand Surgery, Departments of Plastic and Orthopedic Surgery, Rush-Presbyterian-St. Luke's Medical Center, 1725 West Harrison Street, Chicago, IL 60612, U.S.A.

## Discussion

Question: Do these patients have any difficulties in moving or running or walking steps?

*Schenk:* We thought that there would be a loss of extension in the knee, but this did not happen, not at all. So I don't think that using the rectus femoris as a free muscle graft imposes any particular disadvantage on the patient.

# Problems of Direct Neurotization

## H. Millesi and L. Walzer

Department for Plastic and Reconstructive Surgery
of the First Surgical University Clinics of Vienna,
and the Ludwig Boltzmann-Institute for Experimental Plastic Surgery, Vienna, Austria

With 3 Figures

More than 60 years ago it was proved by animal experiments that a denervated skeletal muscle can be re-innervated by implanting a proximal stump of a motor nerve into the area of distribution of the motor end plates (Steindler, 1915; Elsberg, 1917). McCoy and Rubin, repeated these experiments in 1977 with dogs and came to the same conclusion.

Whenever possible an attempt should be made to restore continuity of transected peripheral nerves in order to achieve motor recovery, even if the lesion is very close to the entrance of the muscular branches into the muscle.

But there are cases in which there is extensive destruction and no peripheral stump of muscular branches can be identified. In such circumstances the implantation of the proximal stump of a motor fiber carrying nerve can provide a useful recovery.

## Case Report

A 27-year old female patient suffered a left forearm fracture with extensive soft tissue destruction. The radial nerve was destroyed. The level of the lesion was located peripheral to the branches supplying the brachioradialis and the extensor carpi radialis longus and brevis. The patient was, therefore, able to extend the wrist joint with radial deviation (Fig. 1).

She could not extend the MP-joint of the fingers; there was no active abduction of the thumb and extension of the MP- and IP-joints of the thumb.

The reconstructive operation was performed in July 1974. During the exploration the proximal stump could be well defined, but it was not possible to identify distal stumps. Two segments of the sural nerves were used as nerve grafts and coapted with the proximal stump. The split ends of one graft were

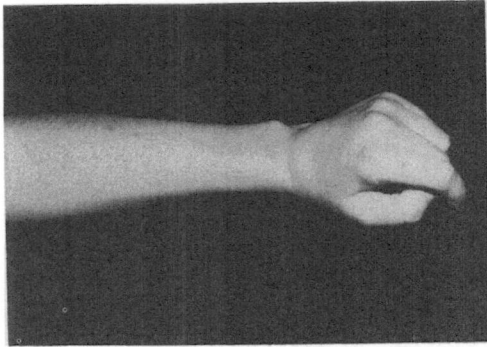

Fig. 1. Peripheral lesion of the radial nerve distal to the branches of the radial wrist extensors. The patient can extend the wrist joint but there is no active extension in the MP-joints of the fingers, the MP- and IP-joint of the thumb and there is no thumb abduction

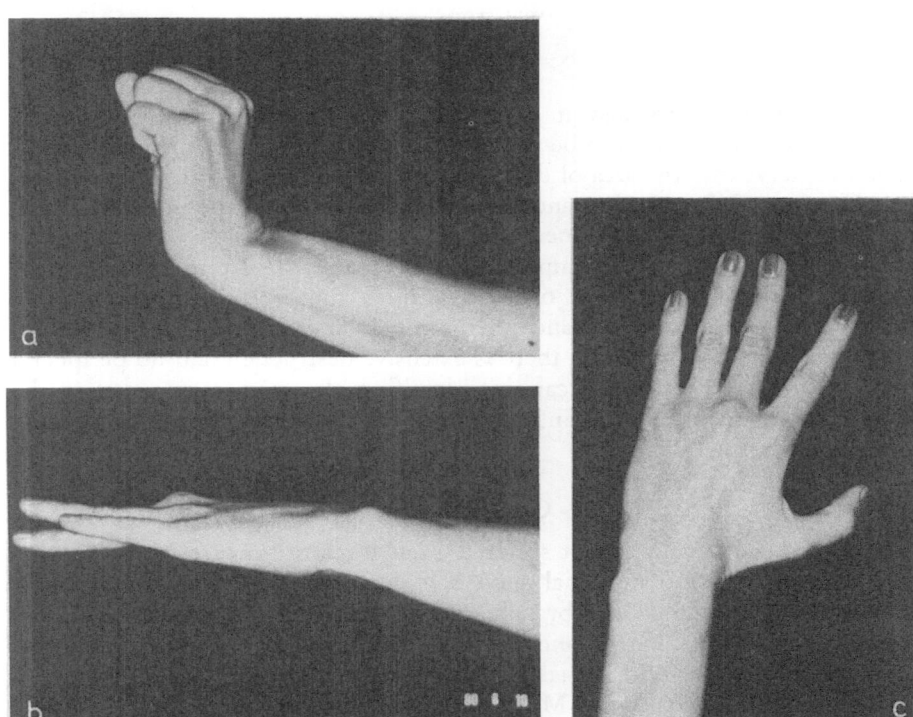

Fig. 2. After direct neurotization there is useful recovery; dorsal flexion is now possible without radial deviation (a). Extension of the fingers is improved for the middle finger and nearly normal for the other fingers (b). Abduction of the thumb is possible (c). Extension of the MP- and the IP-joint of the thumb is improved but not complete

implanted into the extensor digitorum communis and the split ends of the second graft were implanted into the extensor pollicis longus and the abductor pollicis longus. The length of the grafts was 10 cm.

The implantation of the peripheral ends of the graft was performed at the level where the location of the motor end plates of each muscle could be expected. The individual fascicles of the grafts were separated before implantation. No attempt was made to fix the distal ends of the grafts into the muscle. After splitting the perimysium and separation of the muscle bundles, the distal ends of the grafts were simply laid between the muscle bundles. Since the grafts were long enough, there was no longitudinal traction at all and the grafts remained in place. Special attention was paid to *avoid shearing forces* during wound closure. The left upper extremity was immobilized for ten days.

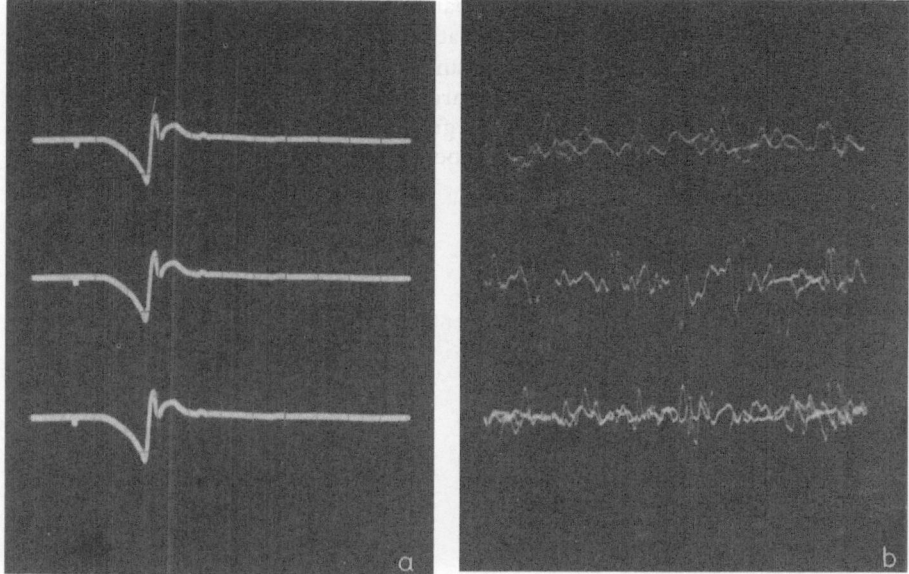

Fig. 3. Indirect stimulation of the abductor pollicis longus muscle (one $\mu$V, 20 mm sec-*a*) and interference pattern during voluntary contraction (1 $\mu$V 20 mm sec-*b*)

Several months after repair, regeneration commenced. The last follow-up study was performed in May 1980, nearly six years after the operation.

Dorsal flexion is now possible without radial deviation (Fig. 2a); the second, fourth and fifth finger achieved full extension of the MP-joint. With the middle there is still lack of full extension (Fig. 2b). Abduction of the thumb is possible in a normal way. MP-extension is nearly normal the IP-extension is now much better but still incomplete (Fig. 2c). Fig. 3 shows the muscle action potential after indirect stimulation (Fig. 3a) and the interference pattern of the abductor pollicis muscle (Fig. 3b).

Successful regeneration by direct neurotization of paralyzed muscles was achieved in three more cases.

### References

Elsberg, C. A.: Experiments on motor nerve regeneration and direct neurotization of paralyzed muscles by their own and foreign nerves. Science *45*, 318–320 (1917).

McCoy, W. H., III., Rubin, L. R.: Nerve-end implantation into denervated muscle. In: Reanimation of the Paralyzed Face (Rubin, L. R., ed.), pp. 166–173. Saint Louis: Mosby. 1977.

Steindler, A.: The method for direct neurotization of paralyzed muscles. Amer. J. Orthop. Surg. *13*, 33–45 (1915).

Author's address: Prof. Dr. H. Millesi, Abteilung für Plastische und Wiederherstellungschirurgie, I. Chirurgische Universitätsklinik, Alser Strasse 4, A-1090 Wien, Austria.

## Discussion

*Brunelli:* We have done experiments on animals in which we get better reinnervation of a muscle graft by separating the nerve in its particles and putting every fascicle of the nerve itself at different points into the muscle. We are using this technique now in human beings and are sure to get better reinnervation by this way of neural neurotisation.

*Millesi:* I think by that way there is a greater contact between the muscle and the nerve and it seems to be a very good idea.

# Direct Neurotization of Severely Damaged and Denervated Muscles

## G. Brunelli

Department of Orthopaedics,
E.U.L.O. University School of Medicine,
Brescia, Italy

With 4 Figures

It is known that a normally innervated muscle cannot be innervated by another nerve but that a denervated muscle has a spread sensitivity to acetylcholine and therefore can accept a new nerve.

Several physiological experiments have been done in the recent past.

In the early seventies we performed experiments on rabbits, demonstrating by means of electron microscopic examination the capacity of the terminal sprouts of a nerve to form new motor end-plates in aneural zones of muscles.

Those experiments were repeated afterwards on rats by removing the tibial nerve and inserting the peroneal nerve in the extreme proximal end of the triceps suralis that normally has no motor end plates (Figs. 1–3).

I improved the surgical technique, dividing the peroneal nerve into fasciculi and inserting these fasciculi in small slits atraumatically made in the muscle, in order to spread the supply of the nerve to the muscle and to increase the number of neurotized muscular fibers.

In order to avoid the release of the nerve, it is fixed to the muscle by means of one stitch taking the epineurium and the muscular fascia.

In the last 6 years I have performed 8 operations on human beings with this procedure, dividing into many fasciculi or fascicular units the grafts sutured to the proximal stump of the nerve in cases in which there was no possibility of suturing the distal part of the grafts to the distal stump or to its branches (Fig. 4).

All of them had very good results as in the best cases of suture of the nerve and all of them are presented.

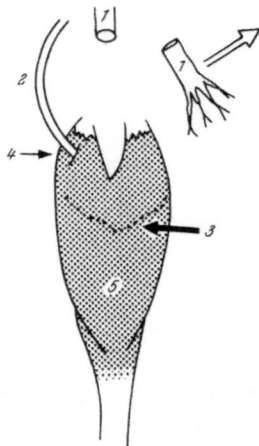

Fig. 1. Scheme of the experiment: the tibial nerve is removed from the triceps muscle and the peroneal nerve is inserted into an aneural zone of this muscle. *1* tibial nerve; *2* peroneal nerve; *3* neural zone (V shaped); *4* aneural zone; *5* triceps muscle

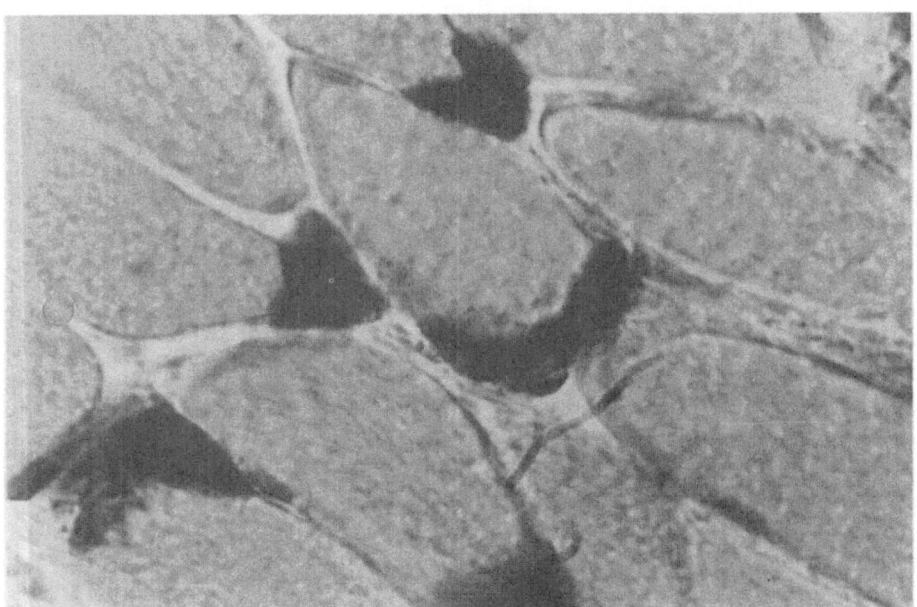

Fig. 2. New formed end motor plates in an aneural zone

## Conclusion and Summary

Previous experiments on rabbits and rats had convinced me of the usefulness of direct neurotization of denervated muscles and has lead me to develop a

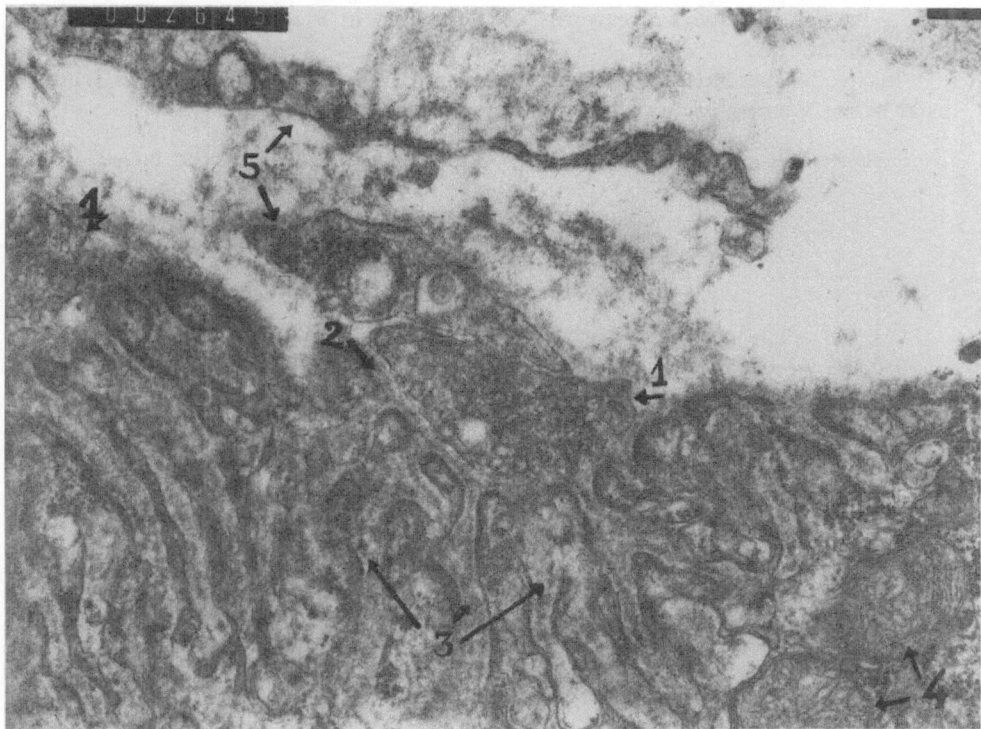

Fig. 3. Newly formed motor endplate in an aneural zone of muscle: *1* bare branches of axon with vesicles; *2* synaptic cleft; *3* typical folding of the muscle membrane; *4* mitochondria; *5* schwann cell cytoplasmic layer

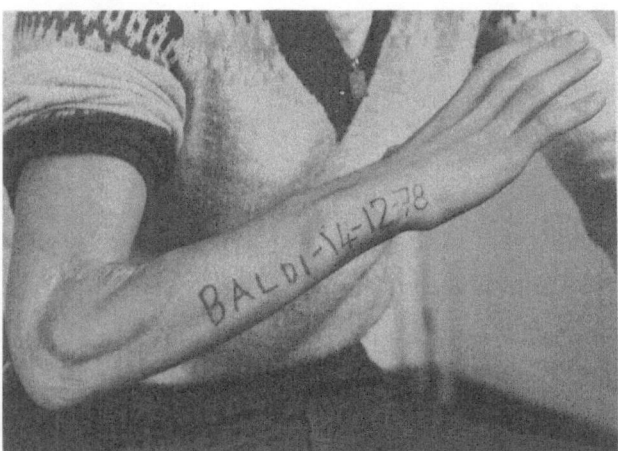

Fig. 4. Result 2 years after direct neurotization of the muscles innervated by radial nerve. The operation had been done 14 months after the trauma that had consisted in total avulsion of the proximal 2 thirds of extensor muscles and in total avulsion of radial nerve with its muscular branches from the distal 4th of the arm, large skin avulsion (previously repaired by means of an abdominal flap) and partial bone avulsion

standardized technique I afterwards used on man in 8 cases, all of which had very good results.

This technique must be kept in mind and used in those muscles in which distal nerve stumps or branches are not available.

Author's address: Prof. Dr. G. Brunelli, 2ª Ortopedia, Spedali Civili, I-25100 Brescia, Italy.

# A Proposal for the Use of the Tensor fasciae latae Muscle as a Free Microneurovascular Graft

G. Brunelli and G. Li Bassi

Department of Orthopaedics,
E.U.L.O. University School of Medicine,
Brescia, Italy

With 3 Figures

The story of free microneurovascular muscle grafts is still at an early stage.
Different muscles have been suggested and some of them have been tested (gracilis, rectus anterior, extensor digitorum brevis for example).

However, when considering a muscle that can be applied to the forearm, it becomes evident that none of the proposed muscles are suitable, mainly because they do not correspond with the muscles in the forearm, the length of the muscle being disproportionate to that of the tendon.

We therefore considered the tensor fasciae latae muscle as a potential muscle donor since it has a muscular venter of about 13–15 cm and tendons of any desired length. We then conducted anatomic research on cadavers and electrophysiological research on patients who were undergoing hip surgery.

The tensor muscle is extremely interesting since it is continuous with the Maissiat band, true tendon in the whole fascia lata, and so great in length that it allows arm grafting with the transmission of action to the hand from the forearm.

This small band is wide, and it can be divided in such a way as to transmit the flexor (or extensor) action to the four fingers and, if necessary, even to the thumb. Anatomic research has proved that the muscular belly of the tensor muscle is on the average 14 cm long, while the tendon can reach 45 cm in tall persons.

Vascularization is provided by an artery which originates in the lateral circumflex femoral artery and which has a diameter of 1.1–1.3 millimeters, a more than reasonable size in microsurgery.

The direction is medial-lateral.

The vein or veins (2 comitantes) are tributaries of the lateral circumflex femoral vein which, when single, can reach 1.5–1.7 mm in diameter and, when double, 0.8–1.2 mm, a size still sufficient to permit a vascular anastomosis well within the safety margin.

The artery and the vein can be separated for a length of about 4–5 cm and, if necessary, their total length can be extended by using parts of the circumflex vessels. The nerve enters the muscle from the superior gluteal nerve in a latero-medial direction, and up to 5 cm of its length can be removed together with the muscle.

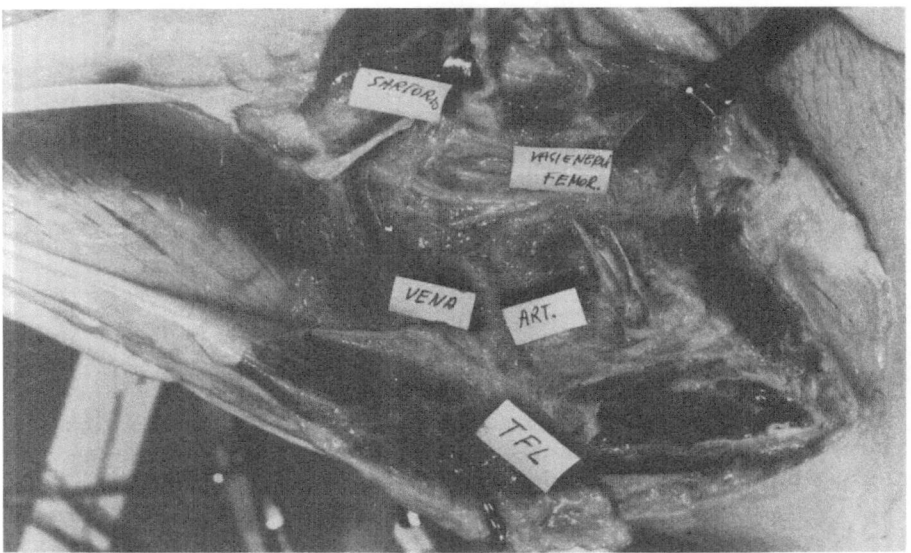

Fig. 1. T.F.L. muscle detached from iliac bone. Artery and vein originates in the lateral circumflex femoral vessels coming from femoral vessels

It is located between the gluteus medius and minimus. We have also studied the type of muscle fibers which, for the most part, are of the slow twitch kind, but this is of no importance, as it is common knowledge that the type of fibers varies with the innervation, and it eventually matches the type of nerve.

The tensor fasciae latae tendon is the most interesting element of this potential free graft, firstly because it can be taken of any desired length and width such as to fully satisfy the requirements of any receiving site and secondly because it can be divided into various small terminal bands (up to five) so as to give movement to the different fingers simultaneously.

The muscles fibers run lengthwise.

The oblique anatomic position (which balances the action of the superficial portion of the glutaeus major) had in early days suggested a semifeather-shaped muscle with an oblique action and a short run.

However, when isolated from the iliac spine it can be aligned with the Maissiat band and have a longitudinal contraction and a far greater run.

Electric stimulation applied to the patient during hip surgery, while keeping muscle in adduction (in tension), indicated a shortening of the muscle up to 3.5 cm.

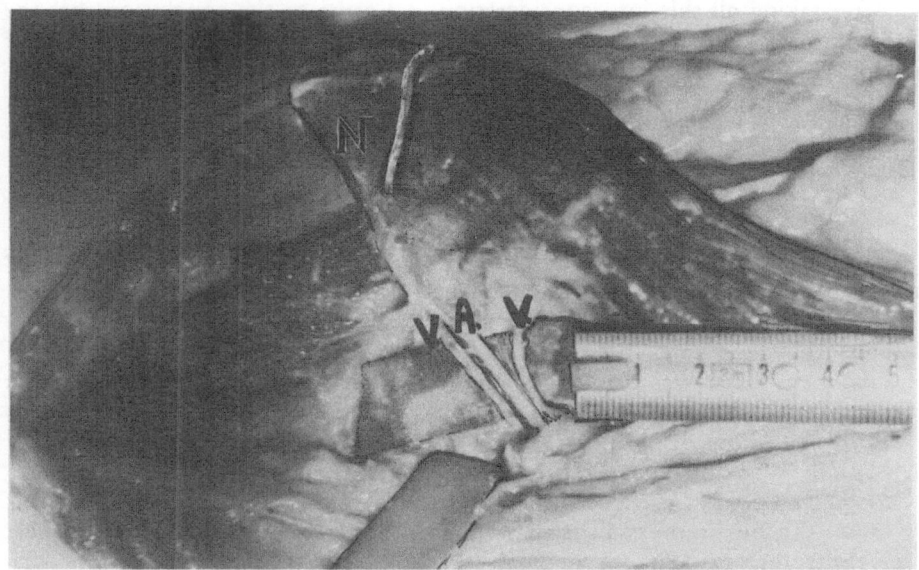

Fig. 2. Detached T.F.L. muscle showing the nerve and the vessels

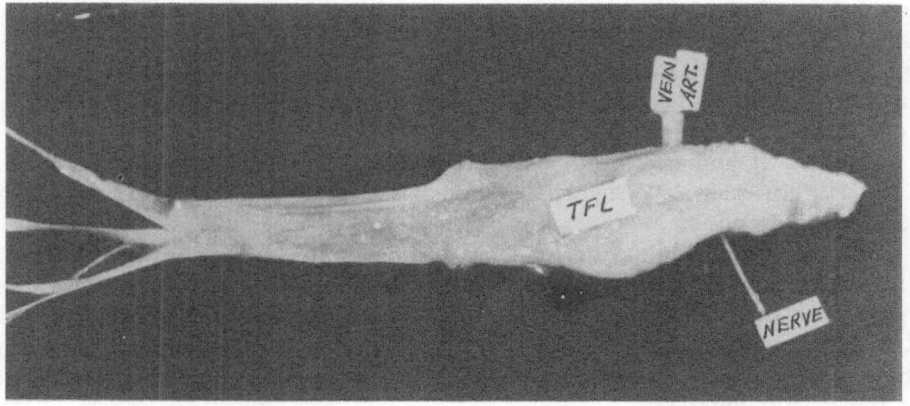

Fig. 3. Removed T.F.L. muscle and division of it tendon as it is required

This run is greater if the muscle is aligned longitudinally with the tendon band.

## Conclusion and Summary

The tensor fasciae latae muscle can easily be taken. Innervation and vascularization are almost constant, and their size is more than reasonable for microsurgery.

Its run is greater than 4 cm when it is in a longitudinal position and it has tendon which can be divided into different strips.

After taking all this into consideration, we came to the conclusion that the tensor fasciae latae is the most suitable muscle for free microneurovascular transplantation as far as the extension and flexion of finger are concerned.

Author's address: Prof. Dr. G. Brunelli, 2ª Ortopedia, Spedali Civili, I-25100 Brescia, Italy.

## Discussion

*Faulkner:* How do you determine if the nerve has been accepted to the muscle by implantation, and have you had any failures?

*Brunelli:* I have shown you our seven cases, where we have not had any failures.

*Faulkner:* What was the longest time after denervation of the muscle, that you implanted the nerve?

*Brunelli:* About 12 months.

*Nicolai:* What do you think of electrotherapy?

*Brunelli:* I always use electrotherapy, but I am not able to say now, what is its value. But our impression is that we have better preservation of the muscle after electrotherapy. But we cannot say that exactly.

*Banièlic:* In a healthy patient we are not happy with a donor side of the tensor fascial flap. What is your opinion about that?

*Harii:* I have some patients with a tensor fascie lata flap. If you can close the donor side without the skin graft, then we have almost no complications after taking off this flap. But if you take some skin grafting, there is depressed scar, and sometimes the patients complain about that. But the tensor fascie lata flap muscle has almost no excursion, no gliding power. So my question: How long is your contracting amplitude?

*Brunelli:* If you take your leg in abduction, the muscle can gain 13.5 cm.

*Harii:* For example, the gracilis muscle has a good gliding power, and gliding contracting amplitude.

*Brunelli:* I don't think, there is a big difference. If you look at the movement of the leg, you see that the gracilis muscle has a longer bundle, but not a long tendon and the movement of the leg is the same in abduction and reduction. I think, the excursion of the tensor fasciae latae muscle is not very different from that of the gracilis. My question to Dr. Harii: what is the maximum extension of the gracilis muscle?

*Harii:* About 17 cm.

# Muscle Plastic in Subcutaneous Mastectomies by Use of the Latissimus dorsi Muscle

## H. G. Bruck

Department of Plastic and Reconstructive Surgery,
Vienna Town Council–Wilhelminenspital, Austria

With 5 Figures

Whilst muscle-tissue transplants and transfers are generally used to provide movement of some kind, other uses have proven advantageous. This very well nourished tissue can be used as the carrier of a blood-supply in so called "musculo-cutaneous flaps" (Mathes) as well as for a cover for major alloplastic implants as used in reconstructive breast-surgery (Jarrett). Here in cases of subcutaneous mastectomies the placing of the prostheses under local muscle plates–like the pectoralis or serratus muscle–has so many advantages that it has become almost a routine procedure in many units.

In secondary or complicated cases these local muscles are not always available in sufficient size or quality, so other possibilities were looked for. Since we have had considerable experience with skin or musculo-cutaneous flaps pedicled on the thoracodorsal artery and vein and containing the latissimus dorsi muscle, or parts of it, this muscle seemed to provide a chance for transferring a new cover-material into the breast area in difficult cases. Here some or even many months after subcutaneous mastectomy and immediate reconstruction the skin in the two lower quadrants of the breast becomes progressively thinner; it takes on a bluish tinge; and the complete extrusion of the implants seems imminent (Fig. 1). Since no local plasties are feasible without severe and conspicuous scarring as their consequence, a new procedure was developed.

## Technique

With the patient under general anaesthesia and in a lateral position on the operating table a 7 to 9 cm long incision is made on the anterior border of the latissimus dorsi muscle about 8 to 10 cm down from the axilla. The skin is than undermined over all the muscle in the dorsum and meticulous hemostasis obtained. With the freeing of the anterior edge of the muscle, its whole plate is

19*

dissected off the thoracic wall in an almost completely bloodless level. Only a few perforating vessels have to be tied. Now the whole of the latissimus dorsi muscle can be cut off from its dorsal and caudal attachments, which is best done with an electric knife to minimize bleeding. Dissecting further upward towards the axilla, the nerve-vessel bundle of the thoracodorsal artery, veins and nerve can be identified, and the muscle itself is transected cranially from the insertion

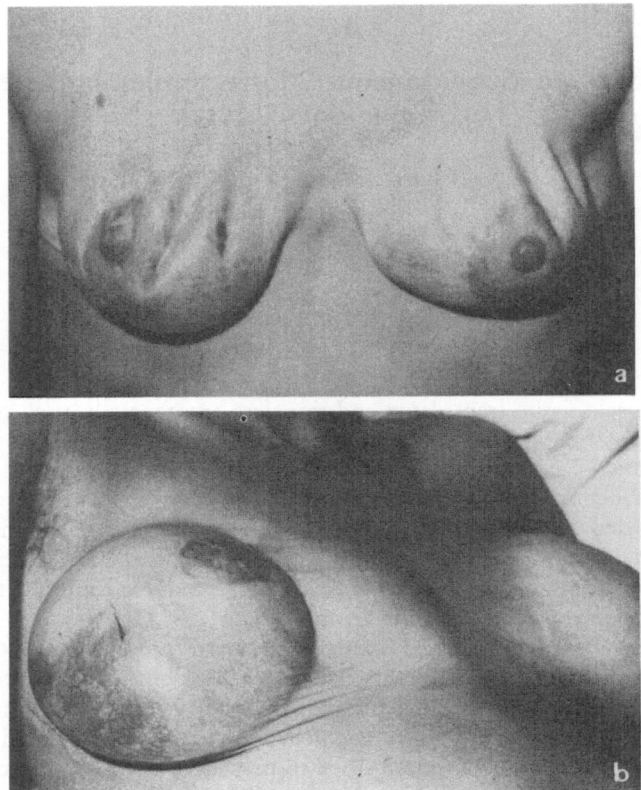

Fig. 1. 37 year-old woman, 6 months after bilateral subcutaneous mastectomy. *a* Note the thinned and discoloured skin especially on the right side. *b* The skin condition becomes even more obvious in a prone position

of this bundle into the muscle itself (Fig. 2). It is important to preserve the nerve, as well, since it carries a considerable amount of nutritional fibres and its intact presence therefore will help to diminish secondary atrophy of this now afunctional muscle plate. The division of the muscle itself lengthens and mobilizes the muscle-plate considerably; it also minimizes any postoperative bulkiness in the axilla. Now a subcutaneous tunnel is made towards the breast and the cavity with the implant is reached. After further checks regarding hemostasis in the big dorsal wound, the muscle is placed in the tunnel towards the breast, a suction drain introduced and the wound closed in layers.

The patient is then rotated in a normal prone position, redraped and the old mastectomy-scars, wherever they may be, are opened and the implant is removed. In the lateral half of the now empty cavity the tip of the muscle can be

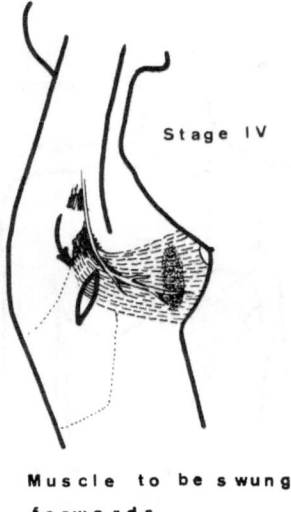

Stage IV

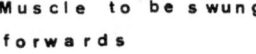

Muscle to be swung
forwards

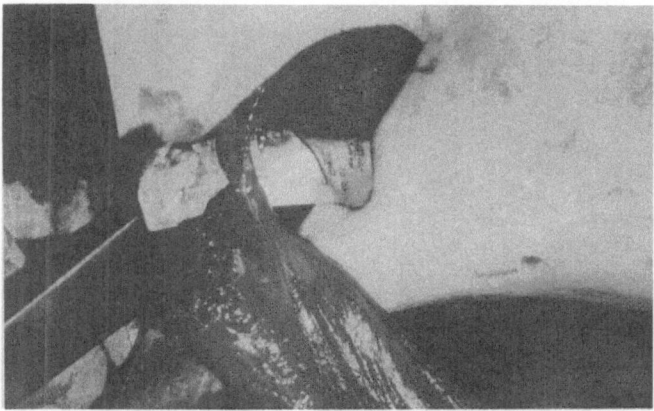

Fig. 2. The muscle on its neurovascular pedicle can easily reach the implantation cavity and cover the whole anterior surface of the prosthesis

identified and the whole plate brought out through the anterior incision (Fig. 3). After ascertaining that the thin neurovascular pedicle has not been twisted, the muscle-plate of the latissimus dorsi muscle is spread over the whole cavity of the former implant, which it partially fills. No attempt is made to remove any parts of the capsule or to dissect and identify any parts of the still remaining local muscles. All these procedures only tend to increase the danger of hemorrhage. The new muscle tissue provides so much safe tissue for cover that no local flaps are required. After spreading out, the free edge of the lat. dorsi muscle is stitched all around the implant-cavity with 3–0 Vicryl sutures. Only a few centimeters are left open under the incision, and through this opening a new prosthesis is introduced under the muscle. It should be considerably smaller–or

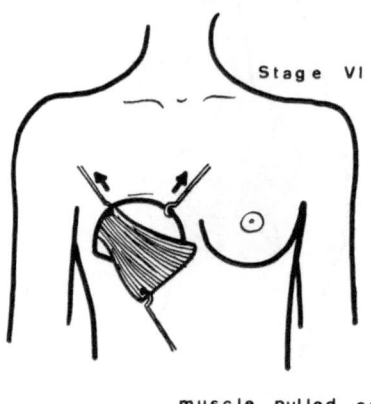

muscle pulled out
and spread

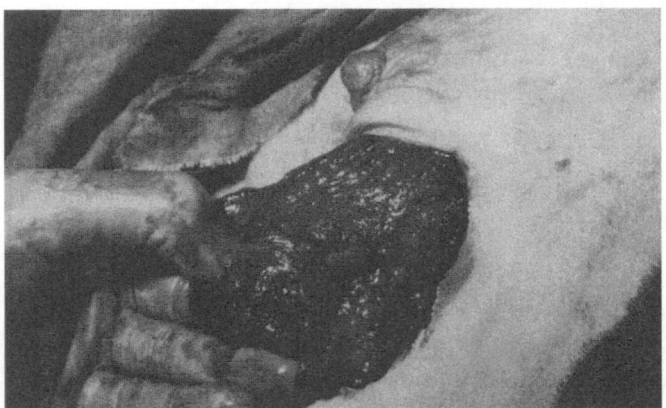

Fig. 3

less filled–than the original, removed one, since the bulk of the muscle adds markedly to the amount of build-up required. When the last sutures to the chest wall are completed, the implant should completely be covered by the new muscle-sheath. The skin wound can than be closed over a second suction drain. Dressing and postoperative care are equivalent to the usual techniques for augmentation mammaplasty.

## Discussion

The latissimus dorsi muscle is an easily expendable muscle, which will leave no disability to speak of, if transfered to other parts of the body (Bostwick). Its nutrition by its axillary blood-supply through the thoraco-dorsal vessels is so

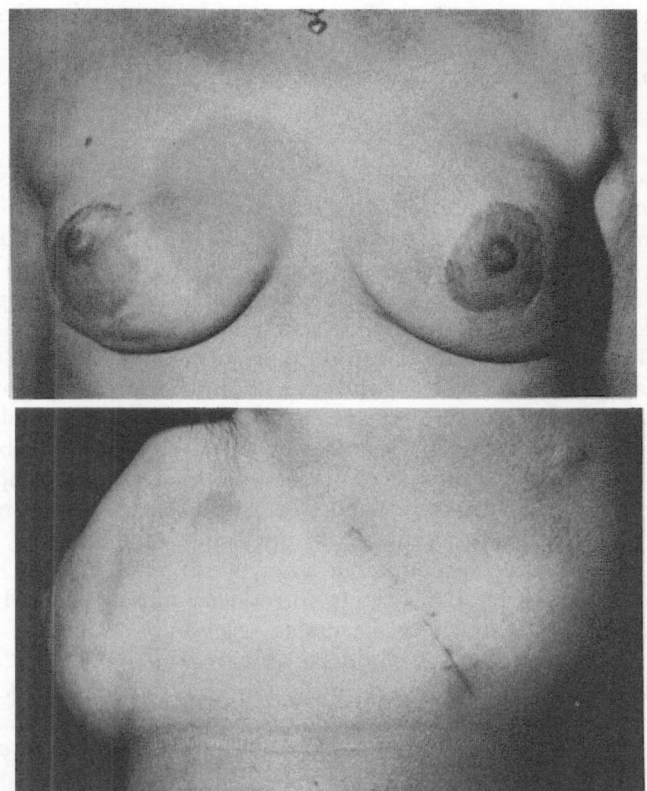

Fig. 4. Same Patient as in Fig. 1, 15 months after the described operation. Mark the retention of shape and the normal appearance of the skin

safe, that it can be used as a carrier for musculo-cutaneous island flaps, which are transfered free and reanastmosed in other parts of the body by microsurgical techniques (Baudet, de Conick). The dissection of the pedicle is comparatively easy even through a smallish incision, and its length is ample to reach the anterior thoracic wall up to the sternum without stretch. The described technique has several advantages:

There is very little additional scarring and it occurs in an area hidden by even a normal-sized brassiere.

The big sheet of latissimus dorsi muscle provides an abundance of well nourished muscle tissue to cover the whole outer aspect of any prosthesis and can easily be wrapped all around it. Especially the two lower quadrants of the breast, where gravity works against the plastic surgeon can so safely be secured against all further misfortunes to the skin.

The slender pedicle crossing the axilla, consisting only of a neurovascular bundle produces no noticeable or conspicous ridge.

The division of all muscle fibres all around prevents any involuntary and sometimes embarassing movements of the breast, whilst secondary atrophy of it is minimized by the retention of the nutritional nerve fibres.

There is practically no loss of movement or function.

## Results

This operation has now been performed on 8 consecutive cases with imminent extrusion of implants after subcutaneous mastectomy and immediate reconstruction of the breast by means of implants. No major postoperative problems were encountered with the exception of the first case, in which the division of the muscle in the axilla was obviously incomplete and the patient tore some fibres loose from their medial attachment in a strong and involuntary movement. The patients could be dismissed from hospital after 10 to 14 days and have remained safe and well-satisfied for up to 18 months by now (Fig. 4).

The newly reconstructed breasts are slightly firmer than normal ones, but compare favorably with other similar cases in which implants have been placed under local muscles of the chest wall. They have all retained their shape well and no major constricting fibrosis could be detected up to now. The cosmetic result was not always perfect, but acceptable to the patient and surgeon, as well.

No problems were ever encountered from the original capsule, which was left behind between skin and the newly introduced muscle-sheet. It seems to resorb spontaneously without any detectable reaction.

The most impressive changes could be observed in the skin of the breast. Without any kind of treatment the previously thin, bluish and angry looking skin returned to a practically normal texture, colour and temperature. These changes took place in a few weeks, but even after some months thermography could still show a slightly raised temperature level over the new muscle-area, as compared to its surroundings. This does prove the high rate of metabolism in the transposed muscle and is a strong proof of the patency of the vessels in the pedicle (Fig. 5).

This method, although not simple, has been a great help with the management of otherwise rather difficult problems. Neither the size of the operation nor the skill required of the performing surgeon should however be underestimated. Since the results obtained were uniformly favorable, it is suggested for trial in other units faced with similar problems.

## Summary

For cases after subcutaneous mastectomy with simultaneous reconstruction, where perforation of the implants via a secondarily malnourished skin seems imminent a new procedure is advocated. The latissimus dorsi muscle is pedicled on its neurovascular bundle and swung forward across the axilla in a subcutaneous tunnel. It can so cover the whole implant-area and has saved the result in our 8 cases, which would have otherwise suffered severe disfigurement.

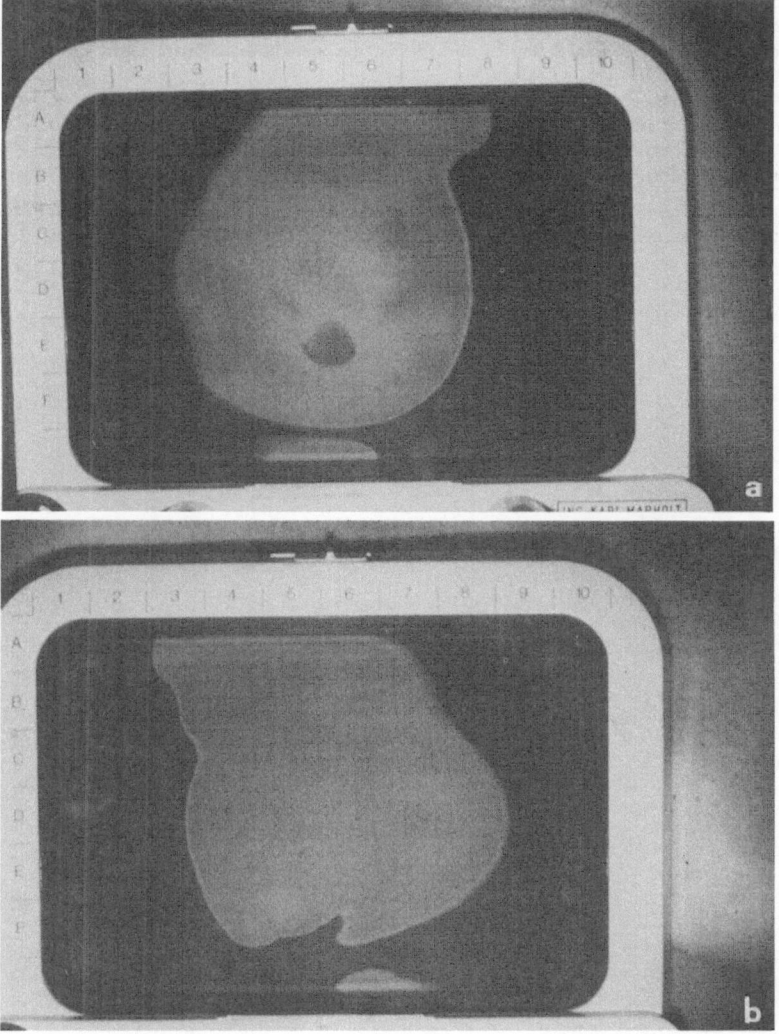

Fig. 5. Thermographies of a patient only unilaterally operated with the described technique 4 months postoperatively. *a* Left (untouched) side. *b* Right (operated) side compares favorably with the untouched side with temperatures slightly above the other

### Acknowledgement

We are indebted to Dr. K. Pflanzer from the Radiologic Department of the Krankenhaus Lainz, Vienna (Chief: Prof. Dr. K. Fochem) for providing us with his thermographic facilities and for helping us in the interpretation of Fig. 5.

## References

Baudet, J., Guimbeteau, J. C., Nascimento, E.: Successful clinic transfer of two free thoracodorsal axillary flaps. Plast. Reconstr. Surg. *58*, 137–141 (1976).

Bostwick, J., Nahai, Foad, Wallace, J. G., Vasconez, L. D.: Sixty latissimus dorsi flaps. Plast. Reconstr. Surg. *63*, 31–41 (1979).

De Conick, A., Vanderlingen, E., Boeckx, W. D.: Thoracodorsal skinflap. New possible donor site in distant transfer of island flap by mikro-vascular anastomosis. Ann. Chir. plast. *20*, 163–172 (1975).

Jarrett, J. R., Cutler, R. G., Teal, D. F.: Subcutaneous mastectomy in small, large or ptotic breasts with immediate submuscular placement of implants. Plast. Reconstr. Surg. *62*, 702–705 (1978).

Mathes, S. J., Nahai, Foad: Clinical Atlas of Muscle and Musculo-Cutaneous Flaps. St. Louis-Toronto-London: Mosby. 1979.

Author's address: Prim. Dr. H. G. Bruck, Abteilung für Plastische und Wiederherstellungschirurgie, Wilhelminenspital der Stadt Wien, Montleartstrasse 4, A-1171 Wien, Austria.

# Pressure Sores and Myocutaneous Flaps

## G. Lupo

Department of Plastic Surgery,
St. Anna Hospital, Como, Italy

With 6 Figures

All surgeons who have examined the problem of pressure sores affirm that the best therapy consists in their prevention. Since this is not always possible, therapy through years has expressed itself thus: from increasingly thicker cutaneous flaps to muscular flaps and, most recently, myocutaneous flaps.

We must make a distinction between: plain muscular flaps, muscular and myocutaneous island flaps, pedicled myocutaneous flaps, free myocutaneous flaps.

The study concerns the second and third topic. We will limit our work to the most frequent pressure sores: the sacral, trochanteric and ischial, highly frequent in 80% of paraplegics. This division tells us through literature which muscles or group of muscles have been used for the different types of pressure sores. The use of musculocutaneous flaps in pressure sores is quite recent (1977) [16], but one cannot ignore the simple preceding muscular flaps, dating since 1947–1948, from whom they derive. The muscles up to now employed to cover these sores (alone or "en bloc" with overlying skin) are:

1. *in sacral sores* (Fig. 1a): gluteus maximus [7, 10, 9, 27, 8, 30, 32, 20, 23, 28, 21, 19], sacrospinalis inferior [15], gracilis [15], semimembranosus [21], tensor fasciae latae [21, 24, 36].

2. *in trochanteric sores* (Fig. 1b): tensor fasciae latae [10, 27, 21, 22, 24, 29, 18, 36], sartorius [9], rectus femoris [9, 15, 28, 2, 21], vastus lateralis [9, 20–23, 21, 22], gluteus maximus [23], biceps femoris [21], semimembranosus [21].

3. *in ischial sores* (Fig. 1c): biceps femoris [13, 4, 3, 7, 10, 5, 31, 25, 6, 20, 33, 15, 28, 1, 21, 22], obturator internus and biceps femoris [3], gluteus maximus [3, 9, 23, 21, 22], semitendinosus [10, 1, 21, 22], gracilis [35, 21, 26, 12, 24, 11, 15], semimembranosus [21], rectus femoris [21], vastus lateralis [21], tensor fasciae latae [18, 24, 36].

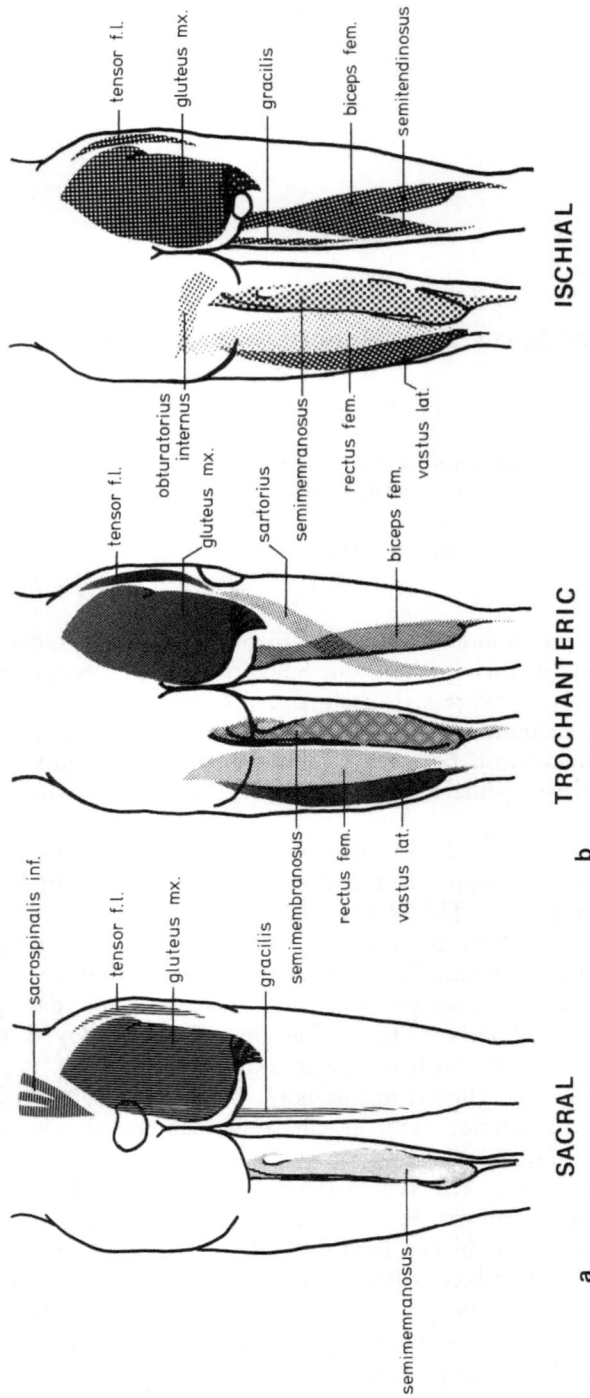

Fig. 1. *a* Scheme of muscle employed in covering sacral pressure sores, *b* Scheme of muscle employed in covering trochanteric pressure sores, *c* Scheme of muscle employed in covering ischial pressure sores

It is interesting to note that the main reconstructive problems come from the ischial pressure sores. Bearing in mind only the myocutaneous flaps, we must consider the following points:

1. *Indications:* these must be related to the seriousness and depth of the sore; its age and recurrence with presence of surrounding scar tissues; the importance of support, the age of the patient and his psychological and general conditions. Some superficial and recent sores, usually not supporting weight (mainly in non-paraplegics), can still be cured with rotation of fat cutaneous flaps with a large pedicle.

2. *Requisites* for a myocutaneous flap can be thus summarized: a) the size of a myocutaneous unit must be large enough to cover the defect which may result after excision of all necrotic and scar tissues, undermined or not; b) the blood supply of muscle (which also provides nutrition to its overlying skin through perforating blood vessels) must be autonomous and axial and the dominant vessels to each flap should be well known [17]; c) the muscle must be accessible; d) the point of rotation of the flap and its arc of rotation are essential in reaching and covering the defect [17]; e) in non-paraplegics, the muscular function must be preserved.

3. *Advantages* of these flaps are: one stage coverage, maximum reliability (due to the vascular pedicle), high healing potential and a greater versatility in flap design. From a surgical point of view they are technically easy and relatively bloodless. Furthermore the problem of non-adherence of skin flaps to underlying structures is minimized, and the support areas are well padded by muscle. Eventually the donor defect is negligible and can often be closed primarily.

4. *Pre-operative care* is most important and it must accustom the patient to the new position through psychological cooperation, test of support points, breathing exercises etc. A good result of the operation is essentially due to a total freedom from weight on the transplanted myocutaneous unit. Optimal general conditions must also be reached through restoration of the haemoglobin level, a high caloric intake, prevention of infection (genito-urinary), control of intestinal function etc.

5. *Surgical Treatment:* a) deep excision must be done of ulcer, scar, bursa, soft tissue calcification and any bone prominence (trochanterectomy, ischiectomy); b) the myocutaneous flap is outlined so that the size of the skin segment is appropriate to the muscle used; c) the muscle is atraumatically dissected, taking care of its vascular pedicle; d) careful hemostasis is essential; e) the flap is rotated, fixing the muscle deeply to the edges of the defect and avoiding all tension; f) U-transfixed cutaneous stitches help to keep the muscle in place filling at distance the surrounding undermined areas; g) a suction drainage placed parallel to the axis of the flap [34] is normal routine; h) the closure of the donor site is done primarily or with a skin graft when the defect is too large.

6. *Post-operative care* consists in avoiding any compression of the flap (a fortnight ventral decubitus) until a good cicatrization occurs. All maceration must be avoided together with new pressure sores in other sites.

7. *Complications: Necrosis* (partial or total) of the flap. It can be avoided thanks to precise knowledge of anatomy [34]. The vascular pedicle must be respected especially in its points of rotation [17], including the deep fascia [17]; all undue traction and tunnelisation must be avoided. It is important to suture the muscle edges to the skin to prevent shearing of the musculocutaneous perforators while the flap is manipulated [17, 34]. One must also take care to put the suction catheters parallel to the axis of the flap [34] (not perpendicular!). *Wound separation* is avoided by suturing without tension. *Hematoma* does not occur with good suction drainage. *Infection* is prevented with antibiotics and maximum hygiene.

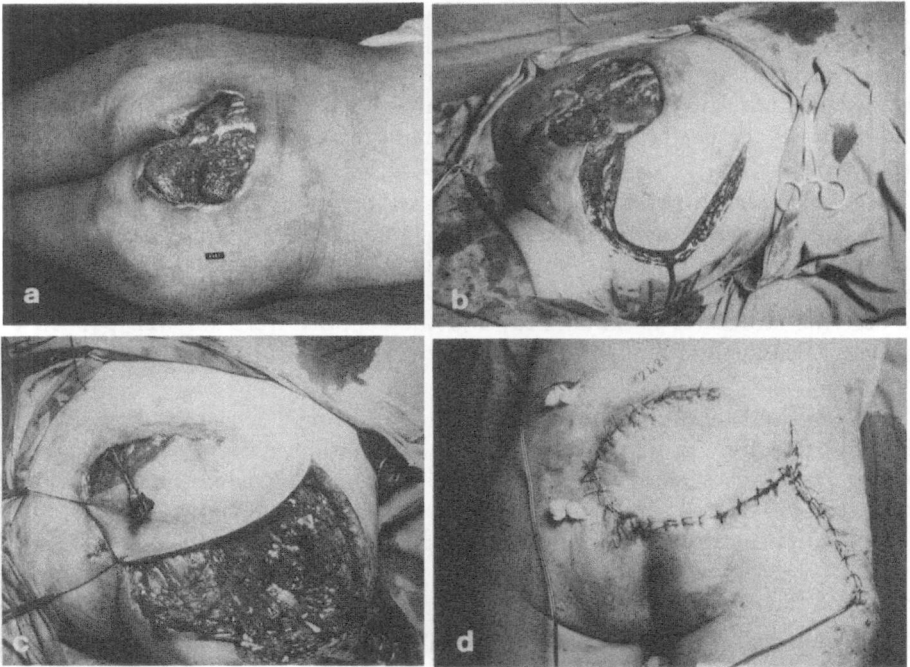

Fig. 2. *a* Sacral pressure sore, *b* Outlining of a myocutaneous flap including gluteus maximus muscle after excision of the sore, *c* Rotation of the myocutaneous flap, *d* Suture of the myocutaneous flap. U-transfixed stitches at a distance. Primarily closure of donor site. Drainage

## Cases

*Sacral pressure sores:* correction by myocutaneous flap including *gluteus maximus*.

Case I–R. R.–Large sacral pressure sore in a 42-year old man seriously ill with acute liver atrophy (Fig. 2a). After radical debridement of the sore a myocutaneous flap including gluteus maximus is outlined (Fig. 2b) and rotated on the defect, fixing the muscle at distance with U-transfixed stitches filling the undermined area (Fig. 2c) (note split metal tube as a guide to transfixed sutures). The donor defect is closed primarily. A double suction drainage is left (Fig. 2d).

*Trochanteric pressure sores:* correction by myocutaneous flap including *gluteux maximus.*

Case 2–P. C.–Pressure sore in a 29-year old paraplegic. The sore is apparently small, but with a large undermined bag (Fig. 3a). The amount of skin needed is small but the muscular need is great to fill all the undermined area, so that the small outlined cutaneous flap may support a large

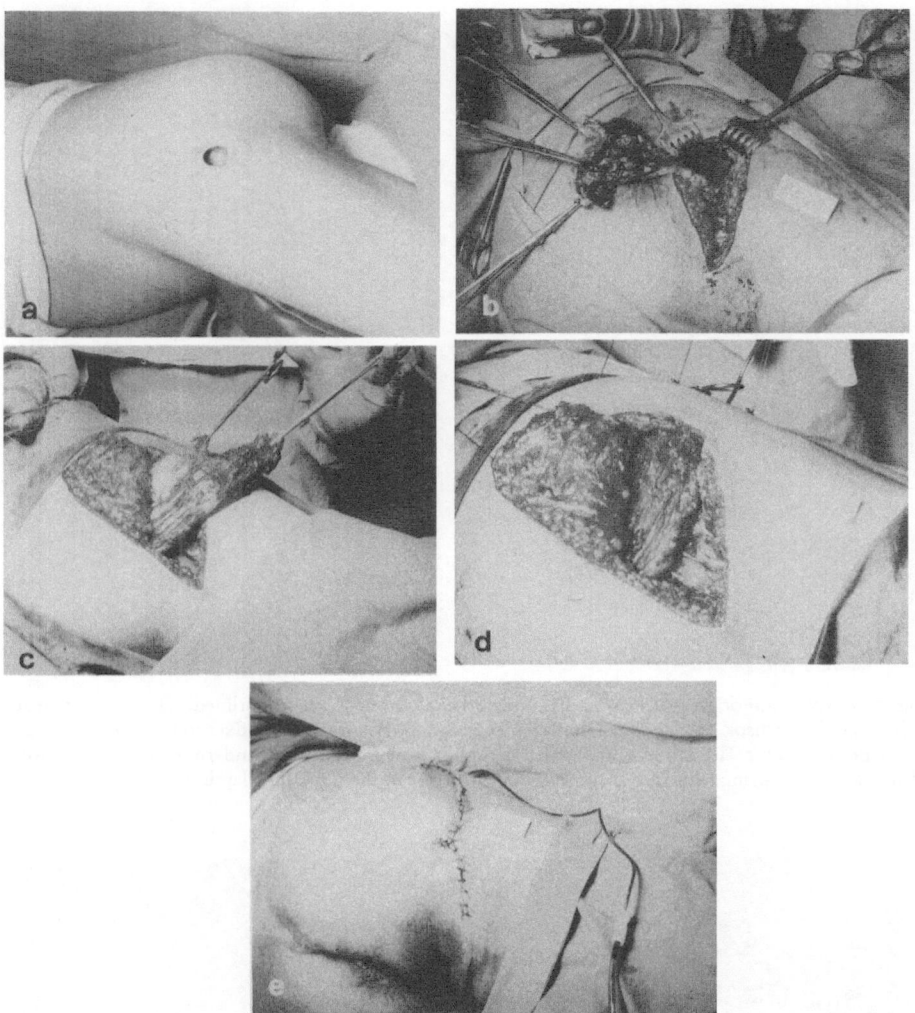

Fig. 3. *a* Trochanteric pressure sore, *b* Radical excision of bursa undermined, *c* Myocutaneous flap of gluteus maximus, *d* Rotation of the flap to fill the undermined region, *e* Closure of the defect

muscular flap of gluteus maximus (three times bigger). The whole bag is excised (Fig. 3b); a trochanterectomy is performed; the gluteus maximus muscle is made free (Fig. 3c) and rotated to fill all the undermined area, fixing it with U-stitches at distance (Fig. 3d). Closure of the defect and drainage (Fig. 3e).

Case 3–P. N.–Correction by myocutaneous flap including *tensor fasciae latae*.

Trochanteric pressure sore, with upward undermined edges in a paraplegic 30 years old (Fig. 4a). The undermined area is outlined. The amount of skin needed is small, but great is the muscular need. Thus a small cutaneous flap is outlined supporting a large flap of tensor fasciae latae (Fig. 4a). The bag is excised, the flap carefully dissected and a good trochanterectomy performed

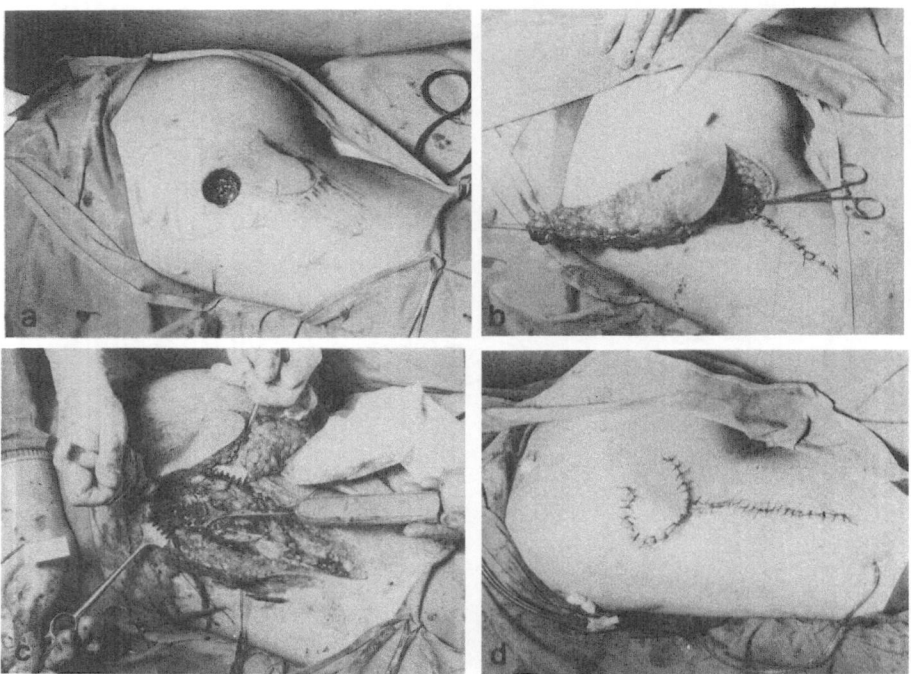

Fig. 4. *a* Trochanteric pressure sore. The upward undermined area is outlined. The myocutaneous flap including tensor fasciae latae muscle is designed downward, *b* Excision of the sore and trochanterectomy, *c* The myocutaneous flap is rotated upward to fill the undermined area, *d* Closure of the donor site primarily. U-transfixed stitches keep firm the muscular flap in the undermined area

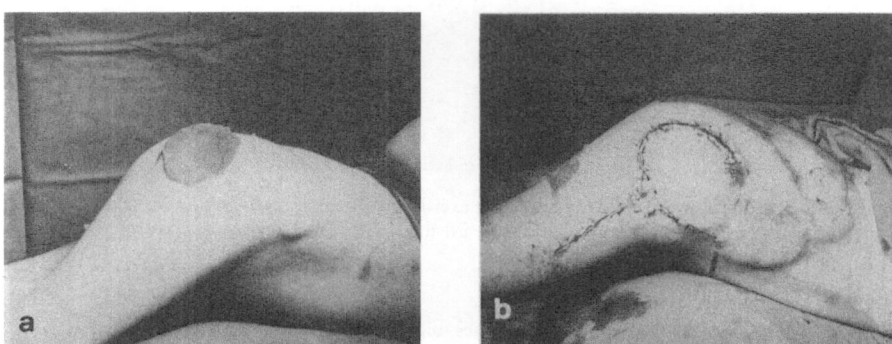

Fig. 5. *a* Severe trochanteric pressure sore with prominence of the bone, *b* Closure with myocutaneous flap including tensor fasciae latae. The donor site is partially closed by a skin graft

(Fig. 4b). The myocutaneous flap is rotated (Fig. 4c) upward and fixed at a distance with U-transfixed stitches. The donor defect is closed primarily (Fig. 4d).

Case 4 – A. M. – Severe trochanteric pressure sore in a 26-year old patient tetraplegic with a large prominence of the trochanter (Fig. 5a). The correction is effected by trochanterectomy, and coverage of the defect by a myocutaneous flap including the tensor fasciae latae. The closure of the donor site is completed by a small cutaneous graft (Fig. 5b).

*Ischial pressure sores:* correction with myocutaneous flap including *gracilis* muscle.

Case 5 – T. P. – Severe bilateral ischial pressure sore in paraplegic 34-year old (Fig. 6a). Excision of the sores in two different times, first on the left side then on the right. Ischiectomy. Large visualization of the area of the myocutaneous flap including the muscle gracilis; careful muscular dissection up its vascular pedicle (Fig. 6b) and rotation of the flap (Fig. 6c). Suture and drainage (Fig. 6d).

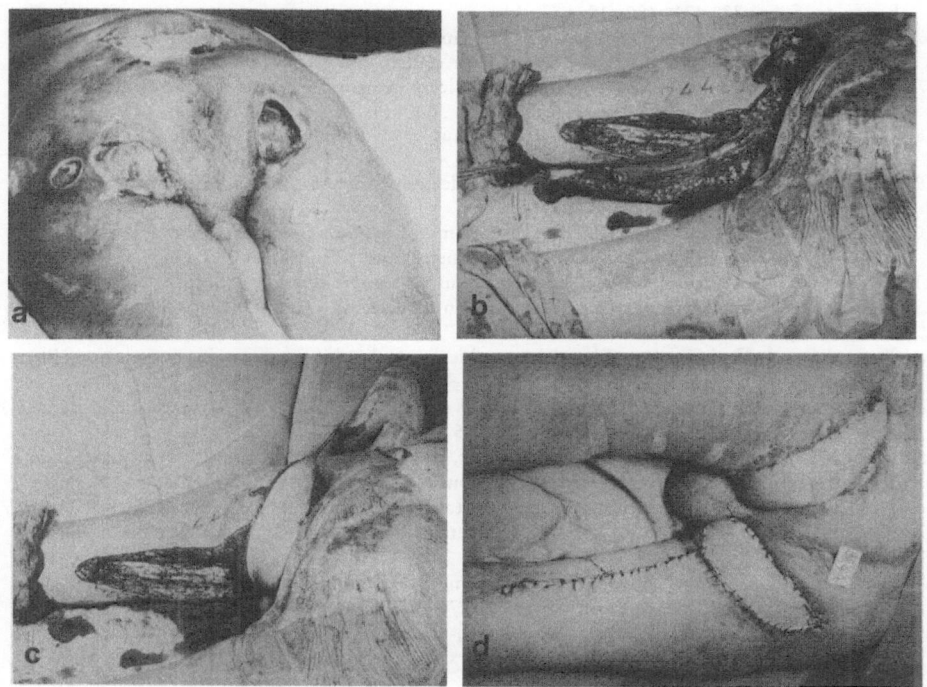

Fig. 6. *a* Ischial bilateral pressure sore, *b* After debridement of the left sore and ischiectomy, dissection of a myocutaneous flap including gracilis muscle, *c* Rotation of the myocutaneous flap, *d* Late result on the left side, and closure of the right side

## Conclusions

Myocutaneous flaps must not be applied thoughtlessly in all pressure sores, but must be seriously considered in each case. Very many pressure sores can still be cured by traditional means. We still think that myocutaneous flaps are fundamental in pressure sores in non-aged paraplegics.

A perfect knowledge of anatomy is essential in carrying out these flaps. Preoperative care is most important. Healing is generally rapid. Support can be tolerated after 15–20 days, but patients must be taught to avoid recurrences, prophylaxis for the future being the essential part of the treatment.

### References

1. Baker, D., Barton, F., Converse, J. M.: A combined biceps and semitendinosus muscle flap in the repair of ischial sores. Brit. J. Plast. Surg. *31*, 26–28 (1978).
2. Bhagwat Bal, M., Pearl, R. M., Laub, D. R.: Uses of the rectus femoris myocutaneous flap. Plast. Reconstr. Surg. *62*, 698–701 (1978).
3. Blocksma, R., Kostrubala, J. G., Greeley, P. W.: The surgical repair of decubitus ulcer in paraplegics: further observations. Plast. Reconstr. Surg. *4*, 123–132 (1949).
4. Bors, E., Comarr, A. E.: Ischial decubitus ulcers. Surgery *24*, 680–694 (1948).
5. Dansereau, J., Conway, H.: Closure of decubits in paraplegics (report on 2000 cases). Plast. Reconstr. Surg. *33*, 474–480 (1964).
6. Dupuis, J. F., Debray, G., Vilain, R.: Traitement des escarres ischiatiques par ischiectomie associée à une plastique musculaire. Ann. Chir. Plast. *18*, 27–30 (1973).
7. Gelb, J.: Plastic surgical closure of decubitus ulcers in paraplegics as result of civilian injuries. Plast. Reconstr. Surg. *9*, 525–542 (1952).
8. Ger, R.: The surgical management of decubitus ulcer by muscle transposition. Surgery *69*, 106–110 (1971).
9. Ger, R., Levine, S. A.: The management of decubitus ulcers by muscle transposition. Plast. Reconstr. Surg. *58*, 419–428 (1976).
10. Griffith, B. H., Schultz, R. C.: The prevention and surgical treatment of recurrent decubitus ulcers in patients with paraplegia. Plast. Reconstr. Surg. *27*, 248–260 (1961).
11. Heckler, F. R.: Gracilis myocutaneous and muscle flaps. Clin. Plast. Surg. *7*, 27–44 (1980).
12. Hentz, V. R.: Management of pressure sores in a speciality center. Plast. Reconstr. Surg. *64*, 683–691 (1979).
13. Kostrubala, J. C., Greeley, Ph.: The problem of decubitus ulcers in paraplegics. Plast. Reconstr. Surg. *2*, 403–412 (1947).
14. Labandter, H. P.: The gracilis muscle flap and musculocutaneous flap in the repair of perineal and ischial defects. Brit. J. Plast. Surg. *33*, 95–98 (1980).
15. McCraw, J. B., Dibbel, D. G., Carraway, J. H.: Clinical definition of independent myocutaneous vascular territories. Plast. Reconstr. Surg. *60*, 341–352 (1977).
16. McCraw, J. B.: The recent history of myocutaneous flaps. Clin. Plast. Surg. *7*, 3–7 (1980).
17. McCraw, J. B., Vasconez, L. O.: Musculocutaneous flaps: principles. Clin. Plast. Surg. *7*, 9–13 (1980).
18. McGregor, J. C., Buchan, A. C.: Our clinical experience with the tensor fasciae latae myocutaneous flap. Brit. J. Plast. Surg. *33*, 270–276 (1980).
19. Maruyama, Y., Nakajima, H., Wada, M., Imai, I., Fujino, T.: A gluteus maximus myocutaneous island flap for the repair of a sacral decubitus ulcer. Brit. J. Plast. Surg. *33*, 150–155 (1980).
20. Mathes, S. J., Vasconez, L. O., Jurkiewicz, M. J.: Extensions and further applications of muscle flap transposition. Plast. Reconstr. Surg. *60*, 6–13 (1977).
21. Mathes, S., Nahai, F.: Clinical Atlas of Muscle and Musculocutaneous Flaps. St. Louis-Toronto-London: Mosby. 1979.
22. Mathes, S. J., Alpert, B.: Advances in muscle and musculocutaneous flaps. Clin. Plast. Surg. *7*, 15–26 (1980).
23. Minami, R. T., Mills, R., Pardoe, R.: Gluteus maximus myocutaneous flaps for repair of pressure sore. Plast. Reconstr. Surg. *60*, 242–249 (1977).
24. Nahai, F.: The tensor fascia lata flap. Clin. Plast. Surg. *7*, 51–56 (1980).
25. Pers, M., Medgyesi, S.: Pedicle muscle flaps and their applications in the surgery of repair. Brit. J. Plast. Surg. *26*, 313–321 (1973).
26. Pers, M., Medgyesi, S., Bolund, S.: Sur les lambeaux cutanés en îlot avec pédicule musculaire. Ann. Chir. Plast. *24*, 187–190 (1979).

27. Sanchez, S., Eamegdool, S., Conway, H.: Surgical treatment of decubitus ulcers in paraplegics. Plast. Reconstr. Surg. *43*, 25–28 (1969).
28. Souyris, F., Dossa, J., Reynaud, J. P., Gary-Bobo, A.: Notre expérience des lambeaux musculaires dans le traitement des escarres chez le paraplégique. Ann. Chir. Plast. *23*, 157–161 (1978).
29. Souyris, F., Gary-Bobo, A., Reynaud, J. P., Charissoux, G.: Lambeau myo-cutané du tenseur du fascia lata. Mises au point anatomique et techniques. (A propos de 10 cas consécutif en 6 mois.) Ann. Chir. Plast. *25*, 159–162 (1980).
30. Stallings, J. O., Delgado, J. P., Converse, J. M.: Turnover island flap of gluteus maximus muscle for the repair of sacral decubitus ulcers. Plast. Reconstr. Surg. *54*, 52–54 (1974).
31. Sundarason, R.: A method of treatment of pressure sores over the ischial tuberosity. Singapore Med. J. *2*, 34 (1970).
32. Vasconez, L., Bostwick, J., McCraw, J.: Coverage of exposed bone by muscle transposition and skin grafting. Plast. Reconstr. Surg. *53*, 526–530 (1974).
33. Vasconez, L., Schneider, W., Jurkiewicz, M.: Pressure sores. Curr. Probl. Surg. *14*, 41 (1977).
34. Vasconez, L. O., McCraw, J. B., Hall, E. J.: Complications of musculocutaneous flaps. Clin. Plast. Surg. *7*, 123–132 (1980).
35. Wingate, G. B., Friedland, J. A.: Repair of ischial pressure ulcers with gracilis myocutaneous island flaps. Plast. Rec. Surg. *62*, 245–248 (1978).
36. Withers, E. H., Franklin, J. D., Madden, jr., J. J., Lynch, J. B.: Further experience with the tensor fascia lata musculocutaneous flap. Ann. Plast. Surg. *4*, 31–36 (1980).

Author's address: Prof. Dr. G. Lupo, Department of Plastic Surgery, St. Anna Hospital, Via Pessina, 12, I-22100 Como, Italy.

# Subject Index